TOWARDS THE LEARNING GRID

Frontiers in Artificial Intelligence and Applications

FAIA covers all aspects of theoretical and applied artificial intelligence research in the form of monographs, doctoral dissertations, textbooks, handbooks and proceedings volumes. The FAIA series contains several sub-series, including "Information Modelling and Knowledge Bases" and "Knowledge-Based Intelligent Engineering Systems". It also includes the biannual ECAI, the European Conference on Artificial Intelligence, proceedings volumes, and other ECCAI – the European Coordinating Committee on Artificial Intelligence – sponsored publications. An editorial panel of internationally well-known scholars is appointed to provide a high quality selection.

Volume 127

Recently published in this series

Vol. 126. J. Cruz, Constraint Reasoning for Differential Models
Vol. 125. C.-K. Looi et al. (Eds.), Artificial Intelligence in Education
Vol. 124. T. Washio et al. (Eds.), Advances in Mining Graphs, Trees and Sequences
Vol. 123. P. Buitelaar et al. (Eds.), Ontology Learning from Text: Methods, Evaluation and Applications
Vol. 122. C. Mancini, Cinematic Hypertext –Investigating a New Paradigm
Vol. 121. Y. Kiyoki et al. (Eds.), Information Modelling and Knowledge Bases XVI
Vol. 120. T.F. Gordon (Ed.), Legal Knowledge and Information Systems – JURIX 2004: The Seventeenth Annual Conference
Vol. 119. S. Nascimento, Fuzzy Clustering via Proportional Membership Model
Vol. 118. J. Barzdins and A. Caplinskas (Eds.), Databases and Information Systems – Selected Papers from the Sixth International Baltic Conference DB&IS'2004
Vol. 117. L. Castillo et al. (Eds.), Planning, Scheduling and Constraint Satisfaction: From Theory to Practice
Vol. 116. O. Corcho, A Layered Declarative Approach to Ontology Translation with Knowledge Preservation
Vol. 115. G.E. Phillips-Wren and L.C. Jain (Eds.), Intelligent Decision Support Systems in Agent-Mediated Environments
Vol. 114. A.C. Varzi and L. Vieu (Eds.), Formal Ontology in Information Systems – Proceedings of the Third International Conference (FOIS-2004)
Vol. 113. J. Vitrià et al. (Eds.), Recent Advances in Artificial Intelligence Research and Development

ISSN 0922-6389

Towards the Learning Grid

Advances in Human Learning Services

Edited by

Pierluigi Ritrovato

Consorzio CRMPA – Centro di Ricerca in Matematica Pura ed Applicata, Fisciano, Italy

Stefano A. Cerri

LIRMM, CNRS & University Montpellier II, Montpellier, France

Saverio Salerno

DIIMA – Dipartimento di Ingegneria dell'Informazione e Matematica Applicata, Università degli Studi di Salerno, Fisciano, Italy

Matteo Gaeta

DIIMA – Dipartimento di Ingegneria dell'Informazione e Matematica Applicata, Università degli Studi di Salerno, Fisciano, Italy

Colin Allison

School of Computer Science, University of St Andrews, Scotland, UK

and

Theo Dimitrakos

BT Group Chief Technology Office, BT Research, Adastral Park, Ipswich, UK

IOS Press

Amsterdam • Berlin • Oxford • Tokyo • Washington, DC

ISBN 1-58603-534-7
Library of Congress Control Number: 2005929743

Publisher
IOS Press
Nieuwe Hemweg 6B
1013 BG Amsterdam
Netherlands
fax: +31 20 687 0019
e-mail: order@iospress.nl

Distributor in the UK and Ireland
IOS Press/Lavis Marketing
73 Lime Walk
Headington
Oxford OX3 7AD
England
fax: +44 1865 750079

Distributor in the USA and Canada
IOS Press, Inc.
4502 Rachael Manor Drive
Fairfax, VA 22032
USA
fax: +1 703 323 3668
e-mail: iosbooks@iospress.com

PRINTED IN THE NETHERLANDS

Towards the Learning Grid
P. Ritrovato et al. (Eds.)
IOS Press, 2005

Preface

This is a book about a paradigm shift in Informatics in general and in technologies enhancing human learning in particular. It is not unexpected that its content is controversial: the debate between the "evolutionaries" – those that wish to optimize and refine current approaches – and the "revolutionaries" – those that support a fundamental change of approach – is quite actual, and probably no solution of the conflict will be reached in the short term. Within the Internet communities, the debate is hidden behind the words "semantic Web" versus "semantic Grid"; within educational technologists between "content/resource centered" and "conversation centered" e-learning, or either between "teaching" and "pedagogy" on the one side, and "learning" and "communities of practice" on the other. In general, in Informatics, the shift from a product-page oriented to a service-conversation oriented view may possibly impact most if not all the foreseen applications, in e-learning, but also in e-science, e-democracy, e-commerce, e-health…

The book emerges from two projects supported by the European Commission: LeGE-WG (http://www.lege-wg.org/) a thematic network within the 5th Framework Programme (2002–2004), and ELeGI (http://www.ELeGI.org/) an Integrated Project within the 6th FP (2004–2007). Both projects involved more than 20 European Institutions, therefore some 100 scientists and technologists. These projects represent the first structured collaborative effort aiming at solving crucial issues in Technology Enhanced human Learning by developing and using Grid services. Further to papers already appeared in preliminary versions in the four LeGE-WG workshops, published by the British Computer Society eWiC electronic site (http://ewic.bcs.org/categories/Gridcomputing.htm) we have invited a few eminent scientists to give a contribution to the subject in the form of a position paper, as described below.

The papers in the book may be classified according to several potential criteria. We have decided to choose a simple one: the approach to Science and Technology in the domain.

Part A of the book is dedicated to *Position papers*: visions about what to do and why to do it in the next years. The remaining parts (B to D) offer partial answers to "how" to do it. Part B concerns what we called: *Content-centered services*, i.e.: a vision of learning systems that privileges knowledge and its structures, standards and their interoperability, storage and retrieval services. The subsequent part C has been called: *Holistic services* to refer to more mature and integrated solutions that address not only content but more generally the creation and management of human Virtual Communities connected on the Grid in order to offer and consume different services facilitating and enhancing human learning. Finally part D is concerned with *new directions in learning services*: papers here propose solutions to non classical, yet stimulating new scenarios: methods, models and tools that are eventually to be realized in the medium term, in synergy with the evolution of concurrent developments on the Semantic Grid.

Hereafter, we will not review all the papers, rather come back to the initial statement – the paradigm shift – by referring to what we may learn from the six position papers (three from external colleagues, three from our project teams) and their challenging but also controversial messages that make our current ELeGI project very exciting and, perhaps, the reading of the book a stimulating intellectual adventure as well.

Bill Clancey's "*Towards On-Line Services Based on a Holistic Analysis of Human Activities*" introduces straight ahead his concept of Service by referring to his vision on Human-Centered Design that privileges the elicitation of services from an in-depth analysis of human real behavior, in context, rather than generating requirements from an idealized consumer's behavior conceived by the producer of the services. The most striking conclusion we may draw from his paper, is that in order to produce an useful automatic Travel Agent service, the last thing to do would be to get inspiration (or acquire specifications) from a human travel agent since the latter is usually not interested in getting the customer satisfied after a pleasant trip, rather just to sell to him/her some airplane tickets or hotel vouchers. Taking this seriously, as it deserves, one may infer that the last persons to ask for guidelines and specifications for automatic learning services are ... the teachers!

Francesco Di Castri, in his "*Access to information and e-learning for local empowerment*" puts clearly the terms and conditions for the development of isolated, fragmented and marginal communities: bidirectional access to digital Information. He is able to demonstrate by means of several real examples, at the planetary scale, through the last 40 years, that empowerment emerges as soon as people have access to Information provided this access is bi-directional (in reading AND in writing). Learning, social and economic development, democracy, the preservation of identity, and many other ones are the side effects of access to Information and empowerment. Once more, transposing the message to human learning scenarios, Di Castri shows that "curricula" and "content" in his depicted potential e-learning contexts (isolated communities) may eventually become the final goal of a long process, certainly are not the starting point. Human communities have first to establish trust and self-consciousness, before even thinking that being connected through technologies may help to better learn, operate and develop. Di Castri reports about a change of paradigm in modern Ecology: from top-down to bottom up. It is needless to say that the main message has been taken on board within ELeGI by injecting a small effort into a quite risky, yet most promising scenario: rural development in an underdeveloped area in Europe by bidirectional access to Information enhanced by Grid services.

Rosa Michaelson's position paper: "*The Challenge of Change*" wisely suggests looking carefully into the reasons why so many failures occurred in past implementations of e-learning initiatives, even if well supported at a large scale. Since the final goal is to enhance human learning by means of new technologies, the message clearly indicates that any significant change for human communities with respect to traditional ways of operating is not just a consequence of performing technologies, rather of human acceptance of the change.

Foster, Jennings and Kesselman in their "*Brain meets Brawn*" paper present their vision for the research agenda in the years to come, concerned with the synergies between Agents and Grid services. A similar vision was adopted at the beginning of the LeGE-WG project by Stefano Cerri, who in his position paper: "*An integrated view of Grid services, Agents and Human Learning*" offers an historical overview of the integration between Software Engineering (Objects, Actors and Agents), Artificial Intelligence and its impact in Human Computer Interaction (Intelligent Tutoring) and the semantic Grid. Both papers seem to concretely set the scene for the subsequent parts of the book, that deal more with the "how" to realize advances within a reasonable time scale and a limited amount of available resources as it is possible in the ELeGI project.

Finally Gaeta, Ritrovato and Salerno in their paper "*Making e-Learning a Service Oriented Utility: The European Learning Grid Infrastructure Project*" present the challenging European ELeGI Integrated Project. Other than the description of the research challenges that will be faced and the integrated approach that will be pursued in order to define and validate a pedagogy-driven, service-oriented software architecture based on Grid technologies for supporting ubiquitous, collaborative, experiential-based, contextualised and personalised learning, they highlight the benefit coming from use of Grid for setting up the future learning scenarios.

The editors of the book wish to thank all the colleagues, within and outside LeGE-WG and ELeGI European projects, for their contribution to the Learning Grid endeavor, as well as the readers of the book for their patience in case some minor slips have escaped from the editorial correction. Yes, the book is work in progress, but if it is possible to hope for a good day from the sun rays in the early morning, we are confident that our pioneering community will reach progressively a level of maturity that will allow us in due time not just to claim the need for a paradigm shift, but to show that it is feasible and useful.

This book includes one of the last papers of Francesco Di Castri, yet unpublished. Francesco left us recently (http://www.unesco.org/mab/news/FDC/tribute.htm). His impact, among others, in Information Sciences and Technologies for human development, has been unanimously recognised as unique in the XXth Century. It is a honour to dedicate the book to his memory.

Inspired by his work, that recently linked the succeeded development of Easter Island with the potential one of isolated areas in the Mediterranean, many professionals have adopted as their primary commitment to make the vision of Francesco Di Castri happen in the years to come, for human development and peace, by means of empowerment through bidirectional access to Information.

October 2005

Pierluigi Ritrovato (Salerno – IT), Stefano A. Cerri (Montpellier – FR), Saverio Salerno (Salerno – IT), Matteo Gaeta (Salerno – IT), Colin Allison (St. Andrews – UK) and Theo Dimitrakos (Ipswich – UK)

Contents

Part C. Holistic Services

Part D. New Direction in Learning Services

Part A

Position Papers

Towards the Learning Grid
P. Ritrovato et al. (Eds.)
IOS Press, 2005

Towards On-Line Services Based on a Holistic Analysis of Human Activities

William J. Clancey
NASA-Ames Research Center
Computational Sciences Division, MS 269-3
Moffett Field, CA 94035
William.J.Clancey@NASA.gov

Introduction

Very often computer scientists view computerization of services in terms of the logistics of human-machine interaction, including establishing a contract, accessing records, and of course designing an interface. But this analysis often moves too quickly to tactical details, failing to frame the entire service in human terms, and not recognizing the mutual learning required to define and relate goals, constraints, and the personalized value of available services. In particular, on-line services that "computerize communication" [15] can be improved by constructing an activity model of what the person is trying to do, not just filtering, comparing, and selling piece-meal services.

For example, from the customer's perspective the task of an on-line travel service is not merely to establish confirmed reservations, but to have a *complete travel plan*, usually integrating many days of transportation, lodging, and recreation into a happy experience. The task of the travel agent is not merely "ticketing," but helping the customer understand what they want and providing services that will connect everything together in an enjoyable way.

The communication process required to provide a travel service is necessarily iterative, based on tentative constraints and plans, and considers long-term business relationships. Indeed, in the case of a computerized travel agent, mimicking human behavior and social customs would be a bad idea—we need to provide much better services than what people currently receive.

Using a web-based travel planning experience as a detailed example, this chapter critiques the approach to computerized interactions suggested by "Elephant 2000" [15] and relates it to the response "Language for Interactions" [4]. The ensuing discussion considers relations to Grid learning [3, 16] and makes recommendations for using activity-based modelling to facilitate mutual learning between computer agents and people. A broad view of educational material and learning is required to realize the potential of Grid computing to provide high-level services, as in the example of a travel agent.

1. Example: Web-Based Travel Reservation

The following example is expressed in first-person form, to emphasize that it was an actual event and to remind the reader of the everyday nature of the situations and problems described here.

In the winter of 2001, I used the WebTravel system (a pseudonym for a free internet service) to specify a flight from San Francisco to Page, Utah. The program told me that there were no planes flying to Page and listed the closest airports. I chose the Grand Canyon, seeing that I could arrive by 2 PM and join my friends who by coincidence would be staying there the previous night and then driving on to Page. After making the plane reservation, I then proceeded to make a rental car reservation. Surprise! There were no rental cars available at the Grand Canyon! This is remarkable given that 2 million visitors come to that area per year. Why didn't the WebTravel program notice this? My remaining itinerary, already input to the program, clearly shows that I am flying from Grand Junction, Colorado to San Francisco—how did the program expect me to get from the Grand Canyon to Grand Junction?

The user experience is even worse than I have described. For the program does not say, "no rental cars are available"—it displays instead that "The car type requested is not available at this location through WebTravel.com at this time. Please select a different car type."

The WebTravel program, as in the Elephant 2000 analysis, focuses not on my *travel*, but myopically only on *reservations*. I indeed now held guaranteed reservations (the emphasis of McCarthy's logic-based approach), but they were worthless to me. My stated goal of "going to Grand Canyon" (which was not even my destination) doesn't capture my overarching *activity*, which is visiting the Page area, driving for a week to Arches, Utah, and then finally flying home via Grand Junction. The program needed to know my *plan*—locations, activities at each location, timing, who was involved (could my wife and I share a ride with friends already at the Grand Canyon?), etc.

Capping this experience, when I sent an email requesting customer support from WebTravel.com, I received the following response (vendor name has been edited):

Subject: Re: computer reserves non-rental car airports (KMM2768689V6442810KM)
Date: Fri, 09 Feb 2001 18:25:58 -0600
From: WebTravel <WebTravel@travel.com>
TO: <BCLANCEY@mail.arc.nasa.gov>

Due to unexpected system errors, we are unable to accept your email at this time. We hope to have the system back up soon. If you have a question regarding a reservation you have made, please call our customer service center at 1-888-709-5983.

Thank you,
WebTravel customer service

Unfortunately, the problem is not just that WebTravel provides no real travel service, but human travel agents fail, too. Here's what happened next. I went to an airline counter at an airport to attempt to resolve my situation. I had already learned that the closest airport to Page, Utah that had rental cars was Flagstaff, Arizona. I wouldn't have to pay the $75 change fee per ticket because the new flights would cost $350 less than the original. However, I wouldn't receive a refund either. I had already looked up the best flights, and presented them. The agent indicated that my preferred flight (to the required stop in Phoenix) was booked, but I could get on a later flight; this would require also changing the flight from Phoenix to Flagstaff. Finally, she handed me the tickets. I remembered that I should read them over before leaving the counter. But I was flustered, trying to find the flight information on the ticket, and then trying to evaluate the revised plan, since all the flight numbers and times were different from what I had carefully determined were best. I checked that the dates and locations were correct, and thanked her. (I was given $200 coupons for future flights as a consolation for the lost $350.)

However, when I was able to sit down and read over the tickets, I discovered something terrible: Not only did we not arrive in Phoenix until 2 PM; there was a wait of more than three hours until the flight to Flagstaff! And we would not arrive at Page until well into dinner time, losing the afternoon activities we had planned for nearby Lake Powell. I found a map and determined that we could *drive* from Phoenix to Page in less time than it would take to fly to Flagstaff and then drive to Page. Knowing all of this, I might have chosen to fly from San Francisco to other locations in Utah that were almost as close as Flagstaff. But once again, the travel agent (remember, an actual human being) engaged in no background discussion about my actual trip—where I was going, when I wanted to get there, my tradeoffs on cost and driving effort and arrival time, etc. Here I had spent more than $500 than was necessary and was faced with a four hour unnecessary car trip, arriving half a day later than I desired!

Ironically, the special flight coupon I received as a consolation gift prominently displays the airline's mantra: "More CARE Plus." Simply caring at all would have been good enough.

2. Holistic Analysis of Travel Semantics

Given the realities of everyday travel planning, computational talk about promising to make a reservation [15] appears silly. Ticketing has very little to do with the customer's perspective of what making reservations is about. A travel agent, properly concerned with my *trip* and not just my individual reservations, would ensure the completeness of my plan (am I ensured of transportation between all points?), timing constraints (is driving faster than flying?), and my activity goals (arriving in time to enjoy Lake Powell during the day; arriving in time for dinner).

A travel agent must understand how people spend time enjoyably—maybe driving is tedious, but are there places I might enjoy photographing along the way? Travel is not all just about cost and time optimization—that's the least of it.

So how would we improve WebTravel and the human travel agent? First, we would reorient how the software system is designed and how the person works. The work system design of people, roles, software, and conversation must reflect that the goal of a service provider is to develop a *travel activity plan*, not merely to reserve transportation tickets. The human travel agent's focus on ticketing is very clear; she has no interest whatsoever in my *vacation*, which is what I am actually needing to discuss. As put by Cerri [4], what is missing is a "shared ontology" used by "communicative agents."

Here the idea of speech acts (Searle, 1969), properly interpreted, is useful: The travel agent must interpret my requests about flights and destinations as being *tentative* articulations, placeholders for specifying what I really need. When I say, "I want to fly to Flagstaff," the travel agent should at least ask, "Is that your final destination for the day?" This simple question would reveal that I don't want to go to Flagstaff at all on that day! The lack of understanding here of my interests, which is a routine deficiency in both human and computer conversations about tickets, is astounding when you think about it. And compounding matters, travellers have been coerced by reservationists to speak using their ontology of "flights," "Saturday stay-over," and "Class Y ticket." Within the software communication and the asymmetric dialog controlled by the airline reservationists, there is virtually no investigation of the traveler's intentions and activities.

A key problem is that customers do not know what questions to ask. I never thought to ask whether Grand Canyon had rental cars. A "non-defective" performance [15] by the travel agent would involve volunteering information about typicality ("Did you realize that the Grand Canyon has no rental car locations?"). The form of communication required here goes well beyond Gricean conventions. The truth of individual assertions about flight availability and timing are meaningless if taking such flights would violate what I am broadly trying to accomplish. Yet ironically, the first level of logical analysis is well within a computer program's capability. WebTravel could ask users, "How will you get from the Grand Canyon to Grand Junction?"

But a radical shift in design is required. Rather than conceiving web services only in terms of logistics—accessing information, interoperability, composing meanings within different ontologies, etc.—we require methods for understanding a person's overall activity. Crucially, this requires techniques for articulating desires and negotiating goals incrementally, within the process of constructing alternative solutions [18]. In other words, we can't first bundle up the "specifications" for the journey, and then produce an optimized plan. Because the traveler's desires are shaped by the travel options available—which may be unavailable, a poor fit for the emerging schedule, or too expensive—each tentative schedule provides an opportunity for the schedule to modify goals, relax constraints, and discover unexpected value (e.g., visiting an Indian reservation for the first time).

How can we design software to do what people don't do well? The solution is of course the essence of artificial intelligence programming—model-based problem solving. The travel agent should construct a model of the traveler's trip. Again, such a model is constructed in the process of searching, filtering, and composing alternative services, such that the model is created, refined, and validated in a conversation that changes the goals, constraints, and how solutions are evaluated.

In summary, mapping stated goals about destinations into guaranteed ticket reservations [15] is an absurd view of the problem to be solved in providing travel services. A joint construction is required, a conversational interaction that bit-by-bit draws out from me what I am trying to do and draws out from the travel agent the space of relevant options [2, 13, 14, 21, 22, 24, 25]. In developing a model, the travel agent learns about my activity plans: lodging, sightseeing, recreation, relaxation, and all the other people involved (children, friends, pets, etc.). A timeline is developed that includes activities of "getting settled," "enjoying a resort," "photographing while driving," eating, sleeping, etc. Notice that these are facts about a *social world,* not just a physical world. This social world is always personal—most travel plans are customized—though they may fit norms and even highly probable routes.

A candidate representational framework for formalizing such a travel activity model is the Brahms multiagent simulation system [5, 19, 20, 12]. Brahms was conceived to complement business process modelling tools by representing how work actually gets done. As a model of practice, in contrast with formal processes, Brahms simulations emphasize circumstantial interactions (e.g., how placement of people and tools affects what information is shared or how long a job takes). People are modelled as located, having multiple group identities, having behaviors that dynamically blend the conventional activities of multiple group memberships, and having perceptual interests coupled to activities.

If a travel agent (computational or person) were to construct a Brahms activity model of the customer's trip, then it might be able to determine transportation options that truly satisfy the customer. However, the agent must use conversational techniques and representational tools (e.g., maps, timelines, and diagrams) to help the customer recognize the implications of how options interact ("No, of course I don't want to fly to Flagstaff if I must wait in Phoenix for over three hours. I'm trying to get to Page by 3 PM!").

The problem involves not only expressing information (e.g., available schedules) in a comprehensible way, but *instructing* the traveler about how services interoperate (e.g., you can move from an airport to rental car provider using a free shuttle bus). In effect, the travel plan has a corresponding procedure that the traveler must learn (e.g., "When you get to the gate, look for the DesertAir representative"). At the same time, the travel agent learns about the traveler's values. As is well-known in instructional research, personalization (as in student modelling, [5]) is aimed at much more than classifying the user and selecting from fixed choices to be delivered as lessons. Rather the modelling process itself is a problem solving endeavor, leading to constructing a potentially quite complex process with causal and temporal constraints, built out of simpler components (cf. classification vs. construction, [7]). More generally, the modelling dialogue must be structured, planned, and negotiated, as revealed in a variety of research from medical diagnosis to design tools, but explored especially well in intelligent tutoring systems [17].

Finally, the travel planning problem can be framed in a yet broader way, viewing over a longer time scale what it means for someone to be a customer. The objective of the travel service is not only to sell a ticket and make a profit, but to secure future business. The travel agent must establish a *relationship* with the customer. That is, the travel agent must consider his or her own identity as a service provider, as viewed by the customer. The idea of speech acts might need to be extended to take into account that service-oriented communications transcend the particular trip being discussed. Each interactive moment is part of an overarching activity in which the customer is conceiving, "You are (or are not) my preferred service provider. This is (or is not) how I will in general construct travel plans." Thus a "successful" speech act [15] is one that accomplishes the broader goal of establishing long-term trust, usually by showing that the travel agent's capabilities are very broad and general—going beyond what is stated by the customer, surprising and delighting him or her.

In our example, by providing coupons as a form of "good will," the airline supervisor showed that she cared about my future business. She didn't merely recite the $75 penalty fee rule or say that I had been amply warned by the computer program about non-refundability. She recognized that I had not been served well and had paid far too much for my flights.

3. Conclusions

Moving from the simple idea of hyperlinks on the internet to web semantics and Grid computing necessarily involves at first an emphasis on the logistics of how to relate diverse, independently created resources. The vision is to make it easier for people to benefit from a vast network of facts, media, presentations, and computing resources. But interposing agents between people and the web replaces one access and interpretation problem by several more: Besides the problem of getting software agents to find and understand web content, we now have the problem of getting the software agents to understand people, just as people now need to understand the agents (Figure 1).

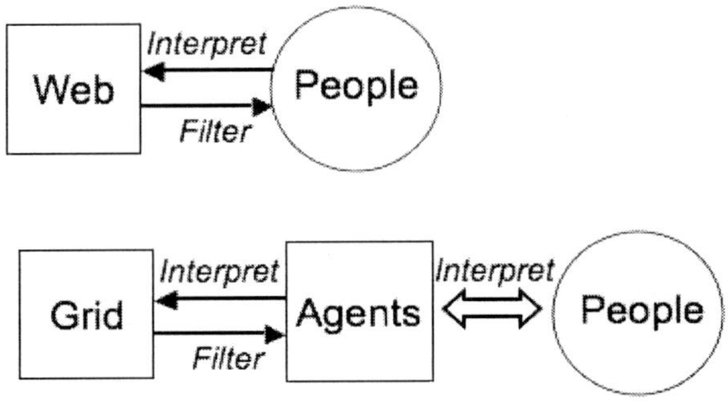

Figure 1 – In the original internet search model (top), people interpret filtered results (web pages, products) retrieved from the web. In the ideal "Grid services" model (bottom), software agents perform these searches and filter functions, while providing higher-level services to people in a conversation requiring mutual learning.

The real-world examples we encounter everyday should be sobering: If trained human agents cannot easily meet our needs, how will computer systems do better? The experience with WebTravel reveals that the service must be conceived in terms of what the person is trying to do (the broader activity and its motives), not the local, and superficial aspects of web transactions. And this requires constructing a model of the person's activity—ironically something a computer program might do more patiently and cost effectively than people today who are travel, real estate, and investment agents.

To summarize the travel agent example, making a reservation is a means, not an end in itself. A distinction must be drawn between providing confirmed tickets at the least cost (a simple view of a web-based transaction) and getting me to my destination in time for dinner with my companions, with consideration for cost, driving distance, rental car expense, etc. (my activity). The problem from the customer's perspective is not merely to hold confirmed *reservations* but to have a complete travel plan that will be a happy experience. The task from the travel agent's perspective is not "ticketing" (as is it is so often described by the airlines), but helping the customer understand what they want and providing services that will connect everything together in an enjoyable way.

Perhaps the most difficult challenge in developing an automated travel planning service is that travel constraints and preferences usually cannot be formulated up front. The process of articulating constraints is necessarily interactive and iterative. A seed goal produces a set of options and tentative plan, which are evaluated for implications that were previously unanticipated. New preferences or constraints are articulated and the options and plan are revised, etc.

What is missing from the method of relating requests and promises, the most common technical approach for coordinating goals and services, is that requests are often just tentative placeholders for unarticulated (non-verbal) beliefs, desires, and concerns. Helping the traveler to describe his or her intentions to create a *good experience* is the actual service required.

The interaction between the person and the travel agent can be phrased as, "Do what I *will prefer* (once I have all the information), not what I say I want now." The program must be proactive to model and understand the person's activities—what they will be doing before, during, and after the transportation event. Reservations for a trip constitute a *total plan*, which cannot be evaluated solely by time or cost optimization.

Relating different ways of framing a situation is the essence of a holistic analysis [25, 8].

Certainly, some of the problems we experience today with human agents stems from inadequate computer tools, which shape how a business views the roles of their workers [23]. The human airline reservationist is using a tool not much different from WebTravel, and is coerced by its design to converse in the ontology of ticketing, not trip planning. A crucial conclusion is that the opportunity and problem for Grid computing and the semantic web community is to not merely replicate what human service providers do, but to discover and address what services people really want to buy. Accordingly, terms like "educational material" and "learning" should be viewed broadly, not just in terms of presentation or explanation, but *what are people trying to accomplish in their lives* by means of the present inquiry. Indeed, a good design heuristic may be to make it possible for a person to interrupt an interaction and express a conflict with what he or she is trying to accomplish and/or introduce a constraint that better defines high-level goals (e.g., "But wait, how will this get me to Page in time for dinner?").

Perhaps the most specific lesson for today's system developers is to beware definitions of "successful performance" that are based on narrowly framing the problem to be solved—especially technical definitions based on legacy software that has produced unsuccessful business practices. Fulfilling reservation commitments, the emphasis of Elephant 2000, is probably the narrowest view of a travel service provider. I had high confidence that the airline would allow me to get onboard the airplanes I reserved for August 3, 2001. But I also knew that I was going to a city where I don't want to go, that I paid $350 too much for the flight, that I would throw my Phoenix-Flagstaff tickets into the garbage, and I would have to drive 4 hours to arrive at my desired destination, arriving too late to enjoy the day.

In artificial intelligence research, people sometimes refer to what is missing in WebTravel and the reservationists I encountered as "common sense." But if the capability and knowledge were so common, we would not be so routinely frustrated and poorly served. Very likely some of the deficiencies in human performance at the airlines stem from an overworked, undertrained work force, and a business model that focuses on moving planes and bodies from place to place, rather than constructing travel plans for loyal customers [23]. A "happy performance" [1] must be one that is helpful and *useful*—one that constructs a plan that will be a happy experience and not just satisfies legal obligations and notions of reservation "correctness."

The analysis presented here does not mean that the mechanics addressed by the "Elephant 2000" or "Language for Interactions" papers and all of the related problems researchers are now handling to develop Grid technologies are unnecessary. Rather a holistic analysis complements the analysis of mechanics, to consider the kind of *content*, the models that such computer programs must develop through interactive communication, in order to know what to search, filter, compose, etc. from available resources. To adapt McCarthy's phrase, "computerizing a communication" should entail viewing the interaction as a process of constructing an activity model. This process is necessarily iterative, based on tentative constraints and plans, and considering larger issues of business relationships. In the case of a computerized travel agent, mimicking human behavior and social customs would be a bad idea—we need to do much better than that.

Acknowledgments

This chapter is based on a paper presented at San Marino Summer School, June 2001, "Semantics and Pragmatics on the Web: Synergies between Philosophy and Computing." Charlotte Linde and Chin Seah provided helpful comments. This work has been supported in part by NASA's Computing, Communications, and Information Technology Program, Intelligent Systems subprogram, Human-Centered Computing element, managed by Mike Shafto at NASA Ames.

References

[1] Austin, J. L. 1962. How to Do Things with Words. Oxford.
[2] Brown, J. S. and Duguid, P. 2000. The social life of information. Boston: Harvard Business School Press.
[3] Cerri, S. A. 2002. Human and artificial agent's conversations on the Grid. In 1st LEGE-WG International Workshop on Educational Models for Grid Based Services, Lausanne, Switzerland. September. Electronic Workshops in Computing (eWiC). http://ewic.bcs.org/conferences/2002/1stlege/session3/paper1.htm
[4] Cerri, S. A., Sallantin, J., Castro, E., Maraschi, D. 2000. Steps towards C+C: a language for interactions. In S. A. Cerri and D. Dochev (eds.), Artificial Intelligence: Methodology, Systems, Applications (AIMSA 2000), Lecture Notes in Artificial Intelligence 1904, Springer Verlag. pp. 33-46.
[5] Clancey, W. J. 1986. Qualitative student models. Annual Review of Computer Science.
[6] Palo Alto: Annual Reviews Inc., pp. 381-450. Also excerpted in J. Self (Ed.), Artificial intelligence and human learning: Intelligent computer-aided instruction, London: Chapman and Hall, 1987, pp. 49-68.
[7] Clancey, W. J. 1992. Model construction operators. Artificial Intelligence, 53(1):1-115.
[8] Clancey, W .J. 1995 Practice cannot be reduced to theory: Knowledge, representations, and change in the workplace. In S. Bagnara, C. Zuccermaglio, and S. Stucky (eds),Organizational learning and technological change. Berlin: Springer-Verlag.
[9] Clancey, W. J., Sachs, P., Sierhuis, M., & van Hoof, R. 1998. Brahms: simulating practice for work systems design. Int. J. Human-Computer Studies, 49, 831-865.
[10] Clancey, W. J. 1997. The conceptual nature of knowledge, situations, and activity. In P. Feltovich, K. Ford, & R. Hoffman (eds.), Human and Machine Expertise in Context, pp. 247–291. Menlo Park, CA: The AAAI Press.
[11] Clancey, W. J. 2002. Simulating activities: Relating motives, deliberation, and attentive coordination. Cognitive Systems Research 3(3):471-499, September.
[12] Clancey, W. J. in press. Cognitive modelling of social behaviors. To appear in R. Sun, Cognition and multi-agent interaction: From cognitive modelling to social simulation. New York: Cambridge University Press.
[13] Gasser, L. 1991. Social conceptions of knowledge and action, Artificial Intelligence, 47(1-3)107-138., January.
[14] Greenbaum, J., and Kyng, M. (Eds.) 1991. Design at work: Cooperative design of computer systems. Hillsdale, NJ: Lawrence Erlbaum Associates.
[15] McCarthy, J. 1998[1989]. Elephant 2000: A programming language based on speech acts. Stanford University unpublished manuscript: http://www-formal.stanford.edu/jmc/elephant/elephant.html, appeared: 6 Nov 1998, written 1989.
[16] Mostow, J. and Tedesco, P. (Eds.). 2004. Grid learning services. Workshop proceedings from ITS 7th International Conference on Intelligent Tutoring Systems, Maceio, Brasil.
[17] Psotka, J., Massey, L. D., Mutter, S. A. (Eds.). 1988. Intelligent tutoring systems: Lessons learned. Hillsdale, NJ: Lawrence Erlbaum Associates.
[18] Schön, D.A. 1987. Educating the reflective practitioner. San Francisco: Jossey-Bass Publishers.
[19] Sierhuis, M. 2001. "Modelling and simulating work practice," Ph.D. thesis, Social Science and Informatics (SWI), Univ. of Amsterdam, SIKS Dissertation Series No. 2001-10, Amsterdam, The Netherlands, ISBN 90-6464-849-2.
[20] Sierhuis, M., W.J. Clancey, Seah, C., and Trimble, J., and Sims, M.H. 2003. Modelling and simulation for mission operations work systems design. Journal of Management Information Systems, 19(4), 85-128.
[21] Suchman, L. A. 1987. Plans and situated actions: The problem of human-machine communication. Cambridge: Cambridge Press.

[22] Vincente, K. J. 1999. Cognitive Work Analysis: Toward safe, productive, and healthy computer-based work. Mahwah, NJ: Erlbaum.
[23] Wales, R., O'Neill, J., and Mirmalek, Z. 2002. Ethnography, customers, and negotiated interactions at the airport. IEEE Intelligent Systems, 17(5): 15-23.
[24] Winograd, T. & Flores, F. 1986. Understanding Computers and Cognition: A New Foundation for Design. Norwood: Ablex.
[25] Wynn, E. 1991. Taking practice seriously. In J. Greenbaum and M. Kyng (Eds.), Design at work: Cooperative design of computer systems. Hillsdale, NJ: Lawrence Erlbaum Associates, pp. 45-64.

Towards the Learning Grid
P. Ritrovato et al. (Eds.)
IOS Press, 2005

Access to information and e-learning for local empowerment: The requisite for human development and environmental protection

Francesco di Castri
Director of Research
National Council of Scientific Research of France (CNRS), Montpellier

Introductory remarks

I am aware that this paper may seem – and probably is - out of context with respect to the technological aspects. First, most activities related to this paper have been developed and are still being promoted out of the European space, and primarily in developing countries. Second, conceptual discussion on this topic has taken place more in North America (Harvard University, MIT, and University of Quebec) than in Europe. Third, I am not an expert in informatics, but an ecologist that has progressively evolved towards community development. I can represent - to a certain extent - the point of view of users rather than that of promoters of a learning infrastructure. Fourth, my main concern and goal are to provide access to information to isolated, fragmented and marginal communities, and to promote an almost spontaneous interaction among them and with the outside world, rather than to establish formal e-learning systems and structures.

1. Conservation and development: changing paradigms

During the last forty years, as an academic ecologist, I have been working on projects related to the conservation of natural and cultural heritage, that is to say of the conservation and valorization of biodiversity [5] and of cultural diversity [2]. This has been done both at the grass-roots community level and as related to the international worldwide organization and coordination of these activities, mainly in the framework of UNESCO and ICSU (International Council for Science).

From the very beginning of these activities, it has become self-evident that this conservation can be meaningfully achieved and can ensure some continuity in time – out of all external regulations, restrictions, management and control - only to the extent that local communities enjoy a minimum, satisfactory level of development, economic wealth and employment. Awareness of the need of conservation, community acceptance of it, and local participation and commitment do not last long in the absence of appropriate development.

This easily understandable – almost obvious - fact was noticed much before the large environmental happenings and event, such as the United Nations Conferences of

Stockholm on the human environment (1972), of Rio de Janeiro on environment and development (1992) and of Johannesburg on sustainable development (2002).

Let's try to retrace historically the evolution of this process of changing paradigms in research and management. In the early seventies, the accepted paradigm was that ecosystems submitted to the same climatic and ecological conditions are similar and converge in their aspect, structure and functioning, whatever be their origin and geographical position. I have then started exploring more in depth the patterns of ecosystem functioning and structure, through comparative research in the five widely separated regions of the world (Mediterranean Basin, California, Chile, South Africa and western and southern Australia) that share a very similar mediterranean-type climate (dry period in summer), but have been originated by largely different and disconnected phylogenetic pools of plants and animals. The result of ten-year international cooperative research was that divergence of ecosystem functioning is at least as important as convergence, the main factor being their different biological and human cultural evolution [29].

There is a kind of *co-evolution* between man - and his old cultural history - and the attributes and functioning of terrestrial ecosystems [1]. The new paradigm has been, accordingly, that ecosystem functioning and biological diversity cannot be studied and understood while disregarding the cultural human evolution -with all its intangible and perceptional patterns - that leads to a multiplicity of cultural diversities and attitudes.

The operational and managerial implication of this paradigm is that biological conservation can no longer be achieved in closed and untouchable areas, protected from any human influence. Human imprinting on ecosystems has already taken place everywhere and forever. Conservation can only be achieved in a sustainable way *"with humans and by humans"* living in the protected areas and outside them. The role and the commitment of local populations appear to the indispensable ingredient for conservation of species, ecosystems and resources, as well as of the tangible and intangible cultural heritage.

This consideration and this new paradigm are at the origin of the launching of the two most important and widespread conservation programs: the international network of biosphere reserves of UNESCO and the Convention on the World's Cultural and Natural Heritage. In both programs, nature and culture, humans and ecosystems are considered, integrated and interacting [28] [30].

Nevertheless, translation into practice and in concrete field situations of these concepts and these principles has very often encountered several difficulties for implementation. The prerequisite of some acceptable level of development for local populations, or the accompanying measure to ensure such development, were frequently missing or discontinued. In many cases, such as in isolated and fragmented situations, where a critical size for development did not exist, development was simply not feasible within the past economic and information patterns.

Furthermore, without local development and endogenous economic incentives, the motivation and commitment of local people for conserving their heritage and their biological and cultural diversity cannot be stimulated. When development is replaced by subsidies and full governmental assistance – as it can happen only in rich countries – local autochthonous populations are not motivated either. Rather they fall in a status of passivity, indifference and total lack of commitment and stimulus for initiatives, as well as in a condition of social and cultural disruption and collapse. This has occurred, and still occurs, with several Amerindian communities in the North of Canada. Contrary to what is usually believed and stated, at least among conservationists from the North, development is a *sine qua non* requisite for conservation. This also represents a new paradigm.

2. The emergence of the information society

The above described situation, that is to say, the practical impossibility to provide conditions for in situ development to local communities and – therefore – to motivate and involve them, was going on for a couple of decades without noticeable change, in spite of the diverse efforts and the distinct phraseology to describe this type of alternative unreachable development (integrated development, endogenous development, ecodevelopment, human development, sustainable development) used by the United Nations [3][6][20].

However, during the last ten years, along with the transition from the industrial society and the emergence of an information, knowledge-based society, opportunities and tools for facilitating an appropriate development to local communities – in accordance with their cultural background and aspirations, and specific to the ecological conditions of their environment – have considerably increased [7][8][12]. This is a kind of development implying full participation, commitment and involvement of local people, promoting progressively their own entrepreneurial capacity, and leading them to the full awareness that their development depends mostly on protection, conservation and valorization of their own cultural and natural heritage [24].

Also the emergence of the current globalization, when it is locally regulated, modulated and filtered by the strength of local cultures, strongly promotes the opening up of isolated communities to the global market, and increases the potential and the diversification of their development [4][5][9][10][11][14].

The five new openings and tools for community development and conservation – as win-win strategies (both development and environment are winners) – facilitated by the information society and globalization, are as follows. All of them are expressed in terms of access by local communities to different kinds of information.

1. The access to the digital information and language with its new bi-directional, transversal and non-hierarchical patterns, including the potential for continuous distance learning.
2. The access to the genetic information and language through biodiversity and biotechnology.
3. The access to the economic information of an equitable international trade, allowing a quality economy and a greater diversification of products.
4. The access to the interactive relational information of the new generation of responsible tourism (cultural tourism, rural tourism, ecotourism, etc.), managed directly by local people themselves, with greater economic return and closer cultural interaction between residents and visitors.
5. The access to the technological information of the new generation of dematerialized, proactive and highly efficient innovation.

3. The access to digital information

The most radical change of the new society is that information can be transversal and highly interactive in nature, and no longer with almost exclusively vertical, top-down flows. Above all, information is bi-directional now. Mostly through the Internet, e-mail and web sites, access to information means at present not only the possibility of receiving it, but also of creating, publicizing and transmitting it freely.

Networks can be accordingly established among persons, communities and enterprises sharing similar interests, aspirations, value systems, even cultures and languages. A network can act as a driving force for development, and often as a trigger for the renaissance and the strengthening of a cultural identity – up to the revival of a language – going along with the protection of natural and cultural heritage that represents the founding part of that identity [21].

This new access to information allows a much more decentralized utilization of it – less hierarchical in nature – and stimulates local participation and actions. Isolated, fragmented, marginal and small populations - sharing similar development aspirations and often common cultural and natural heritage – can therefore be connected through electronic communication tools, so that they reach a critical size for diversification of products and services, and establish more reliable market distribution channels (di Castri 2000 a). Through the new sense of initiative and responsibility acquired in this form, dependent communities (mostly in islands) can be entitled to a highest degree of administrative and political autonomy in decision-making processes [25].

In addition, new relations exist now between urban and rural environments. Information can be equally available and usable in both environments, providing almost equal job opportunities and continuous learning. There is no longer the pressing need of a large rural exodus [16]. The countryside can remain inhabited, valorised and economically wealthy, through the introduction – thanks to the new availability of information – of a mosaic of secondary activities of elaboration and industry, tertiary activities of services (cultural, financial, informatics and, above all, tourism services), a quality forestry [17] and a quality agriculture - with high added value - and labelled and origin-certified products for export [18].

4. The access to genetic information

In addition to the possibility of discovering and commercializing their own biological diversity, through principles defined by the Convention on Biological Diversity, local populations can be greatly favored by progress in biotechnology, based on the opening of genetic systems and their management [15]. The second generation of transgenic plants permits to considerably decrease the use of pesticides and fertilizers in agriculture, then reducing or preventing water and soil pollution, in addition to lowering production costs. Cultivation of arid lands becomes also feasible, including by poor local farmers [35].

Furthermore, research and creation of small enterprises in biotechnology require investments, laboratories and know-how that are accessible in most developing countries. Countries of the South could therefore export patents and products of high added value, to reach the necessary stage of development that is not solely based on the exploitation of local natural resources, but with a greater investment on human resources. The technological and methodological similarities in the handling and managing of both the genetic and the digital information should also be emphasized [33].

5. The access to the economic information of the international trade

Trade represents the most ancient and relevant human adaptation to overcome the limitations of space heterogeneity (lands with different agriculture and production potential) and of time heterogeneity (strong seasonality, unfavourable years), through exchanges among different peoples, regions and countries.

An equitable international trade (but it is not always the case) can help promoting community development and protecting heritage in at least four aspects. First, it can prevent or limit subsidies and artificial price fixation that have had a perverse effect – since old Roman times – on the environment, the biodiversity, the protection of heritage and even on human societies [19]. Second, it allows escaping from the constraints of a forced food self-reliance that usually leads to the destruction of fragile and arid lands, up to massive desertification processes. Third, it permits a much larger diffusion of quality agricultural products, often based on local specificity and diversity, and promotes a great diversification of export products [18]. Fourth, through the export of innovative industrial products (for instance, microprocessors in Malaysia), it decreases human pressure on fragile landscapes and safeguard heritage. It should be emphasized how much all these exchanges, including appropriate international marketing and benchmarking, are promoted by access to information, the establishment of networks and continuous learning. It is practically a sine qua non for success[36].

6. The access to the interactive information of international tourism

Tourism is – at present – the economic and social sector of the greatest importance in the world as regards international exchanges and creation of new jobs. Its management is potentially the most decentralized one up to the level of local, including native, populations and micro-enterprises, often of a family size. It is therefore the economic sector most germane to the main transversal flows and networks of the information society [21][26][27]. Furthermore, tourism is likely to become the main driving force of cultural exchange, leading to a greater understanding of the differences and diversity among people and cultures – a stimulus for increasing tolerance [37].

Of course, all these considerations refer to the "quality tourism" (from cultural tourism to ecotourism) that has been even differentially promoted and supported after the crisis of 11 September 2001 [22].

The *resources* for quality tourism are the biological and cultural diversities, the heritages derived from the biological and cultural evolution, the local identities. This tourism consists in the marketing – rational and sustainable – of these diversities. It is also, therefore, the economic sector most linked to and most dependent on the protection and valorization of natural and cultural heritage.

The *mean* for developing this tourism is mostly the direct electronic communication between these small operators and the potential tourists, through a very attractive web page stimulating the imaginary perception of the area and the culture, so that the action of middlemen and large tourism operators are restricted as much as possible.

Patterns of this tourism are particularly appropriate for and applicable to physically fragmented areas, as for instance the Andes and the sub-Arctic zones, but with special emphasis on small islands. Access to information that stimulates both tourism and the maintenance of local agriculture and fishery activities is the only way – at present – to break the cycle of poverty in marginal and isolated populations [20][21][22][23]. In some regions of the world, for instance Polynesia including Easter Island (Rapa Nui), a tourism adopting the paradigm symbolized by the trilogy *culture-environment-information* has changed in a short time the living conditions, the economic income and the entrepreneurial capacity of local populations [23]. These are the so-called **digital islands**, now largely connected among them and open to the world thanks to electronic communication.

Furthermore, most local communities find again – as a kind of cultural renaissance – the pride of their history, their language, their diversity and identity, and of their environment that is part of it. They become fully aware that their economic and cultural development and expansion depend on two conditions: a wise management and protection of their natural and cultural heritage, and the opening up to the world through information, interaction and continuous learning.

This community culture-driven development leads also to great diversification, especially in this time of globalization. In my network of 28 Polynesian islands [23], nearly all of them apply a different mode of development, the single one consistent with their own will and aspirations.

The best example – almost the symbol – of this digitally- and culturally-driven development is Easter Island (called at present Rapa Nui in Polynesian language), the most isolated island of the world. In less than a decade, local people and small native entrepreneurs have increased the number to their connections to the Internet from 3 to more than 280, for an active population of less than 2.000 persons [13][25][34]. From the condition of having been the poorest zone of Chile, Easter Island is now – as an average – economically much wealthier than continental Chile. Thanks to its cultural and economic development, this island is again *Te Pito o Te Henua*, the navel of the world, as it was its oldest name.

7. The access to the technological information of a proactive innovation

There is now a multiplicity of new technologies that emphasize the precision and efficiency on resource utilization, the economy of energy and the use of renewable energies, the increased dematerialization of industrial products and the prevention of impacts on the environment. Efficiency, proactiveness and – above all – prevention are the key words. For some of these technologies, the objective is to approach as much as possible the "zero-waste" goal, by an almost complete utilization of the resource. They act at the beginning, and not at the end, of the industrial cycle process, thus minimizing pollution and reducing costs. Others, such as precision agriculture, represent a real information revolution in agriculture. Among the many miniaturized technologies inspired by space research and satellites utilization, Geographic Information Systems (GIS), Global Positioning Systems (GPS), Geographic Mark-up Language (GML) and Web Mapping Interface (WMI) are indispensable tools for development, as well as for inventorying and monitoring biodiversity and natural heritage. Emerging approaching and tools for development in the context of the information society are reviewed by di [14].

8. Potential and constraints of access to information and e-learning

The below considerations correspond just too some empirical observations based on my own experience, and do not pretend at all to generalize principles of action.

The first major constraint exists when energy is not available in a given area, or is too discontinuous and unreliable. A program is being planned – mostly to be applied in some African countries – and has been called "Energy for Information".

Learning the elementary techniques for the use of a computer and access to the Internet has proved to be much easier and stimulating than expected. In India, for instance, women from poor rural villages have a particular skill and interest to be involved in information technology and to ensure the links for a network.

The computer and the connection to the Internet – at this stage – have to be rather advanced and universal in nature; the user has to be able to send and receive e-mail and heavy attachments everywhere in the world, and to construct and frequently update an attractive web page with several interconnections. Computer dictionaries in several languages (usually English, French, Italian and Spanish) play an important role to facilitate contacts with the most important potential tourists or trade partners. The most advanced and automatic anti-virus system is a main asset to avoid temporary interruptions or collapse of communications that have usually a character of urgency and the need for a prompt reply (as in the case of tourism). Admittedly, all this use does not imply more than 10 % of the computer capacity, so that the possibility for some simplification can be welcomed, as it is tried to be achieved by some computer specialists from India. The demand is not for more speed, but for a more robust and easily manageable system.

The problem of distance learning is a tricky one. Of course, most of these populations have already been exposed in the past and has had access to distance learning by radio and television. This has been rather inadequate for the purpose of community development, since it has been – much too often - too general in nature, non-interactive, culturally biased or delivered by incompetent or obsolete bureaucracies, as it has been very often the case in India, Africa and Latin America. The requisite of *culturally appropriate and environmental specific information for development* is difficult to be met, considering the infinite diversity of cultures and ecosystems. Furthermore, several universities and research organizations – particularly in Europe – are too compartmentalized, and even disconnected or not interested in development issues, to be able to provide usable knowledge in these topics. This is a problem of relevant content rather than of advanced technique.

E-learning, if not properly planned taking into account the main requirement and aspiration of local communities for specificity, relevance and appropriateness in its content, could lead to the same unsatisfactory results. Of course, there are more general aspects that suffer less from a generalized approach, as alphabetization or continuous up-dating on technical matters.

As far as I am concerned in my activities, e-learning is almost an autonomous, user-originated process, where learning is achieved by local communities through constant and expanding interactions with other communities having solved a given problem with different approaches, or having had a different range of experiences – during this overall process of trial and error. These spontaneous interactions, as well as the stimulating and constructive interaction between small tourist operators and friend tourists from different nationalities and backgrounds, construct progressively a body of usable knowledge on tourism development, much more than the contacts with the university and research bodies dealing with development in a rather academic, general and inapplicable way. In particular this kind of very interactive and responsible e-learning, where learning applies at the two end of the knowledge-acquiring chain, is also an indispensable ingredient towards local empowerment.

9. Local empowerment

The interaction of these different accesses to information – in order to promote community development – has been successfully tested during the ICSU-SCOPE international program "Environment in a Global Information Society (EGIS). Field situations where myself and my associates workers have developed their Research & Development activities are in largely separated islands (mostly in Polynesia, with special emphasis on Easter Island), in the Canadian Arctic, in the Chilean Andes and Patagonia, along the Argentinean coasts, in squatter settlements of Argentina and Brazil, and in villages of South India, as well as in coastal and mountain zones of Italy, Spain and France. In several cases, they have contributed breaking the cycle of poverty through information and communication, and specially by launching tourism and quality agriculture micro-enterprises with access to possibilities of micro-capitalization and micro-investment.

In addition, observations from all continents show that the ideal condition for this kind of rapid development that is also in accordance with the protection of natural and cultural heritage occurs when the following three patterns are reached.

- **Diversification** of economic activities, and not monocultures, including at a community level and referring to different economic sectors.
- **Connectivity** (both internal and external) of the system and its opening up to the world (closing the system, under present circumstances, leads to economic and cultural collapse).
- And, above all, **local empowerment** (see also [23]).

Local empowerment implies a cultural control and modulation of development by local communities themselves through capacity building, habilitation and other enabling backups, access to information and knowledge, continuous education including by e-learning, decision-making autonomy and local decentralized initiative to search for specific and appropriate solutions and innovations - the most adapted to face globalization as a winner. This process is much facilitated when local communities master the information technology by them.

Local empowerment leads also to cultural pride and identity, while accepting with no complex and with tolerance the diversity of the others in an open world, stimulates initiatives and entrepreneurial capacity, and valorizes and protects natural and cultural heritage as the main elements for their development.

10. Cultural adaptation to change for sustainability

In a globalized world characterized by very rapid, repeated and unforeseeable change, sustainability of development depends – above all – on the capacity and willingness of *cultural adaptation to change*. Local communities have all the right to face this change with all enabling knowledge and tools. They should face it with specificity, not renouncing to their diversity, identity and their evolutionary roots; on the contrary, taking strength from their roots for a better adaptation to change.

Diversity in all its expressions, from biological to cultural to economic diversity, has always been in evolutionary terms, and still is, the essential strategy for adaptation to unforeseeable change. Cultural adaptation and control (the so-called culturally-driven development) is the base for the diversification of cultures and development patterns. It is the only way for local community to build up their destiny and their future.

The new paradigm for community development comprises, therefore, two elements: local empowerment for a better and voluntary (not passive) adaptation to change, and access to interactive information - at a worldwide basis - as the indispensable requisite to acquire such empowerment.

References

[1] di Castri F. 1981. Mediterranean-type shrublands of the world. In: di Castri F., Goodall D.W. and Specht R.L. (Eds.), Mediterranean-type shrublands. Ecosystems of the World 11. Elsevier Scientific Publ., Amsterdam: 1-52.

[2] di Castri F. 1995 a. Diversité biologique et diversité culturelle. Les fondements de l'universel. In: Sitter-Liver B. and Sitter-Liver B. (Eds.). Culture with nature. Culture dans la nature. Swiss Academy of Humanities and UNESCO. Wiese Publ., Basel: 295-311.

[3] di Castri F. 1995 b. The chair of sustainable development. Nature and Resources 31 (3): 2-7.

[4] di Castri F. 1995 c. 1492-1992. Searching for signal and consequences of globalization. In: Turner B.L. II, Gomez A., Gonzalez F. and di Castri F. (Eds.), Global Land Use Change: A Perspective from the Columbian Encounter. CSIC, Madrid: 109-130.

[5] di Castri F. 1996. Keeping the course between globalization and diversities. ECODECISION 21: 17-22.

[6] di Castri F. 1998 a. Le développement durable dans un monde ouvert. In: Dufour J. (Ed.), NIKAN, Les territoires du développement durable, héritage et enjeu pour demain. Université de Québec, Chicoutimi: 87-104.

[7] di Castri F. 1998 b. Environment in a global information society. Nature and Resources 34 (2): 4-7.

[8] di Castri 1998 c. L'environnement dans la société globale de l'information. In: Delisle C.E. and Bouchard M.A. (Eds.), Evaluation d'impacts et participation publique. Tendances dans le monde francophone. IAIA and Université de Montréal, Montreal: 21-61.

[9] di Castri F. 1998 d. Ecology in a Global Economy. In: Gopal B., Pathak P.S. and Saxena K.G. (Eds.), Ecology Today: An Anthology of Contemporary Ecological Research. International Scientific Publications, New Delhi: 1-17.

[10] di Castri F. 1998 e. Politics and environment in Mediterranean-climate regions. In: Rundel P.W., Montenegro G. and Jaksic F. (Eds.), Landscape disturbance and biodiversity in mediterranean-type ecosystems. Ecological Studies 136. Springer-Verlag, Heidelberg: 407-432.

[11] di Castri F. 1998 f. The interactive chain of globalizations: From the economic to the ecological one. In: Theys J. (Ed.), L'environnement au XXIe siècle. GERMES, Paris: 65-85.

[12] di Castri F. 1999 a. La société globale de l'information: atout ou risque pour l'environnement? Groupe Miollis, UNESCO, Paris, 75 p.

[13] di Castri F. 1999 b. Scenarios of tourism development in Easter Island. INSULA, International Journal of Island Affairs 8 (3): 27-39.

[14] di Castri F. 2000 a. Ecology in a context of economic globalization. BioScience 50 (4): 321-332.

[15] di Castri F. 2000 b. La diversité comme ressource et comme service dans la société de l'information (Biodiversité, Biotechnologie, Information). In: Nachhaltige Nutzung natürlicher Ressourcen. Schweizerischen Akademie der Naturwissenschaften 7, Luzern: 55-66.

[16] di Castri F. 2001 a. Urban-Rural Interactions. Introduction. In: Solbrig O.T, Paarlberg R. and di Castri F. (Eds.), Globalization and the Rural Environment. The David Rockefeller Center on Latin American Studies. Harvard University Press, Cambridge, MA: 413-417.

[17] di Castri F. 2001 b. Forestry in the context of the information society. Unasylva 52: 16-17.

[18] di Castri F. 2001 c. Rural values and the European view of agriculture. In: Solbrig O.T., Paarlberg R. and di Castri F. (Eds.), Globalization and the Rural Environment. The David Rockefeller Center on Latin American Studies. Harvard University Press, Cambridge, MA: 483-513.

[19] di Castri F. 2001 d. Développement, environnement et science dans la société post-industrielle de l'information. Bulletin de l'Académie des Sciences et Lettres de Montpellier 32: 113-128.

[20] di Castri F. 2002 a. Le développement durable, entre théorie et pratique, entre rêve et réalité. Liaison Energie-Francophonie. Numéro spécial Sommet de Johannesburg. 55-57: 38-45.

[21] di Castri F. 2002 b. The trilogy of the knowledge-based, post-industrial society: Information, Biodiversity and Tourism. In: di Castri F. and Balagy V. (Eds.), Tourism, Biodiversity and Information. Backhuys Publishers, Leiden: 7-24.

[22] di Castri F. 2002 c. Tourism revisited after 11 September 2001. In: di Castri F. and Balaji V. (Eds.), Tourism, Biodiversity and Information. Backhuys Publishers, Leiden: 483-488.

[23] di Castri F. 2002 d. Diversification, connectivity and local empowerment for tourism sustainability in South Pacific Islands - A network from French Polynesia to Easter Island. In: di Castri F. and Balaji V. (Eds.), Tourism, Biodiversity and Information. Backhuys Publishers, Leiden: 257-284.

[24] di Castri F. 2003 a. Access to information and local empowerment as a paradigm for conciliating conservation and development. In: Vigier F. (Ed.), Protecting cultural and natural heritage in the Western Hemisphere: Lessons from the past; Looking to the future. Center for Urban Development Studies, Harvard University, Cambridge, MA: 1-6.

[25] di Castri F. 2003 b. The dynamic future of Rapa Nui. Rapa Nui Journal 16 (in press).

[26] di Castri F. and Balaji V. 2002 a. Tourism, Biodiversity and Information. Annals of Tourism Research 29 (1): 269-270.

[27] di Castri F and Balaji V. (Eds.). 2002 b. Tourism, Biodiversity and Information. Backhuys Publishers, Leiden, 502 p.
[28] di Castri F. and Loope L. 1977. Biosphere reserves: theory and practice. Nature and Resources 13 (1): 2-7.
[29] di Castri F. and Mooney H.A. (Eds.). 1973. Mediterranean Type Ecosystems: Origin and Structure. Ecological Studies 7. Springer Verlag, Heidelberg, 405 p.
[30] di Castri F. and Robertson J. 1982. The Biosphere Reserve concept: 10 years after. Parks 6 (4): 1-6.
[31] di Castri F. and Younès T. (Eds.). 1996. Biodiversity, Science and Development. Towards a new partnership. CAB International, Wallingford, UK, 646 p.
[32] di Castri F., Sheldon P., Conlin M., Boniface P. and Balaji V. 2002. Introduction to Section VI: Information, Communication and Education for Tourism Development. In: di Castri F. and Balaji V. (Eds.), Tourism, Biodiversity and Information. Backhuys Publishers, Leiden: 423-429.
[33] Enriquez J. 2001. Technology, Gene Research, and National Competitiveness. In: Solbrig O.T., Paarlberg R. and di Castri F. (Eds.), Globalization and the Rural Environment. The David Rockefeller Center on Latin American Studies, Harvard University Press, Cambridge, MA: 225-254.
[34] Hereveri E. 2002. Internet and Culture for the Sustainable Development of Easter Island. In: di Castri F. and Balaji V. (Eds.), Tourism, Biodiversity, Information. Backhuys Publishers, Leiden: 282-284.
[35] Houdebine L.M. 2000. OGM. Le vrai et le faux. Le Pommier-Fayard, Paris, 204 p.
[36] Solbrig O.T., Paarlberg R. and di Castri F. (Eds.). 2001. Globalization and the Rural Environment. The David Rockefeller Center on Latin American Studies, Harvard University Press, Cambridge, MA, 535 p.
[37] UNESCO 1997. Culture, tourism, development: crucial issues for the XXIst century. UNESCO, Paris.

Towards the Learning Grid
P. Ritrovato et al. (Eds.)
IOS Press, 2005

The Challenge of Change: reducing conflict in implementing e-learning

Rosa MICHAELSON
Accountancy & Business Finance, University of Dundee, DD1 4HN, Scotland.

Abstract. This paper calls for the design of the European Grid for Learning to take note of important issues which have arisen in previous e-learning cycles in the UK. In particular, low take-up of products and services by lecturers has been explained in terms of techno-fear, or ignorance of e-learning potential. These claims are unsubstantiated. Other explanations are possible for the observed resistance of the educational specialist to the use of educational technology. Rather than ignore possible areas of conflict, or to assume (after Foucault) that any change results in shifts of power which produce inevitable counter-balances from a threatened group, it is possible to use resistance to change as an important part of the design process. To this end, I discuss the findings of an analysis of recent UK-wide initiatives in C&IT and e-learning. The issues raised by participants of the many different groups involved have implications for the take-up of future Grid-based learning. In particular, the needs of educators are identified as crucial to the effective deployment of e-learning.

Keywords. e-learning; design focus for Grid technologies; teacher's rights; Information Systems methodologies; managing change.

Background

In the UK Higher Education sector online learning has been greeted with enthusiasm by many. For example, the UK-wide e-University was launched in 2000 to meet a suggested lack in HE online provision for lifelong learning, and in response to perceived threats of other global educational projects [1]. The growth of the virtual university, such as the global conglomerates Fathom and Cardean University, based on Unext.com, has been perceived as a threat to standard university education [2], [3]. Many such ambitious e-learning projects have failed, most recently the UKeU [4] [5].

Evaluation of large Information Systems (IS) implementation, and in particular of IS failure, leads to the understanding of the importance of counter-implementation and resistance to change, informing methods which reduce conflict and improve design processes [6], [7]. In order to inform the effective design of a European Grid for Learning we need to consider possible problem areas which might be of concern to the lectures and teachers who will use Grid-enabled applications.

This paper outlines issues that arose in two UK-wide initiatives which have deployed C & IT in Higher and Further Education. The first initiative of interest was the Teaching and Learning Technologies Project (TLTP). This initiative ended in 2001, after 10 years of funding. The first phases of the TLTP consisted of 72 subject-specific projects, many of which produced multimedia resources. More recent projects focused on web-based delivery of these products, and other forms of networked education. The cost of the TLTP was in the order of £90 Million [8].

The second initiative, which has been promoted by JISC (the Joint Information Systems Committee), concerns the use of Learning Environments (LE). Within UK higher and further education there are now many users of web-based applications variously described as virtual learning environments (VLE) including First Class, WebCT and BlackBoard. Many institutions are also using locally developed VLE such as TAGS, COSE and Merlin [9], [10], [11]. More recently managed learning environments (MLE) – the integration of VLE with the institutions MIS - have been the main funding focus for JISC supported projects [12].

1. Important issues

An analysis of the above initiatives has identified the following issues as problematic for e-learning [11], [8]:

- Cost
- Evaluation
- Sustainability
- Focus
- Standards
- Social Learning
- De-skilling
- Acceptance and take-up

Many of the above have implications for those who are intended to use the new educational technologies, namely the lecturers and teachers. The next section details the problems that were identified in the analysis of reports and papers generated by the initiatives.

2. Impact of e-learning issues

2.1. Cost

The actual cost of networked learning is contentious. Many claim cost-benefits for e-learning. The main assumption is that there is no extra cost, or comparable costs, in using educational technology. This was expressed as the need to show efficiency gains during the TLTP period. There are those who claim that they know about the cost of developing C&IT, but assumptions concerning economies of scale or time-scale of use adjust the true cost downwards [13]. It is unusual for infrastructure and maintenance costs (which are of great importance for e-learning service provision) to be explicitly included in cost-benefit analysis. Cost is also an issue for creating e-learning standards, discussed below.

2.2. Evaluation

What is evaluated? There seems confusion over how to evaluate learning efficacy via educational technology. The focus of evaluation varies from usability issues, type of application, software functionality [14], 'soft' studies of student attitudes, and as suggested above, cost. There are few evaluations of the UK-wide impact of particular programmes for C&IT [15], [11]. A recent scoping report for JISC found that the time-scale for MLE adoption in UK universities was in the order of 5 years, but did not look at pedagogical concerns [16].

2.3. Sustainability

Sustainability has been a persistent theme for the last 30 years of C&IT in education, as it has for computing in general. Timeliness of adoption of new technologies by a community has a far-reaching effect on sustainability: by the time a novel technology has been taken up in the wider educational community it is out of date. In addition, the research efforts of those who test a particular technology are often ignored because managers wish to use *off-the-shelf* commercial solutions. The paradox of research and development in educational technologies is that during the lifetime of the project there is already some other technology on the horizon which will supersede or replace the focus of the current enthusiasm. These replacement technologies often over-stretch the existing infrastructure requirements.

2.4. Focus

An important issue for the success of any IS project is focus. However, educational or pedagogic objectives are rarely discussed by those who drive initiatives. It is often the case that the originators of change promote the idea that a particular problem will be solved by the application of technology, even if there is no evidence for such an outcome. For example, in the UK the wider access agenda is often expected to be solved by e-learning, thereby ignoring the costs to the individual, and the high drop-out rates of distance learning.

2.5. Social Learning

E-learning blurs the distinction between Distance Learning versus campus-based learning. There is an assumed equivalence of these models which needs to be carefully considered. Networked learning institutes are often given the name ‘university’ but are more akin to distance learning establishments, such as the UK Open University, than the majority of campus-based institutions. What are the implications for the teacher's role when such blurring occurs? How does this affect the role of the social in learning? Distance Learning requires a division of labour (those who develop a course are not the delivers or administrators of the course), and courses and materials must persist for several years if it is to be cost effective [17], [18].

2.6. The Threat of De-skilling

Is the objective of e-learning the replacement of the educator? Threats to the educator’s professionalism include unbundling and interoperability. The concept of unbundling follows the division of labour needs of Distance Learning discussed above. Patel and Franklin's report to JISC on MLE states:

“Unbundling the delivery of HE courses is a key issue in the provision of a national learning infrastructure. Currently the delivery of courses in HE is bundled i.e. the same people design develop and deliver courses and materials and deliver and conduct assessment and courses are studied as a whole at one institution.” [19]

Thus the professional role of the lecturer or teacher in controlling their own materials is directly challenged by the impetus of networked learning. There has also been, in the UK, an unpredicted growth of 'specialised' support - the Learning Technologist with as yet no formal or professional status within the sector. Some propose that learning technologists are vital to re-introduce the social learning aspects to e-learning [20]. What is the new role of the lecturer if learning technologists or e-moderators are required to make e-learning work?

2.7. Standards

In the case of web-based learning the need for interoperability of systems translates into a quest for meta-data or classification systems for educational content. Here content is talked about in terms of 'learning objects' or 'chunks' which may have wider application than a specific course and are seen as the key to material being created in one system and being transferable between different systems. There are still unresolved issues of quality and consistency associated with this view. In addition the management of learning is seen only in terms of the production of small enough 'chunks'. Unfortunately there is as yet no single definition of what constitutes a 'learning object'. Freisen has identified three problems with learning objects: firstly, the problem of identifying a precise definition for the term and the implications of such imprecision; secondly, the way that learning is not considered when discussion of e-learning standards arise; and thirdly, that some of the possible standards under consideration arise from US military training, leading to probable conflicts in identifying appropriate forms for higher and public education [21]. Many vendors are creating their own definitions with little recourse to the diversity of practise among educators. Hence there are competing standards, some of which emerge from training in the US (e.g. SCORM, ADL). This also raises issues concerning cultural differences in education. There is already work to show that expectations of the way teachers use material have proved incorrect [22]. The costs of metadata classification are well documented, as are issues with the quality of the metadata classification process [23].

2.8. Acceptance and Take-up

By the end of the TLTP initiative it was discovered that very few products were in use. Those employed were generally for pre-university education – often used to bring students up to a particular level of achievement. The common consensus from those involved in the projects was that to increase use staff needed to be taught about C&IT. The concept of possible replacement of staff by new technologies, and hence cost-benefits, were rejected. The technology was seen as an addition to range of techniques available for lecturers and teachers. This had an additional effect on take-up, also noted in the LE initiative. Lectures noted that this addition of technology increased the individual workload tremendously. In the case of production of content for LE this may seem so overwhelming, given that staff continues to teach with traditional methods, that they cannot easily include LE in their teaching practice.

3. Possible reasons for conflict

Those who are not educators, or enthusiasts for particular applications, tend to explain resistance to using new technologies as being based on lack of staff-development or lack of management support for the champions of e-learning. Other explanations also include the claim that lecturers are scared of new technology. In fact, most lecturers in HE have assimilated computing technology as part of their everyday work – the production of overhead slides, the administration of student records, the use of e-mail for communicating with colleagues, students and research collaborators, the use of the

Internet as an additional resource – all of these are common in UK academic life. It is difficult for those with involvement in research and development of novel educational technology to understand that they may have ignored the diverse educational styles and objectives of professional staff. They do not acknowledge that they may have designed unusable applications.

Another factor in the effective take-up of new technologies is that enthusiasm for C&IT deployment in education produces a subsequent, often unrecognised; growth in IT infra-structure since all C&IT is dependent on increased IT resources. This increases the influence that technologists have on the educational process, without engaging the educationalist.

In addition, Managerialism in e-learning manifests itself in ideas of cost-effectiveness; the replacement of the lecturer by technology; the introduction of the specialist technology moderator (the threat of de-skilling the educator); concepts of unbundling and granularity of content; the down-grading of pedagogy; assumptions of metadata classification by the non-specialist; and the intervention of IT support and administration into teaching style (as in the MLE program). Can these types of conflict be avoided by possible future Grid technologies?

4. Conclusion

I would argue, in the light of these issues that in order to design effective Grid-based e-learning the current processes of education must be more fully understood. Educational objectives must be a focus for the design, as must the wishes and needs of the educators. The idea of radical change, brought about by new technologies, cannot be realised without understanding possible points of conflict such as those identified in previous initiatives.

References

[1] *ICT in Higher Education*, **1**, 5. Times Higher Education Supplement, 7 February 2003.

[2] Kirschner, A. (2000) Fathom: the global university. *LSE Magazine*, Winter, London.

[3] Rosenfield, A. (2000) unxt.com (founder, chairman and CEO of unxt.com), *LSE magazine*, Winter, London.

[4] Ryan, Y. (2002*) Emerging indicators of success and failure in borderless higher education*, Report for The Observatory on Borderless Education, The Association for Commonwealth Universities. http://www.obhe.ac.uk/products/reports/pdf/February2002.pdf (6/04/02)

[5] HEFCE (2004) *HEFCE discusses restructuring of e-Universities' activities,* 27 February 2004. www.hefce.ac.uk/news/hefce/2004/euni/

[6] Keen, P. G. W. (1981) Information Systems and Organizational Change. *Communications of the ACM (CACM)*, **24**, 1, 24-33.

[7] Beynon-Davies, P. (1999) Human error and information systems failure: the case of the London ambulance service computer-aided despatch system project. *Interacting with Computers*, **11**, 699 - 720.

[8] Michaelson, R. (2001) Learning from our mistakes: 10 years of UK-wide C&IT initiatives, *BAA Accounting Education SIG*, Glamorgan.

[9] Allison, C., Bain, A., McKechan, D., Michaelson, R. (2000) "Using TAGS for Distributed IT Project Management" in *Proceedings of the LTSN-ICS 1st Annual Conference*, Heriot-Watt University, Edinburgh, 23 - 25 August.

[10] COSE (2001) http://cetis.bangor.ac.uk/co3/cose.html

[11] Merlin (1999) http://www.hull.ac.uk/merlin

[12] Michaelson, R. (2002) Let's get real: Virtual or Managed Learning Environments, *LTSN-Best 2nd Conference for Business, Management and Accounting*, Edinburgh, April 2002.

[13] Bacsich, P., Ash, C., Boniwell, K., Kaplan, L., Mardell, J., Cavan-Atack, A. (1999) *The cost of networked learning*. A report for JCALT. Sheffield Hallam University, JISC. October.
[14] Britain, S. & Liber O. (1999) *A Framework for Pedagogical Evaluation of Virtual Learning Environments*. JTAP Report, October. www.jtap.ac.uk/reports/htm/jtap-041.html (26/03/01).
[15] Selwyn, N. (2000). Researching computers and education - glimpses of the wider picture. *Computers and Education*, **34** (2000), 93-101.
[16] JISC/MLEScope (2003) Managed Learning Environment Activity in Further and Higher Education in the UK: A Supporting Study for the Joint Information Systems Committee (JISC) and the Universities and Colleges Information Systems Association (UCISA), The Social Informatics Research Unit, University of Brighton, Education for Change Ltd, The Research Partnership. August/December 2003. www.jisc.ac.uk/uploaded_documents/mle-study-final-report.pdf
[17] Peters, O. (1989) "The iceberg has not melted: further reflections on the concept of industrialisation and distance teaching". *Open Learning*, 4, 3, 3-8. Harlow: Longman Group.
[18] Brown, J. S., Duguid, P. (2002) *The Social Life of Information*, Harvard Business School Press.
[19] Patel, D., Franklin, T. (2001) *Summary Briefing Paper on issues for the development and implementation of MLE*, JISC Report, 4 June 2001. www.jisc.ac.uk/mle/reps/paper-1.htm
[20] Salmon, G. (2000) *E-moderating: the key to teaching and learning online*, Kogan-Page.
[21] Friesen, N. (2004). "Three Objections to Learning Objects" in McGreal, R. (Ed.). *Online Education Using Learning Objects*. London: Routledge/Falmer. See phenom.educ.ualberta.ca/~nfriesen
[22] Monthienvichienchai, R., Sasse, A., Wheeldon, R. (2001) Educational Metadata: Teacher's Friend or Foe? in *Euro CSCL 2001, the proceedings of European Perspectives on Computer-supported Collaborative Learning*. Dillenbourg, P., Eurelings, A., Hakkarainen, K., eds. March 22-24, University of Maastricht, 508-519.
[23] Currier, S. (2004) "Metadata Quality in e-Learning: Garbage In - Garbage Out?", CETIS, April 02, 2004. www.cetis.ac.uk/content2/20040402013222

Towards the Learning Grid
P. Ritrovato et al. (Eds.)
IOS Press, 2005

Brain Meets Brawn: Why Grid and Agents Need Each Other[1]

Ian Foster [a], Nicholas R. Jennings [b], Carl Kesselman [c]
[a] *Argonne National Laboratory& University of Chicago foster@mcs.anl.gov*
[b] *Electronics & Comp. Science University of Southampton nrj@ecs.soton.ac.uk*
[c] *Information Sciences Institute University of Southern Californiacarl@isi.edu*

Abstract. The Grid and agent communities both develop concepts and mechanisms for open distributed systems, albeit from different perspectives. The Grid community has historically focused cn "brawn": infrastructure, tools, and applications for reliable and secure resource sharing within dynamic and geographically distributed virtual organizations. In contrast, the agent's community has focused on "brain": autonomous problem solvers that can act flexibly in uncertain and dynamic environments. Yet as the scale and ambition of both Grid and agent deployments increase, we see a convergence of interests, with agent systems requiring robust infrastructure and Grid systems requiring autonomous, flexible behaviors. Motivated by this convergence of interests, we review the current state of the art in both areas, review the challenges that concern the two communities, and propose research and technology development activities that can allow for mutually supportive efforts.

Keywords: Grid technology, Virtual Organisations, agent systems, service oriented architecture,

Introduction

In open distributed systems, independent components cooperate to achieve individual and shared goals. Both individual components and the system as a whole are designed to cope with change and evolution in the number and nature of the participating entities. Such systems are important in many contexts, from large scientific collaborations to enterprise systems and sensor networks.

The Grid and agent communities are both pursuing the development of such open distributed systems, albeit from different perspectives. The Grid community [12] has historically focused on what we refer to here as "brawn": interoperable infrastructure and tools for secure and reliable resource sharing within dynamic and geographically distributed virtual organizations (VOs) [14], and applications of the same to various resource federation scenarios. In contrast, those working on agents have focused on "brains," i.e., on the development of concepts, methodologies, and algorithms for autonomous problem solvers that can act flexibly in uncertain and dynamic environments in order to achieve their aims and objectives [21]. A key component of this research is motivated by the fact that such agents are often required to form themselves into collectives (i.e., VOs) and act in a coordinated manner. This need to support aggregation has, in turn, led to much research into rich and flexible mechanisms for managing such interactions.

---

[1] Reprinted from the Proceedings of the 2000 Conference on Autonomous Agents and Multi Agent Systems (AAMAS 2004).

As these two communities mature and turn their attention to fundamental problems of scope, both are encountering challenging problems in terms of scale and application. This maturation process is causing an increasing overlap in the problems that they address. Specifically, current Grid systems are somewhat rigid and inflexible in terms of their interoperation and their interactions, while agent systems are typically not engineered as serious distributed systems that need to scale, that are robust, and that are secure [34]. Nevertheless, each is working its way towards the others' territory, as Grids seek to become more flexible and agile, and agent systems seek to be more reliable and scaleable.

Given this background, it is fruitful to examine work in these two domains, first to communicate to each community what has been done by the other, and second to identify opportunities for cross fertilization. We seek to take a first step towards that goal in this paper. To this end, we first review the state of the art in Grids and agents (Sections 2 and 3), compare and contrast the two approaches (Section 4), present a common vision of service-oriented architecture (Section 5), and conclude with a list of significant research challenges (Section 6).

Limited time and space require that we restrict ourselves in this article to the work being performed within the Grid and agents communities. Thus, we do not cover the highly relevant and interesting work pertaining to open distributed systems that can be found in other domains, including robotics, peer-to-peer networking, semantic web, distributed systems, artificial intelligence, and autonomic systems.

1. Grids

Grids aim to enable "resource sharing and coordinated problem solving in dynamic, multi-institutional VOs" [12]. In other words, Grids provide an infrastructure for federated resource sharing across trust domains. Much like the Internet on which they build, current Grids define protocols and middleware that can mediate access provided by this layer to discover, aggregate, and harness resources. These applications span a wide spectrum. Moreover, the standardization of the protocols and interfaces used to construct systems is an important part of the overall research and development program.

1.1. Technologies

Grid technologies have evolved through at least three distinct generations: early ad hoc solutions, de facto standards based on the Globus Toolkit (GT), and the current emergence of more formal Web services (WS)-based standards within the context of the Open Grid Services Architecture (OGSA) [13].

OGSA adopts WS standards such as Web Services Description Language (WSDL) as a basis for a service-oriented architecture within which arbitrary services can be defined, discovered, and invoked in terms of their interfaces rather than their implementations. This approach provides a basis for virtualization, interoperability, and composition.

The Grid community has participated in, and in some cases led, the development of WS specifications that address other Grid requirements. The WS-Resource Framework (WSRF) defines uniform mechanisms for defining, inspecting, and managing remote state, a crucial concern in many settings. WSRF mechanisms underlie work on service management (WSDM, in OASIS) and negotiation (WS-Agreement, in GGF), efforts that are crucial to the Grid vision of large-scale, reliable, and interoperable Grid applications and services. Other relevant efforts are aimed at standardizing interfaces to data, computers, and other classes of resources.

Work on Grid-related standards is driven by, and influences, the work of a vibrant open source community. GT (in its most recent instantiation, Web services-based and WSRF-compliant) provides basic middleware to create VOs, addressing such issues as specification and enforcement of VO wide policy, discovery, provisioning and management of services and resources, and federation, replication, discovery, and movement of data. At deployment, depending on available resources and planned applications, specific service implementations can be chosen and deployed, often in conjunction with other GT-based components.

Grid technology R&D has produced specifications and technologies for realizing service-oriented architectures according to robust distributed system principles. Global control mechanisms able to deal reliably with failure and adapt to changing environmental conditions and application concerns have been a lesser concern.

1.2. Applications

Early application drivers were largely from scientific computing [6, 10, 19], and included large-scale distributed computing [2, 15] (federation of computers), integration of large-scale data repositories (data Grids [7]), collaboration [31], and tele-instrumentation [23, 26]. More recently, the technology has seen considerable uptake in industry as a means of addressing issues of virtualization and distributed system management [13].

GT is in production use across VOs integrating resources from 20-50 sites with thousands of computational and data resources, and is expected to scale to 100s of sites with 1000s of sites as a future goal. In the remainder of this section, we list a few examples to show the range and scope of Grid deployments.

The U.S. Network for Earthquake Engineering Simulation Grid (NEESGrid) connects experimental facilities (e.g., shake tables), data archives, computers, and a user community of earthquake engineers. Its service-oriented architecture defines standard interfaces for telepresence, monitoring, and control of remote scientific instruments, and for publishing, discovering, and accessing data produced by these instruments [26]. NEESGrid experiments have linked facilities at three sites and more than 50 remote participants.

Grid2003 [15] links 28 sites with clusters totalling some 3000 processors. These resources are used by science communities from high energy physics, astronomy, biology, chemistry, and computer science for large-scale simulation and data analysis computations.

In contrast, Access Grid [31] is focused on interpersonal communication, via sharing of audio, video, and applications within collaborative spaces. Grid technologies are used in Access Grid for such purposes as security, discovery, and resource management.

Butterfly.net is creating a GT-based provisioning infrastructure for multiplayer online games, in which the demands for computation, storage, and network resources can vary dramatically as the popularity of games changes over time [24]. As a second example of a commercial Grid deployment, GlobeXplorer is using GT to support integration and processing of satellite image data [17].

Experiences with such applications reveal issues that must be addressed if Grids are to be scaled to larger communities, more diverse resources, and more complex applications. We review those challenges in Section 6.

2. Agent-Based Computing

An agent "is an encapsulated computer system that is situated in some environment, and that is capable of flexible, autonomous action in that environment in order to meet its design objectives" [33]. In more detail [21], agents are: (i) clearly identifiable problem solving entities with well-defined boundaries and interfaces; (ii) situated (embedded) in a particular environment—they receive inputs related to the state of their environment through sensors and they act on the environment through effectors; (iii) designed to fulfil a specific role—they have particular objectives to achieve and have particular problem solving capabilities (services) that they can bring to bear to this end; (iv) autonomous—they have control both over their internal state and over their own behavior; and (v) capable of exhibiting flexible problem solving behavior in pursuit of their design objectives—they need to be both reactive (able to respond in a timely fashion to changes that occur in their environment) and proactive (able to opportunistically adopt goals and take the initiative).

When adopting an agent-oriented view of the world, it soon becomes apparent that most problems require or involve multiple agents: to represent the decentralized nature of the problem, multiple loci of control, multiple perspectives, or competing interests. Moreover, these agents need to interact, either to achieve their individual objectives or to manage the dependencies that ensue from being situated in a common environment. Thus, in any given system there may be both cooperative and selfish agents whose aims are, respectively, to maximize the social welfare of the system and to maximize their own individual return. These interactions are built on some form of semantic integration (Section 2.3), may well involve trust relationships, and also include the traditional service discovery and invocation discussed above, as well as the more sophisticated social interactions related to the ability to cooperate, coordinate and negotiate about which services are performed by which agents at what time.

In the majority of cases, agents act to achieve objectives either on behalf of individuals (or companies) or as part of some wider problem solving initiative. (Note the similarity to the VO concept.) Thus, when agents interact there is typically some underpinning organizational context that defines the relationship among them. For example, agents may be peers working together in a team or one may be the manager of the other agents. To capture such links, agent systems typically have explicit constructs for modelling organizational relationships or roles such as peer, manager, or team member. In many cases, these relationships are subject to ongoing change: social interaction means existing relationships evolve (e.g., a team of peers may elect a leader) and new relations are created (e.g., a number of agents may form a VO to deliver a particular service that no one individual can offer). The temporal extent of these relationships can also vary enormously: from just long enough to deliver a particular service once, to a permanent bond.

Whatever the nature of the social process, there are two points that qualitatively differentiate agent interactions from those that occur in other computational models. First, agent-oriented interactions tend to be more sophisticated than in other contexts, dealing, for example, with notions of cooperation, coordination, and negotiation. Second, agents are flexible problem solvers, operating in an environment over which they have only partial control and observability. Thus, interactions need to be handled in a similarly flexible manner, and agents need the computational apparatus to make context-dependent decisions about the nature and scope of their interactions and to initiate (and respond to) interactions that were not foreseen at design time. The downside of this autonomy and flexibility, however, is that it is difficult to ensure that desirable global behaviors emerge. To this end, a range of techniques (such as reinforcement learning, mechanism design, and electronic institutions) are often deployed to try and impose greater order.

Drawing these points together, **Figure 1** shows that adopting an agent-oriented approach to system engineering means decomposing the problem into multiple, interacting, autonomous components that have particular objectives to achieve and are capable of performing particular services. The key abstraction models that define the agent-oriented mindset are agents, interactions and organizations. Finally, explicit structures and mechanisms are often used to describe and manage the complex and changing web of organizational relationships that exist between the agents.

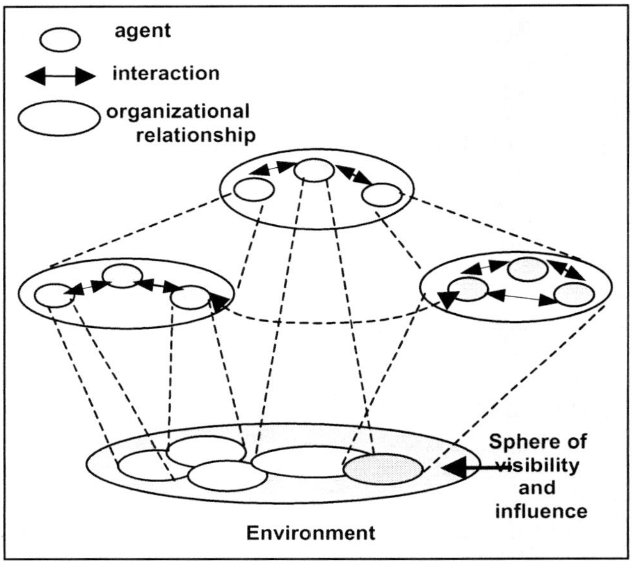

Figure 1: Canonical view of a multiagent system

2.1. Technologies

In contrast to Grid computing, there is less focus on identifiable agent technologies that can be used off the shelf to build applications. Traditionally, more attention has been given to theories and models of how agents can be developed and how they can communicate, cooperate, and negotiate. This work has resulted in the development of a range of algorithms that can be used both to build individual agents and to manage their interactions. In the former case, algorithms and architectures have been developed that enable an agent to plan an effective course of action to achieve a goal in uncertain and unpredictable environments, to adapt its behavior to its prevailing circumstances, and to strike an effective balance between being too responsive (and continually changing its aim such that no task is ever completed) and too committed to its present course of action (such that more important activities are not dealt with in a timely fashion). In the latter case, algorithms have been developed that agents can use to achieve efficient negotiation outcomes, to form teams composed of the optimal set of parties, and to determine the degree of trust that should be placed in a particular agent, based upon its social and organizational relationships.

There has recently been an increasing trend towards making agent technology a serious basis for building complex, distributed systems. Several agent development environments support specific agent architectures and provide libraries of interaction protocols (e.g., JACK, JADE, Cougaar, and ZEUS), software engineering methodologies have been devised to analyze and design agent-based systems (e.g., Gaia, Tropos, and AUML), and there have been efforts to standardize various aspects of agent systems, such as inter-agent communication (e.g., FIPA, KQML). Moreover, as in the Grid community, there is an increasingly reliance on Web services and semantic web technologies for providing the computational infrastructure for such systems and an increasing acceptance of the importance of trust as a central issue in interaction.

2.2. Applications

Agent technology has been deployed in a number of isolated applications over the past ten years. However in the past few years the number and range of applications have increased significantly. In particular, many large companies are now interested in developing applications using agent technologies, and deployed applications exist for domains such as manufacturing, electronic commerce, process control, telecommunication systems, traffic and transportation management, information filtering and gathering, business process management, defence, entertainment and medical care [25].

3. Brains and Brawn

We see that a common thread underlies both agents and Grids, namely, the creation of communities or VOs bound together by a common goal or cause. Yet the two communities have focused on different aspects of this common problem. In the case of Grids, the primary concern has been the mechanisms by which communities form and operate. Thus, we see much effort devoted to how community standards are represented via explicit policy, how policy is enforced, how community members identify one another, how actions within the community are implemented, and how commitments by community members are specified, monitored and enforced. On the other hand, our understanding of how to use these mechanisms to create large-scale systems with stable collective behavior is less mature. For example, commonly used Grid tools provide uniform mechanisms for accessing data on different storage systems, but not for the semantic integration of that data; for accessing service and resource state, but not for anticipating, detecting, and diagnosing problems implied by changes to that state; and for securely authenticating users and services, but not for inferring whether or not specific users or services can be trusted to perform specific actions. To this extent, Grids are all brawn and no brain.

Agents also focus on creating community. Out of the flexible local decision making of system components, sensible community wide behaviors emerge through rich social interactions and explicit organizational structures. However in building all this flexibility and sophistication, scant attention has been paid to how these tasks should be performed in realistic distributed environments. For example, agent frameworks provide sophisticated internal reasoning capabilities, but offer no support for secure interaction or service discovery; cooperation algorithms produce socially optimal outcomes, but assume the agents have complete knowledge of all outcomes that any potential grouping can produce; and negotiation algorithms achieve optimal outcomes for the participating agents, but assume that all parties in the system are known at the outset of the negotiation and will not change during the system's operation. Thus, one may say that agents are all brain and no brawn.

Clearly, neither situation is ideal: for Grids to be effective in their goals, they must be imbued with flexible, decentralized decision making capabilities. Likewise, agents need a robust distributed computing platform that allows them to discover, acquire, federate, and manage the capabilities necessary to execute their decisions. In other words, there are good opportunities for exploiting synergies between Grid and agents.

One approach to exploiting such synergies might be a simple layering of the technologies, i.e., to implement agent systems on top of Grid mechanisms. However, it seems more likely that the true benefits of an integrated Grid/agent approach will only be achieved via a more fine-grain intertwining of the two technologies, with Grid technologies becoming more agent-like and agent-based systems becoming more Grid-like.

As an early example of such a tighter coupling, we point to work on agent-based resource selection, in which re-enforcement-based learning is used to drive the assignment of tasks to resources [16]. In this case, the "agent" (i.e., the logic used to make the task assignment decisions) uses Grid functions for status monitoring, resource discovery, and task submission. The agent, in turn, provides a valuable Grid function, with the collection of agents implementing a robust global resource management behavior that might not otherwise be achieved. A second example is the use of automated negotiation techniques (specifically, various forms of auctions) to allocate resources in Grid systems [32]. Here, designers evaluate the effectiveness of both commodity market and Vickery auction protocols to the problem of allocating resources within a distributed system. This example also shows how techniques familiar to agents' researchers can be integrated with other more standard components within Grid architecture.

This level of integration will undoubtedly create new challenges for both agents and Grids. However, the result could be frameworks for constructing robust, large-scale, agile distributed systems that are qualitatively and quantitatively superior to the best current practice today.

4. Robust Agile Service-Oriented Systems

Having described key agent and Grid concepts, we now draw the two parallel lines of research together to highlight their commonalities and complementarities.

4.1. Autonomous Services

A core unifying concept that underlies Grids and agent systems is that of a *service*: an entity that provides a capability to a *client* via a well-defined message exchange [4]. Within third-generation Grids, service interactions are structured via Web service mechanisms, and thus all entities are services. However, while every agent can be considered a service (in that it interacts with other agents and its environment via message exchanges), we might reasonably state that not every Grid service is necessarily an agent (in that it may not participate in message exchanges that exhibit flexible autonomous actions).

This notion of *autonomous action* is thus central to the question of how agents and Grids can interoperate. To illustrate the issues, let us consider a service that encapsulates a database. In a local area network, we might find a version of this service that responds to requests to "read a record" or "write a record." Such an implementation does not exhibit autonomous behavior.

On the other hand, in a more distributed, administratively heterogeneous, and failure-prone environment, the implementation of such a service might exhibit more sophisticated behavior. For example, the database might be replicated, with the number of replicas determined dynamically by knowledge-based models of system reliability and performance. Distributed negotiation protocols might be used to establish the query throughput achievable on individual copies, such that community throughput is optimized. Finally, distributed planning and scheduling algorithms might be used to map queries to specific database replicas so as to minimize the latency of user requests. In all these cases, a robust database service, designed to operate in an open distributed system, is exhibiting flexible autonomous actions (in the sense that its behaviors are not driven solely by a client request, but also by other considerations, including local policies and the outcomes of negotiations with the client). In short, such services will exhibit agent behavior.

4.2. Rich Service Models

Both agent and Grid systems consist of *dynamic* and *stateful* services. The underlying service model is dynamic in that new services can be created and destroyed over the lifetime of the system. Here an important contribution of Grid technologies is a robust lifetime and naming model for dynamic services [13]. Implicit in this model are the notion of service failure and the definition of scalable distributed systems semantics. In contrast, agent-based systems rarely consider such issues, but they could clearly benefit from exploiting this approach to representing and managing dynamic services.

Statefulness is another important aspect of the service model. A stateful service (or, more-or-less equivalently, a *resource* [11]) has internal state that persists over multiple interactions. It can often be useful to make this state externally visible, so that, for example, another participant in a distributed system can determine the current load on a server, the policies that govern access to a service, and/or the schema(s) supported by a database. Again, Grid technologies have addressed this issue, defining a general model for representing and querying service state [11]. This model includes mechanisms for describing state "lifetime", as well as a means of specifying and enforcing policy with respect to access and modification.

The Grid state model defines how state is represented and accessed, but does not speak to the structure or semantics of the state that is thus exposed. Typical practice is to define state in terms of fixed schema or attributes. In contrast, agent systems address semantics but do not provide a consistent state model. An integrated approach can allow for the publication of richer semantic information within the Grid state model, thus enhancing the ability of applications to discover, configure, and manage services in an interoperable manner [18].

4.3. Negotiation and Service Contracts

Negotiation is emblematic of the brain/brawn schism between current Grid and agent systems. In general, it cannot be assumed that a service will actually provide a particular capability to a user: a provider may be unable or unwilling to provide the service to a putative consumer. Hence, if the system is to have any type of predictable behavior, it becomes necessary to obtain commitments (contracts) about the willingness to provide a service and the characteristics, or quality, of its provision.

Given the ability to provision a resource to provide a desired level of service, we are faced with the question of exactly what levels of service can and should be obtained. The process by which this is determined will necessarily be some form of negotiation, since the autonomous entities involved need to come to a mutually acceptable agreement on the matter. If this negotiation is successful (i.e., both parties come to an agreement) then the outcome of the procurement is a contract (service level agreement) between the service provider and the service consumer.

This negotiation can be arranged in many different ways; there are millions of protocols, with varying properties, and agent researchers have invested significant effort in determining which protocols are appropriate in which circumstances [9]. In this context, the negotiation is driven by the operational policy of both the service provider and the service consumer. Specifically, policy terms to be considered may involve aspects such as the current load, the identity and reputation of the requestor, and the requestor's ability to pay.

The use of negotiation as a means of establishing service contracts is a topic of considerable interest in both the agent [22] and Grid [8] communities. One promising approach within Grids has been to represent agreement as the creation of a shared policy statement and to define robust extensible protocols for exchanging and agreeing to policy terms. Creating these agreements in the face of a Byzantine failure model can be complex. Having designed such protocols, the next step is to determine the strategy that the system components should adopt to achieve their policy objectives. Strategies can vary from the simple (e.g., an agent bidding its true valuation for a service) to the complex (reasoning about the other participants and their likely strategies).

4.4. Virtual Organization Management

A common interaction modality in both Grid and agent systems occurs when several agents come together to form a new VO. Such VOs can be viewed as a form of dynamic service composition: a number of initially distinct entities come together, under a set of operating conditions, to form a new entity that offers a new service. In such cases, one of the key challenges is for the participating agents to determine who else should be involved in the coalition and what their various roles and responsibilities should be. Again, this activity typically involves negotiation among participants, in this case to determine a mutually acceptable agreement concerning the division of labor and responsibilities.

Dynamic creation also raises the issue of service discovery. Experience in the Grid community indicates that this discovery should not simply be on the basis of service type, but rather should incorporate notions of service state and should be based on an understanding of the capabilities of the service (i.e., semantics). While Grid technologies provide the means for describing and grouping services, these higher level matchmaking and discovery capabilities are not currently part of Grid infrastructure. Fortunately, this is an area where much work has been done in the space of agents, and thus incorporation of this technology would do much to improve matters. This integration may have an impact on how state is represented and how services are organized.

4.5. Authentication, Trust, and Policy

As discussed in Section 5.2, the association of identity with dynamically created services has long been an integral part of Grid infrastructure. A common approach to this problem is to map identities into a global namespace and then apply delegation as a means for building federated namespaces for dynamically created entities. More recent work has focused on the application of richer policy statements and the creation of community based authorization and assertion authorities [27].

Also fundamental to the creation of collaboration and community, and building upon the aforementioned notions of authentication, are notions of trust. The effective management of trust and policy within a community, like VO formation, requires flexible, autonomous mechanisms able to consider, when organizing communities, not only the semantics of policy statements but also the ability to negotiate policy terms and to manage restricted delegation of rights.

As with other aspects of agents and Grids, we expect to see the adaptation of agent algorithms and technologies as they incorporate policy specification and enforcement into their basic operations and we expect to see Grid algorithms make use of some of the richness of the various agent trust and reputation models that have been developed [28]. We also expect that the types of policy statements made, along with how they are disseminated and applied, will evolve as agent-based techniques become more completely integrated into Grids. For example, reputation-based authentication mechanisms, which lend themselves to agent-based implementations, show great promise in the Grid environment.

5. Ten Research Problems

We conclude by outlining ten areas (in no particular order) in which research is needed to realize an integrated agent-Grid approach to open distributed systems.

Service architecture. The convergence of agent and Grid concepts and technologies will be accelerated if we can define an integrated service architecture providing a robust foundation for autonomous behaviors. This architecture would define baseline interfaces and behaviors supporting dynamic and stateful services, and a suite of higher-level interfaces and services codifying important negotiation, monitoring, and management patterns. The definition of an appropriate set of such architectural elements is an important research goal in its own right, and, in addition, can facilitate the creation, reuse, and composition of interoperable components.

Trust negotiation and management. All but the most trivial distributed systems involve interactions with entities (services) with whom one does not have perfect trust. Thus, authorization decisions must often be made in the absence of strong existing trust relationships. Grid middleware addresses secure authentication, but not the far harder problems of establishing, monitoring, and managing trust in a dynamic, open, multi-valent system. We need new techniques for expressing and reasoning about trust. Reputation mechanisms [29] and the ability to integrate assertions from multiple authorities ("A says M can do X, but B disagrees") will be important in many contexts, with the identity and/or prior actions of an entity requesting some action or asserting some fact being as important as other metrics, such as location or willingness to pay. Trust issues can also impinge on data integration, in that our confidence in the "data" provided by an entity may depend on our trust in that entity, so that, for example, our confidence in an assertion "A says M is green" depends on our past experiences with A.

System management and troubleshooting. Grid technologies make it feasible to access large numbers of resources securely, reliably, and uniformly. However, the coordinated management of these resources requires new abstractions, mechanisms, and standards for the quasi-automated ("autonomic" [20]) management of the ensemble—despite multiple, perhaps competing, objectives from different parties, and complex failure scenarios. A closely related problem is troubleshooting, i.e., detecting, diagnosing, and ultimately responding to the unexpected behavior of an individual component in a distributed system, or indeed of the system as a whole. This requirement will motivate the development of robust and secure logging and auditing mechanisms. The registration, discovery, monitoring, and management of available logging points, and the development of techniques for detecting and responding to "trouble" (e.g., overload or fraud), remain open problems. We also require advances in the summarization and explanation (e.g., visualization) of large-scale distributed systems.

Negotiation. We have already discussed negotiation at some length; here we simply note that major open problems remain in this vital area.

Service composition. The realization of a specific user or VO requirement may require the dynamic composition of multiple services. Web service technologies define conventions for describing service interfaces and workflows, and WSRF provides mechanisms for inspecting service state and organizing service collections. Yet we need far more powerful techniques for describing, discovering, composing, monitoring, managing, and adapting such service collections.

VO formation and management. While the notion of a VO seems to be intuitive and natural, we still do not have clear definitions of what constitutes a VO or well-defined procedures for deciding when a new VO should be formed, who should be in that VO, what they should do, when the VO should be changed, and when the VO should ultimately be disbanded.

System predictability. While open distributed systems are inherently unpredictable, it can be important to provide guarantees about system performance (e.g., liveness or safety properties, or stochastic performance boundaries). However, such guarantees require a deeper understanding of emergent behavior in complex systems.

Human-computer collaboration. Many VOs will be hybrids in which some problem solving is undertaken by humans and some by programs. These components must interwork in a seamless fashion to achieve their aims. New collaboration models are necessary to capture the rich social interplay in such hybrid teams.

Evaluation. Meaningful comparison of new approaches and technologies requires the definition of appropriate benchmarks and challenge problems and the creation of environments in which realistic evaluation can occur. Perhaps the single most effective means of advancing agent-Grid integration might be the definition of appropriately attractive challenge problems. Such problems should demand both the brawn of Grid and the brains of agents, and define rigorous metrics that can be used to drive the development in both areas. Potential challenge problems might include the distributed monitoring and management of large-scale Grids, and robust and long-lived operation of agent applications.

Evaluation can occur in both simulated and physical environments. Rapid progress has been made in simulation systems for both agents and Grids (e.g., [30]). Production deployments such as Grid3 [15], TeraGrid [5], and NEESGrid [26], and testbeds such as PlanetLab [1], are potentially available as experimental platforms for the evaluation of converged systems, for example within the context of the challenge problems just mentioned.

Semantic integration. Open distributed systems involve multiple stakeholders that interact to procure and deliver services. Meaningful interactions are difficult to achieve in any open system because different entities typically have distinct information models. Advances are required in such interrelated areas as ontology definition, schema mediation, and semantic mediation [3]. Again, issues of trust and cost have vital roles to play.

Acknowledgments

The work of the first author was supported in part by the Mathematical, Information, and Computational Sciences Division subprogram of the Office of Advanced Scientific Computing Research, U.S. Department of Energy, under Contract W-31-109-Eng-38. The second author acknowledges the support of the EPSRC project "Virtual organisations for e-Science" (GR/S62710/01).

References

1. Bavier, A., Bowman, M., Chun, B., Culler, D., Karlin, S., Muir, S., Peterson, L., Roscoe, T., Spalink, T. and Wawrzoniak, M., Operating System Support for Planetary-Scale Network Services. *Networking Systems Design and Implementation (NSDI)*, 2004.
2. Beiriger, J., Johnson, W., Bivens, H., Humphreys, S. and Rhea, R., Constructing the ASCI Grid. *9th IEEE International Symposium on High Performance Distributed Computing*, 2000, IEEE Computer Society Press.
3. Berners-Lee, T., Hendler, J. and Lassila, O. The Semantic Web. *Scientific American, 284* (5). 34-43. 2001.
4. Booth, D., Haas, H., McCabe, F., Newcomer, E., Champion, M., Ferris, C. and Orchard, D. Web Services Architecture. W3C, Working Draft http://www.w3.org/TR/2003/WD-ws-arch-20030808/, 2003.
5. Catlett, C. The TeraGrid: A Primer, 2002. www.teraGrid.org.
6. Catlett, C. and Smarr, L. Metacomputing. *Communications of the ACM, 35* (6). 44-52. 1992.
7. Chervenak, A., Foster, I., Kesselman, C., Salisbury, C. and Tuecke, S. The Data Grid: Towards an Architecture for the Distributed Management and Analysis of Large Scientific Data Sets. *J. Network and Computer Applications, 23* (3). 187-200. 2000.
8. Czajkowski, K., Foster, I. and Kesselman, C. Resource and Service Management. *The Grid: Blueprint for a New Computing Infrastructure (2nd Edition)*, 2004.
9. Dash, R.K., Parkes, D.C. and Jennings, N.R. Computational Mechanism Design: A Call to Arms. *IEEE Intelligent Systems, 18* (6). 40-47. 2003.
10. DeFanti, T., Foster, I., Papka, M., Stevens, R. and Kuhfuss, T. Overview of the I-WAY: Wide Area Visual Supercomputing. *International Journal of Supercomputer Applications, 10* (2). 123-130. 1996.
11. Foster, I., Frey, J., Graham, S., Tuecke, S., Czajkowski, K., Ferguson, D., Leymann, F., Nally, M., Storey, T. and Weerawaranna, S. Modeling Stateful Resources with Web Services. Globus Alliance, 2004.
12. Foster, I. and Kesselman, C. (eds.). *The Grid: Blueprint for a New Computing Infrastructure (2nd Edition)*. Morgan Kaufmann, 2004.
13. Foster, I., Kesselman, C., Nick, J.M. and Tuecke, S. Grid Services for Distributed Systems Integration. *IEEE Computer, 35* (6). 37-46. 2002.
14. Foster, I., Kesselman, C. and Tuecke, S. The Anatomy of the Grid: Enabling Scalable Virtual Organizations. *International Journal of Supercomputer Applications, 15* (3). 200-222. 2001.
15. Foster, I. and others, The Grid2003 Production Grid: Principles and Practice. *IEEE International Symposium on High Performance Distributed Computing*, 2004, IEEE Computer Science Press.
16. Galstyan, A., Czajkowski, K. and Lerman, K., Resource Allocation in the Grid Using Reinforcement Learning. *International Conference on Autonomous Agents and Multiagent Systems*, 2004.
17. Gentzsch, W. Enterprise Resource Management: Applications in Research and Industry. *The Grid: Blueprint for a New Computing Infrastructure (2nd Edition)*, Morgan Kaufmann, 2004.
18. Goble, C.A., De Roure, D., Shadbolt, N.R. and Fernandes, A. Enhancing Services and Applications with Knowledge and Semantics. *The Grid: Blueprint for a New Computing Infrastructure (2nd Edition)*, Morgan-Kaufmann, 2004.
19. Grimshaw, A., Weissman, J., West, E. and E. Lyot, J. Metasystems: An Approach Combining Parallel Processing and Heterogeneous Distributed Computing Systems. *Journal of Parallel and Distributed Computing, 21* (3). 257-270. 1994.
20. Horn, P. The IBM Vision for Autonomic Computing. IBM, 2001. www.research.ibm.com/autonomic/manifesto.
21. Jennings, N.R. An agent-based approach for building complex software systems. *Communications of the ACM, 44* (4). 35-41. 2001.
22. Jennings, N.R., Faratin, P., Lomuscio, A.R., Parsons, S., Sierra, C. and Wooldridge, M. Automated negotiation: prospects, methods and challenges. *Intl. J. of Group Decision and Negotiation, 10* (2). 199-215. 2001.

23. Johnston, W. Realtime Widely Distributed Instrumentation Systems. Foster, I. and Kesselman, C. eds. *The Grid: Blueprint for a New Computing Infrastructure*, Morgan Kaufmann, 1999, 75-103.
24. Levine, D. and Wirt, M. Interactivity with Scalability: Infrastructure for Multiplayer Games. *The Grid: Blueprint for a New Computing Infrastructure (2nd Edition)*, Morgan Kaufmann, 2004.
25. Luck, M., McBurney, P. and Preist, C. Agent technology: Enabling Next Generation Computing. *AgentLink*. 2003.
26. Pearlman, L., Kesselman, C., Gullapalli, S., Spencer, B.F., Futrelle, J., Ricker, K., Foster, I., Hubbard, P. and Severance, C., Distributed Hybrid Earthquake Engineering Experiments: Experiences with a Ground-Shaking Grid Application. *13th IEEE International Symposium on High Performance Distributed Computing*, 2004, NEESGrid.
27. Pearlman, L., Welch, V., Foster, I., Kesselman, C. and Tuecke, S., A Community Authorization Service for Group Collaboration. *IEEE 3rd International Workshop on Policies for Distributed Systems and Networks*, 2002.
28. Ramchurn, S.D., Huynh, D. and Jennings, N.R. Trust in Multiagent Systems. *The Knowledge Engineering Review*. 2004.
29. Resnick, P., Zeckhauser, R., Friedman, E. and Kuwabara, K. Reputation Systems. *Communications of the ACM, 43* (12). 45-48. 2000.
30. Song, H., Liu, X., Jakobsen, D., Bhagwan, R., Zhang, X., K., Taura and Chien, A., The MicroGrid: A Scientific Tool for Modeling Computational Grids. *SC 2000*, 2000, IEEE Computer Society Press.
31. Stevens, R. Group-Oriented Collaboration: The Access Grid Collaboration System. *The Grid: Blueprint for a New Computing Infrastructure (2nd Edition)*, Morgan Kaufmann, 2004.
32. Wolski, R., Brevik, J., Plank, J. and Bryan, T. Grid Resource Allocation and Control Using Computational Economies. Berman, F., Fox, G. and Hey, T. eds. *Grid Computing: Making the Global Infrastructure a Reality*, Wiley and Sons, 2003, 747-772.
33. Wooldridge, M. Agent-based software engineering. *IEE Proc. Software Engineering, 144*. 26-37. 1997.
34. Wooldridge, M. and Jennings, N.R. Software Engineering with Agents: Pitfalls and Pratfalls. *IEEE Internet Computing, 3* (3). 20-27. 1999.

Towards the Learning Grid
P. Ritrovato et al. (Eds.)
IOS Press, 2005

An integrated view of Grid services, Agents and Human Learning

Stefano A. CERRI[2]
LIRMM: CNRS & University Montpellier II

Abstract. The contribution reports on three aspects of our research activities on Grid services, Agents and Human learning: an integrated vision, a statement of intentions concerning a relatively new life cycle for Service Engineering and a review of achieved results, presented by embedding remarks and quotations in the relevant points. The essence of the contribution lies in the concept of service that is considered to be intrinsically conversational both during its dynamic definition and during its delivery. It is shown that Agents are the most promising abstractions (and technologies) offering a concrete approximation for future conversational Grid services and that Human learning is a quite suitable context for including the Human in the loop of the higher level services to be developed for mixed Virtual Organizations on future Grid networks.

Keywords. Grid services, Agents, Technology Enhanced Human Learning, Virtual Organizations, Service Engineering, Open Grid Human Service Architecture.

Introduction

Current research results in Informatics can be metaphorically depicted as a forest. Understanding and using the opportunities offered by discoveries as well as inventions available in the forest - where trees, and families of all sorts of plants often allow to evaluate the details, but paradoxically hide their essential contribution to the overall scene - becomes quite hard if not impossible due to the complexities both of the demand - requirements for solutions of very complex problems - and of the offer - multiple and sophisticated technologies and standards continuously evolving and competing with each other -. The only way to "understand" and "choose" seems to be, in the metaphor, to try to fly a bit above the forest and a bit behind in time: evaluating not only the results but also the historical processes as well as the reasons that have produced those results, with a continuous effort of integration and forecast for future research directions offering potential solutions in the years to come.

This paper presents the author's vision on the integration of advances in Agent technologies within Technology Enhanced Learning scenarios such as those emerging from the availability of Grid services [1-4]. The vision has been in part adopted within the ELeGI project[3]. Sections 2, 3 and 4 actualize previous reports on the pair wise intersection between the cited concepts.

Further, Section 5 highlights:

---

[2] Author: Stefano A. Cerri, LIRMM, 161, rue Ada; F-34392 Montpellier cedex 5; E-Mail: cerri@lirmm.fr
[3] www.ELeGI.org

- the proposed Service Engineering life cycle such as it has been intended within the SEES: Scenarios dedicated to Service Elicitation, Exploitation and Evaluation for Informal Learning as well as
- The necessity for including the human in the Grid architecture, by extending the Open Grid Service Architecture to Human services (OGHSA).

Finally, the research advances as they are documented by other papers and software experiments produced by the author and/or collaborating members of the team are inserted in the text when convenient.

A conclusion rounds off the paper.

1. e-Learning versus Grid Services[4]

1.1. Introduction

While e-Learning is a quite established concept, to be traced back in its roots in the 60ties (the PLATO and TICCIT experiences in the US), the Grid notion is considered as the evolution of the WWW and therefore is quite novel both as a technological solution and as its associated opportunities.

The ELeGI project is an important effort that aims to anticipate the conditions for an effective diffusion of the Grid, i.e.: by identifying design constraints that will fit a large significant class of expected uses of the Grid, those around e-Learning. Therefore, it seems to us important to point out where e-Learning and the Grid may eventually cross, i.e.: why e-Learning's traditional problems may find adequate solutions from developments around the Grid and, vice versa, what kind of developments on Grid ' s properties will be required by e-Learning needs.

In order to identify the link between Grid's potential technological innovations and e-Learning, one has first to agree about a few basic assumptions concerning the Grid and e-Learning.

1.2. Assumptions about the Grid

As to our current knowledge, the most important aspect of the Grid concept consists in going beyond the client-server model of one-to-one communication between software applications for a peer-to-peer one, many-to-many and distributed. The same principle has been for years a major objective of autonomous Agent's technologies, even if one may still ask how many multi-agent systems indeed are equipped with a peer-to-peer communication model and thus whether software Agents are really autonomous.

This view of the Grid as the large scale embodiment of autonomous Agent's concepts has recently found an authoritative support [4]. However, in the cited paper the roadmap from Agents to Grid services and vice versa is still in its infancy: we will comment on that roadmap in section 4. By now, we will assume in a first approximation that the Grid will consist of technologies allowing autonomous Agents to perform computations and to communicate on the Net in an optimal way, i.e.: exploiting resources where they are available in a fashion transparent for the Agent user. In the following, a few remarks on how we came to this conclusion.

Looking more deeply into the Grid fundamental notion (movement of processes in order to optimize resource allocation) one indeed discovers that, in order the movement

[4] This section actualizes the previously published paper [5] .

to be useful (effectively optimizing), it has to be decided and executed dynamically. This dynamicity has as a consequence that

a) we have to shift to the Grid the responsibility to execute the movement at run time;
b) we have to assign to each process the responsibility to propose to Grid at run time such an optimizing event.

Processes, therefore, have to decide autonomously (at least for what concerns their potential reallocation) taking into account the expected workload, their proximity to other processes, etc. The decision process, within each computational process on the Grid, may be very complex - as well as very useful -. Processes, being autonomous on the issue, have to be granted the liberty to formulate requests to other processes about Information necessary for them to decide. Conversations among processes become necessary, initiated by any process and addressing, in principle, any other process. The client-server model is thus insufficient.

Once processes may take the initiative to trigger conversations, they may arrive to the conclusion that it would be good to move to a more suited computational resource to perform optimally their task. This movement has then been decided dynamically by the process as a result of conversations. If we consider that the relocation of processes for optimizing the workload of processors in a distributed environment is a typical service asked to the network, the conclusion is that a service is dynamically generated by processes, thanks to previous autonomous conversations.

If a service may be generated dynamically, many other services do, as they would use a similar technology (autonomy of taking an initiative, conducting adequate conversations with peers, deciding and finally asking the Grid to deliver the physical transfer service). One comes to the conclusion of Foster et al. [1,2] that what initially was conceived for supercomputing and optimization may offer a new generation of models, tools and infrastructures for any activity on the Grid, including e-Commerce, where the dynamic generation of service from conversations is a necessary step for credible transactions. One immediately realizes also that the Web, as it is, has its major shortcoming in the lack of state of the HTTP protocol, thus the lack of persistency of conversations.

Indeed, we share the following vision of Grid computing [3]: "The Grid metaphor intuitively gives rise to the view of the e-Science infrastructure as a set of services that are provided by particular individuals or institutions for consumption by others. Given this, and coupled with the fact that many research and standards activities are embracing a similar view, we adopt a service-oriented view of the Grid throughout this document …. This view is based upon the notion of various entities providing services to one another under various forms of contract (or service level agreement)."

Shifting from a product-oriented to a service-oriented view of the Network is a challenging goal that has necessarily to pass through the analysis, definition and implementation of dynamic conversation protocols.

1.3. Assumptions about e-Learning

There is currently much interest on e-Learning. We will not survey here the reasons for this interest (see, for instance, the Introduction to [6]).

However, in spite of the apparently massive growth of the offer of e-Learning products and services, and, in principle, of the demand for human learning as it is expressed at individual, institutional and corporate level, we are not convinced at all that the offer and the demand meet in an acceptable way. There are exceptions, but the rule holds those effective, large scale applications of e-Learning are rare.

Our primary interpretation of this paradox concerns the quite simple observation that e-Learning requires a profound transformation of an established practice, for individuals and for Institutions. In e-Learning the three axiomatic assumptions for traditional educational settings: same content, same times, same location, are not valid. Even if we keep the "same content", yet e-Learning implies asynchronous interactions at a distance. These properties are claimed to be the value added to e-Learning with respect to traditional Education, but may also represent a constraint for its wide acceptance.

Historically, distance learning has been implemented and studied since many years[5]. From those studies, as well as from our own experience in the domain, the lesson we have learned is that we cannot consider e-Learning as an electronic variant of classical Education. That is indeed the problem. Not only the conditions of the educational offer are totally different, but also the cognitive and social attitude of humans require a completely dedicated analysis that most of the times has no precedents and thus requires a research attitude.

e-Learning is therefore not an application of technologies to human learning, in the sense that assuming to know what to apply (the technologies) and how (the pedagogy) one puts things together and the result will be a success (people learn). On the contrary, each serious effort has to be considered unique in the sense that it requires specific technologies and specific pedagogical principles to be developed and applied in a trial and error fashion within a specific context. This is the fundamental challenge of e-Learning: services and products have to be combined differently each time, according to each e-Learning situation.

We believe that the major obstacles for e-Learning are bound to the innovative nature for individuals and Institutions of the asynchronous distance interactions among humans and electronic resources. Surprisingly, the available technical tools are quite sophisticated and ripe, in many respects (for instance, looking at the recent Intelligent Tutoring Systems or AI in Education Conferences one may notice the progress). Perhaps one may better even more the offer by putting efforts in the integration, or in the dialogue management, that is yet poor in real situations. However, we believe that the bottleneck is more to be found on the human motivation and trust for engaging in e-Learning practices. By "human" we encompass any role: learners, teachers, managers, experts, ... as well as combinations thereof, i.e.: societies (classes, groups of teachers, etc.). One of the reasons for a lack of motivation in learners is the difficulty for certification of their learning when is has occurred at a distance. Another is the relative lack of friendliness of systems (when I'm stuck: who helps me?). The list of problems continues, yet human motivation and confidence is crucial in order technologies to be successfully introduced in human social practices.

1.4. Requirements

If the above outlined assumptions about the Grid and about e-Learning are correct, our priorities should be consequent. Hereafter a few consequences.

The technological research priorities for the Learning Grid concern the integration of simple yet very powerful tools supporting the communication in virtual human communities in such a way that the concerned human Agents feel safe are motivated and trust the effectiveness of the learning process in which they engage. Included in this confidence we may consider the effectiveness of heavy computational processes, when required, such as video streaming, simulations, virtual reality. However, very

[5] For an impressive list of contradictory scientific reports on pro's and con's of technologies in Education in the last century, see: http://teleeducation.nb.ca/nosignificantdifference .

large potential audiences for e-Learning are far from even envisioning those applications, as they are not convinced that e-Learning helps them to solve their problems. In order to avoid the Grid to become a set of solutions in search of the problems (as it has been sometimes the case for Web technologies in e-Commerce a few years ago: once more people overestimated short term effects of innovation and underestimated long term ones), we should give the priority to the motivation of humans for e-Learning, we should assume a human-centered or - better - social view of system design. The peer-to-peer model of human learning by focused conversations with teachers, experts and the like (for instance: the pragmatics of dialogues as it is currently expressed in a rudimentary way by Agent Communication Languages and Speech Act Theory) may become a fundamental inspiration for autonomous Agent's software technologies to be developed in order to realize the Grid. Complex standards for interoperability of educational documents - such as SCORM, IMS, EML and the like - may be considered as a technology push attitude, complementary to the social-user-pull one outlined in these pages. The last deserves a priority as it is relatively immature and at the same time crucial for success. The Semantic Grid will emerge insofar the technologies for Agent-to-Agent conversations and their pragmatic layers will be realized.

The strategic priorities for the Learning Grid concern with the evaluation and certification of learning effects. Traditional Institutions (in particular: teachers) do not trust e-Learning unless in a quite trivial utilitarian fashion. Teachers do not have the right to consider their e-Learning activities as part of their pedagogical duties. Traditional Institutions are not prepared to certify the knowledge and skills of learners independently from the way they have acquired them (in presence). Retrospectively, in spite of the recommendations to teachers and Institutions, the practice of e-Learning is rare because no one sees his or her interest in investing into a fundamental modification of traditional behaviours. One may show any impressive result of e-Learning experiments, but unless the practice is considered useful by the delegated people and Institutions (the teachers), as a consequence of a reformed statute, it will not be accepted at a large scale as a serious complement to traditional Education. Most probably, it is useful to look for non institutional potential users, having sincere learning needs (as we do within the Informal SEES, addressed in section 5 hereafter), instead of pushing technologies into reluctant Institutions.

The tactical choices for the Learning Grid should be guided by an experimental, socially oriented and evolutionary view of the infrastructure supporting generic virtual communities. Dialogues are central. Any human collaborative activity requires and implies human learning. Initially the Grid technologies may be dedicated to facilitate mainly human-to-human dialogues (by written, by voice, by video and voice); considering that artificial Agents (our Grid services) may incrementally be introduced, once the communities are stable and motivated, in order to enhance learning effects in suitable conditions. The Learning Grid will be a success when communities of users will eventually testimony their positive experiences, not just when communities of producers will advertise their performing solutions. The challenge will be to transform curiosity driven virtual communities into performing virtual organizations.

2. Agents versus Human Learning[6]

2.1. The historical emergence of Agents

From the seminal work of Newell concerning the Knowledge Level in Knowledge Based Systems [8], we know how to separate the analysis and synthesis of Knowledge from the ways it may be implemented at the Symbol level. Different approaches may be adopted, e.g. Description Languages that assume as an hypothesis the availability of Ontologies and identify methods for deducing Facts, Relations and Rules from interoperable multiple descriptions [9]. An orthogonal approach based on Propositionalisation, instead, uses Terms, Constraints and Machine Learning for inducing and revising Ontologies in interactions among Agents [10, 46].

As Informatics is the art of transforming semantics into syntax, evaluating results of syntactic processing, and mapping them back to semantics; the historical challenge in Informatics consisted of relating syntactic structures to their semantics with respect to meanings in the real world. Semantics denotes here the real world concepts, not just the "world of the Computer" at in the case of Denotation, Operational or Algebraic semantics of programming languages.

Due to the availability of the Web, the process is currently more and more conversational, between and among "abstract computational entities", human or artificial ones, called Agents, on the Web. As a consequence, people are more concerned with conversations on the Web, their semantics, their pragmatics. Among existing conversations, and those that are envisioned to occur in the next future with an impressive growth rate, we consider commercial transactions in e-commerce and intellectual transactions in e-learning to be pivotal for crucial developments. We also assume as intuitive the idea that e-learning and e-commerce, as well as, in general, e-work conversations, share a similar nature and therefore are characterized by similar requirements.

It may therefore be useful to evaluate if and how these developments may integrate different areas of Computing and Artificial Intelligence under a common manifesto, allowing identifying a shared research agenda. In the following, we will mainly concentrate on relations between technologies for human learning and Agents, but we will show that similar arguments hold for distributed systems, software engineering, programming languages and Human-Computer Interaction research. The section is therefore an attempt to unify views in modern Informatics research, apparently diversified, substantially convergent in a Web-centered, Knowledge Communication vision of problem solving [11].

2.2. From Computing as Control to Human-Computer studies: the User in the loop

The essential "conversational" aspect of solving problems by humans and machines is not new, it existed all the time. What is relatively new is the massive impact of Communication Technologies on everyday life. Communication Technologies have not raised new scientific problems; they just have shifted our focus of attention by offering us totally new tools for communicating.

Previously, Computing consisted in its essence of humans conceiving, designing and implementing programs able to activate processes according to well defined algorithms; the result of these processes was back interpreted by humans. This vision

[6] This section actualizes the previously published paper [7] .

of Computing, in order to be useful, required one to adopt many important assumptions. Let us briefly review them hereafter. We will call the User a human or a society of humans interested to solve a problem; the Computer an artefact, or a set of artefacts constructed to perform computations.

c) User was supposed to have a need and to have identified the problem(s) the solution of which would help in satisfying the need;
d) User was supposed to be unable to solve alone the problem;
e) User was supposed to have the intention to use the Computer to help him/her to solve the problem(s);
f) User was supposed to know how to decompose the goal associated to the problem into tasks; design alternative methods able to execute tasks, each of which would generate sub-goals, linked to subtasks and so on. The decomposition of a problem into trees of Tasks and Methods was in itself an issue: is that decomposition possible independently from the application domain [12], or are the two intertwined (as Clancey showed to be the case in GUIDON [13])?

All these assumptions were taken as granted.

g) Once a. through d. was valid assumptions, User was supposed to be able to code his/her representation of the problem and of the problem solution in a formal language that was known for the Computer. In the case of misunderstandings by the Computer, User was supposed to be able to remediate his/her coding until the Computer showed no apparent error.
h) User was supposed to activate the processes in the Computer associated to the code produced; these processes were supposed to terminate with "results" that User was supposed to be able to map against the expected solution so that a judgment was possible, namely if the solution obtained would satisfy his/her need. In the positive case, the process ended; in the negative one: User was supposed to modify the code and/or the abstract problem description until the obtained results from the activated Computer processes would satisfy his/her need.

Clearly, such a scenario for Computing seems ad-hoc constructed in order to support some claim. It is so: "traditional" Computing focused mainly on Computer behaviors by leaving open many important questions concerning the User. We all developed through the years many complexes, sophisticated, powerful Computer languages and studied accordingly in depth the properties of Computation - mainly seen as Control - disregarding the simple fact that Computers are for helping Humans, and not the reverse; and that they do that by means of Conversations. We were not interested in how a human comes to the code [14], and how he/she interprets the results. Elliot Soloway, for instance, tried for years to model novice programmer's errors in order to make "skilled debuggers" or Intelligent Tutoring Systems able to remediate programming misconceptions (e.g.: [15]). One of those misconceptions may originate thousands of errors in the millions of lines of Ada code for the US DoD. The work was hard and not really supported; it was stopped in spite of the encouraging results around PROUST.

We were not interested in the Communication component of the Wiener manifesto on Cybernetics [16]. Computers were considered control systems transforming symbols into symbols according to (possibly terminating and efficient) algorithms. Communication issues were transformed into Transmission concerns.

Artificial Intelligence first, and Human-Computer Studies later have put humans in the loop [17]. They have recognized that two major issues were neglected in Computing:

- how people transform a need into a problem description then into some code in a formal language;
- how people interpret the results of computations with respect to the real world need.

AI and HCI studies stand to Computing in the same way as Statistics stands to Probability. It is not the concern of Probability to make claims on the real world pertinence of the assumed probabilities of elementary events, nor of the computed probabilities of complex events. Those concerns regard Statistics (constructing formal models of real world problems including random variables and interpreting results emerging when "running" or simulating the models). Similarly, AI and HCI have been mainly concerned with defining models and interpreting their resulting deductions.

2.3. From Computer Agents as Servers of a single Client, to Actors and Operating Systems

If we assume that the human-computer communication loop is the object of study, then we should adopt the view that in the loop, two Agents are operating, exchanging messages, evaluating and judging. Two Agents are hardly to be reduced to a single one; insofar they are behaving autonomously [18].

However, for years the loop metaphor of Human Problem Solving with the help of Computers was strongly influenced by a single viewpoint: even if the autonomy of the User was not discussed, the Computer was considered a slave, a server for an important client: the User. With a few notable exceptions, most studies on Interactive Systems were bound to a Client-Server model of Interaction. The most important interactive applicative domains at the time (Information Systems and CAD-CAM or Programming Environments) were developed under this view.

Exceptions consisted on research efforts around Intelligent Tutoring Systems. As an example, from the very beginning, Carbonell, in his foundational paper [19] clarified the quite simple idea that a realistic teacher-student interaction would be neither purely student-driven (as in Information Systems, where the user takes all the initiatives with respect to the system, considered as a server of information, or in CAD-CAM and Programming Environments, where the User commands the Computer to do things for him/her) nor teacher-driven (as it has been the case in most Computer Aided Instruction or Computer-Based Training for decades) but instead should allow mixed initiatives in the course of conversations. After more than 30 years, the "mixed initiative" view of conversations is again considered necessary for modelling realistic Agent-to-Agent conversations [20].

In Intelligent Tutoring Systems, the Computer Agent was designed to "guide" the User to acquire knowledge and expertise (see, for instance, the impressive achievements described in [21]). Most studies on Instructional Design represent explorations concerning the pro-active, autonomous behavior of the Computer Agent in Tutoring Systems that is currently required in Agent languages and applications.

Similarly, Student models were considered necessary in order to personalize the simulated teacher's behavior with respect to the student since the 70ties. Currently, User models are introduced in interactive applications for the same purpose.

As the Computer is a symbol processing device, one may say that the human art of solving problems by using Computers consisted for the User in transforming into symbols (the syntactic-symbolic level) the meanings linked to the problem (the semantic-knowledge level) and back from the symbols-results reconstruct meanings. The syntactic work was left to the machine, the semantic one to the human. Knowledge representation systems and - later - Ontologies were conceived in order to help humans in their semantic task, delegating part of it to the Computer. It is questionable to evaluate their concrete achievements, what is certain is that almost no attention was dedicated to the pragmatics of conversations, again with the exception of studies in Intelligent Tutoring or AI in Education [22,23].

In these conversations between the User and the Computer the "time dependent external world", also called "context" in the Agent's literature, was not considered: during the conversations, the User was not supposed to change his/her mind; s/he was just supposed to "implement" the specifications . In such a scenario, modifications of the state of the Computer were only possible as a consequence of some action (message) of the partner. Such a single-user Computer, therefore, "knows" only what the User said. As a consequence of this single client - single server view, we could deduce that a closed world assumption was adopted in the temporal evolution of the early software Agents.

It is evident that human Users evolve as a result of communicating with the outside world. Therefore, an initial plan (sequence of tasks) may be modified during the conversation [20, 24]. Users do not have static plans; in fact they generate one move at a time, as a consequence of their local judgment of the state of the conversation. At least for the User, a closed world assumption is not realistic. However, this lack of attention to the User's evolving context, and evolving state, was not previously perceived as a good reason for modifying in their essence the fashionable assumptions about the software life cycle. Other phenomena did. Once more, a change of focus of attention in the scientific community was originated by technical, economical needs and not by scientific reflections.

Constructing Computer programs able to satisfy User needs is a costly endeavor. Once you have done it properly, you like to reuse it several times, and perhaps abstract and generalize to other domains. Software engineering was and is concerned with that. If a service delivered by a Computer artefact satisfies a client User, you wish this service to be exploited by as many users in as many different domains as possible. Assuming the service is a function, and the different domains are associated to different data types, reusing the service for different domains implies to develop generic functions (functions applicable to data instances, belonging to several types known only at run time). As the developments around Object Oriented Programming have been originated by the necessity of managing knowledge in order to build generic functions, we may conclude that Computer Agents - initially simple programmed functions - evolved to Objects.

The next step was to offer concurrently functionalities to many potential Clients. Operating Systems fulfil that property: they offer one or many Users the services corresponding to many available functionality, keeping track of the state of each service for each User. They allow capitalizing heavily upon the efforts spent in order to implement a problem solution, offering to reuse the solution constructed. The needs for reuse have dominated the developments in Computing in the last decades, and still motivate most of them. The issue for us, then, becomes how to integrate these developments into more advanced (and realistic) Agent architectures.

In a multi-process, multi-user scenario such as that offered by Actors [25] or Operating Systems, the conversational cycles assume the "autonomy of human Users" and introduce some liberty for the Computer: for instance the autonomy to suspend autonomously a process in a round-robin loop in order to dedicate resources to another process. Yet, the Computer is still a server for clients; its autonomy is restricted to facilitate services but does not rely on any shared knowledge at the application level. You would be surprised if an Operating System would say: "please, excuse me but the conversation I have with your colleague Jean, who just connected from Paris, is so important for me that I wish to dedicate my time to him; please come back tomorrow". Only the owner of the OS, as an Operating System's Manager, would be entitled to explicitly give a priority to Jean's processes. The autonomy of Actors and Operating Systems is limited to the knowledge, available for them, dedicated to how to serve many clients in the "best" way, i.e. the "most efficient" way. All scheduling algorithms are of this, rather "syntactic", nature. The "semantics" yet remains in the autonomy of human Users and is eventually made available to the Computer at the level of each conversational application, under the convention that the Computer is not entitled to autonomously use the knowledge obtained in one conversation in order to manage other conversations.

2.4. From Actors to Agents

The Agent metaphor comes into the scene exactly at this point. Agents are supposed to be autonomous, i.e. to evaluate what to do and how with respect to the current state, as denoted by the multiple conversations ongoing. In order to be autonomous, one needs to have a proprietary goal, or intention in order to decide among actions what to do next in order to reach the goal. No autonomy without the right to decide, no decision without alternatives, no choice criterion among alternatives without an evaluated "distance" of each alternative with respect to a goal. Control theory, cybernetics, and the like have taught us that.

The Agent metaphor therefore gives an equal status to Human and Artificial Agents: that of autonomy in conversational behavior. In our approach, we have outlined a model - and a set of methods and tools - that realize conversational Agents showing autonomous behavior [24, 26]. At the same time other authors [27] have chosen a similar approach concerning how to realize autonomy.

The issue comes into the scenario, if the symbolic representations in machines are sufficient, or even necessary to represent - at least in a primitive way - realistic social behaviors such as those addressed by the community of Situated Cognition. William Clancey is a testimony of such a radical shift: from years of recognized activity in Intelligent Tutoring, AI and Cognition [28], the lessons learned are critical and profound, supporting a synergy but not a confusion between "classical" work at the symbol and the knowledge level on the one side, and more realistic approaches that privilege action and social interactions on the other. The question posed concretely is if the focus of Agent computations should remain in processing networks of symbols, or if we better should concentrate in the social aspects of multiple conversations as a source of Agent's actions and behavior. This shift is not incompatible with our thesis: if we better understand Communication among Autonomous Agents and the social aspects of coherent conversations within a holistic model of human activity, we may be able to better approximate the adequate social behavior described in [29].

Unfortunately, there is a lack of usable, Symbol level models that deal with conversations, i.e. the Pragmatic or Knowledge Communication level[7]. On the contrary, there are important advances on modelling of problem solving methods (see, e.g.: [30, 31]). Insofar problem solving methods and their formal representations will deal with distributed reasoning, including conversations among Agents; they will be foundational not only for the Semantic Web – as it is the case now – but also for the Semantic Grid.

---

[7] Some linguists call it Dynamic Semantics.

This Knowledge Communication level is the fundamental glue missing in most situations, where, we believe, behavior is generated from messages and not the contrary.

3. Agents vs. Grid services[8]

The relations between Grid and Agent research and applications are preliminarily described in [4]: we will annotate hereafter some crucial statements on the light of our recent work and try to show that their considerations (the what to do and why to do it) may receive partial answers (how to do it) within our current research efforts in ELeGI and outside.

Ten Research Problems[9]
We conclude by outlining ten areas (in no particular order) in which research is needed to realize an integrated agent-Grid approach to open distributed systems.

3.1. Service[10] architecture.

The convergence of agent and Grid concepts and technologies will be accelerated if we can define an integrated service architecture providing a robust foundation for autonomous behaviours[11]. This architecture would define baseline interfaces and behaviours supporting dynamic and stateful services[12], and a suite of higher-level interfaces and services codifying important negotiation, monitoring, and management[13] patterns. The definition of an appropriate set of such architectural elements is an important research goal in its own right, and, in addition, can facilitate the creation, reuse, and composition of interoperable components.

3.2. Trust negotiation and management

All but the most trivial distributed systems involve interactions with entities (services) with whom one does not have perfect trust. Thus, authorization decisions must often be made in the absence of strong existing trust relationships. Grid middleware addresses secure authentication, but not the far harder problems of establishing, monitoring, and managing trust in a dynamic, open, multi-valent system. We need new techniques for expressing and reasoning about trust[14]. Reputation mechanisms [...] and the ability to integrate assertions from multiple authorities ("A says M can do X, but B disagrees") will be important in many contexts, with the identity and/or prior actions of an entity requesting some action or asserting some fact being as important as other metrics, such as location or willingness to pay. Trust issues can also impinge on data integration, in that our confidence in the "data" provided by an entity may depend on our trust in that

[8] This section actualizes part of the ELeGI deliverable D12 [32]
[9] The original conclusion section (n. 6 of [4]) is hereafter pasted in Italic; annotations are in the footnotes.
[10] The concept of service is central. Differently from most authors, we distinguish it from the one of product not according to its "type" (e.g: a Web service is an active procedure, different from a static datum) but in terms of its behavior (a service is conversational both at define and at run time).
[11] Integration and autonomy are paradoxically at odd. One may say that Agents privilege autonomy, while Grid services privilege integration.
[12] For an account of our current view on how to model the state in conversational Agents, see [33] .
[13] A quite simple, yet very promising contribution to model the centralized control – including security – of movement and interaction services in a distributed, open, dynamic multi-agent environment is reported in [45] .
[14] Trust is important in Virtual Organizations (VOs) within the current OGSA, where services are delivered by software. In VOs that include Humans, such as ours, trust is fundamental: it is the basis for motivation.

entity, so that, for example, our confidence in an assertion "A says M is green" depends on our past experiences with A.

3.3. System management and troubleshooting

Grid technologies make it feasible to access large numbers of resources securely, reliably, and uniformly. However, the coordinated management of these resources requires new abstractions, mechanisms, and standards for the quasi-automated ("autonomic" [...]) management of the ensemble—despite multiple, perhaps competing, objectives from different parties, and complex failure scenarios[15]. A closely related problem is troubleshooting, i.e., detecting, diagnosing, and ultimately responding to the unexpected behaviour of an individual component in a distributed system, or indeed of the system as a whole. This requirement will motivate the development of robust and secure logging and auditing mechanisms. The registration, discovery, monitoring, and management of available logging points, and the development of techniques for detecting and responding to "trouble" (e.g., overload or fraud), remain open problems. We also require advances in the summarization and explanation (e.g., visualization[16]) of large-scale distributed systems.

3.4. Negotiation

We have already discussed negotiation at some length; here we simply note that major open problems remain in this vital area.

3.5. Service composition

The realization of a specific user or VO requirement may require the dynamic composition of multiple services[17]. Web service technologies define conventions for describing service interfaces and workflows, and WS-ResourceFramework (WSRF) provides mechanisms for inspecting service state and organizing service collections. Yet we need far more powerful techniques for describing, discovering, composing, monitoring, managing, and adapting such service collections.

3.6. VO formation and management

While the notion of a VO seems to be intuitive and natural, we still do not have clear definitions of what constitutes a VO[18] or well-defined procedures for deciding when a new VO should be formed, who should be in that VO, what they should do, when the VO should be changed, and when the VO should ultimately be disbanded .

---

[15] While in complex artificial systems "failure" is an enemy, in complex human VOs misconceptions, contradictions and paradoxes may become a source of learning, when associated to adequate remedial procedures (or services) [34] .

[16] Visualization of networks of resources, when part of them are human resources, comes down to Enhanced Presence, one of the major research endeavors in ELeGI [32] .

[17] Service composition is a "new" engineering challenge, assuming that most services are stateful and intrinsically conversational. Our approach foresees bottom-up composition of lower-level services into more complex ones as well as top-down decomposition of higher level services into simpler ones (see section 5).

[18] In our human learning scenarios, the very first step for humans to be helped by technologies consists in entering an adequate Virtual Community, then facilitating its progressive mutation into a Virtual Organization (see section 5).

3.7. System predictability

While open distributed systems are inherently unpredictable, it can be important to provide guarantees about system performance (e.g., liveness or safety properties, or stochastic performance boundaries). However, such guarantees require a deeper understanding of emergent behaviour[19] in complex systems.

3.8. Human-computer collaboration

Many VOs will be hybrids in which some problem solving is undertaken by humans and some by programs[20]. These components must interwork in a seamless fashion to achieve their aims. New collaboration models are necessary to capture the rich social interplay in such hybrid teams.

3.9. Evaluation

Meaningful comparison of new approaches and technologies requires the definition of appropriate benchmarks and challenge problems and the creation of environments in which realistic evaluation[21] can occur. Perhaps the single most effective means of advancing agent-Grid integration might be the definition of appropriately attractive challenge problems. Such problems should demand both the brawn of Grid and the brains of agents, and define rigorous metrics that can be used to drive the development in both areas. Potential challenge problems might include the distributed monitoring and management of large-scale Grids, and robust and long-lived operation of agent applications. Evaluation can occur in both simulated and physical environments. Rapid progress has been made in simulation systems for both agents and Grids (e.g. [...]). Production deployments such as Grid3 [...], TeraGrid [...], and NEESGrid [...], and testbeds such as PlanetLab [...], are potentially available as experimental platforms for the evaluation of converged systems, for example within the context of the challenge problems just mentioned.

3.10. Semantic integration

Open distributed systems involve multiple stakeholders that interact to procure and deliver services. Meaningful interactions are difficult to achieve in any open system because different entities typically have distinct information models. Advances are required in such interrelated areas as ontology definition, schema mediation, and semantic mediation[22] [...].

---

[19] This is absolutely true for artificial systems. Having put the human in the loop, we may argue that humans are much better as machines to predict emergent behaviors. We insist on the concept of "smooth integration" of the artificial services into VOs, initially consistent of connected human services, in order to avoid unforeseen failures or at least facilitate the human control of unforeseen behaviors. In particular, the goal of "one click human help", necessary for most end users communities, should minimize the risks in our mixed VOs. The issue raised on unpredictability of open distributed systems, however, should also favor machine learning studies: Grid services should perform "better" as a consequence of previous experiences. We have started to investigate the feasibility of inducing patterns (rules or even protocols) from real Human conversations in Virtual Organizations: preliminary results are available in: [47] .

[20] This seems a rewriting of the goal of Open Grid Human Service Architecture within ELeGI.

[21] Our SEES (cf: section 5) have been conceived exactly for this purpose.

[22] The integration of semantics, in our view, will focus on the semantics of distributed problem solving methods by Agents in VOs (see, eg: [30,31]) as a prerequisite for exploiting the semantics of pedagogical documents [35]. In the last case, the approach was to allow remote authors to attribute semantics to

4. Where do we want to go? [23]

4.1. Introduction

The evolution of the technological offer associated to the Grid [1 - 4] induces one to reflect on its consequences on the entire life cycle of the new generation of applications on the Internet. In the following, we highlight our understanding of the core of the OGSA concept and we derive our convictions on a new life cycle for Grid technical (infrastructural) developments and Grid applications.

4.2. OGSA: Open Grid Service Architecture

The notion of a service is radically different from the one of a product, even if there may be a smooth transition between the two viewpoints. Assuming typical products to be cars, washing machines, DMBS or Web sites consisting of collections of static HTML pages, typical services may be represented by legal, financial, medical, educational or advising services of many different kinds, including electronic services complementary to and integrated with human services. In order to simplify our subsequent arguments, we will consider "providers" and "consumers" of services, both called Agents, irrespectively on their human or artificial (software + hardware + network) nature.

In order to set the stage, hereafter a few considerations on the differences:

- a product is developed by the producer with a clearly predefined goal for the potential consumer, a service is offered within a service domain – or competence area, yet the consumer-specific objectives have to be defined during the initial conversations between the provider and the consumer of the service;
- a product is supposed to be in correspondence with a well established and a clearly identified need; a service often anticipates to the customer combinations of needs that were not clearly recognized as such by him/her before;
- a product is most often designed and prototypically developed once, produced many times; the value added by a product increases with the number of copies effectively distributed; a service must be conceived, designed, developed and distributed once for all, as it is custom made for a specific customer with specific needs; the value added by a service increases proportionally with the customer's satisfaction that entails an indirect publicity for the service producer and generates new customers ready to invest resources in order to have similar services;
- a product's evolution is slow, as it requires modifications in the conception, design and development; shortly; a revision of the whole life cycle. A service evolves naturally as it is a combination of basic services and products on the fly as a consequence of a service definition and tuning during the conversations with a customer;
- a product is often chosen as a solution for an established need, even when the customer does not really "trust" the producer's performance (e.g.: even if I dislike cars and prefer a car-less city center, I need one for very practical

---

documents by means of a Web based XML editor – called DYXWEB - helped by Ontologies caring for adapting the document structure and meaning to the user's profile.

[23] This section actualizes the previously published paper [36].

reasons, and I choose the cheapest one because I plan to use it as little as possible); a service requires trust by the customer on the producer (e.g.: I do not go to a dentist or a lawyer unless I believe s/he is trustable).

In general, it is quite hard – some say it is even impossible - to clearly cut the difference between a product and a service. Most probably, the same "object" may be seen on turn as a product or as a service, depending on the viewpoint, the context. Probably, the distinction is not an ontological one, but an epistemological: in relation to the "object's behavior" in a specific context of use.

A few considerations seem to help to start a reflection on ICT services with respect to ICT products. Let us consider the most classical ICT application, i.e.: an Information System, and let us reflect on a paradigm shift: from product to service – for future Information Systems.

Typical Information Systems were developed to satisfy the needs of accurate, well organized, timely updated and trustable Information. This Information is necessary in order to take decisions.

In all the cases where the Information evolves dynamically, as well as the informative needs from the customer evolve continuously; the "Information management system" has to account for both evolutions.

A classical DBMS performs very well under static assumptions, such as the persistence of the logical and physical schemes of the DBMS and of the informative needs of the user. A classical DBMS, and its application for a specific Information system, is much like a "product": developed once and used for years. Any evolution requires heavy resources to redesign the schemas, and import the old as well as the new data.

Now, suppose neither the Information available to the Information system is stable, nor the information needs by the user. In this situation, more and more frequent in our organizations, the value added by an Information system becomes directly dependent from its flexibility, adaptability, dynamicity.

Let us now consider a classical query to an Information system. The success of the query depends of many assumptions, including the following three:

- the querier knows exactly what s/he needs;
- the querier knows that the system's information may satisfy his/her need;
- the querier knows how to formulate the need.

Current daily situations are far from respecting the above outlined assumptions. Users of Information Systems, as well as navigators on the Web, for any purpose – including eCommerce – do not have a well defined need, do not know if and how the system may satisfy their need, do not know how to formulate a query correctly. The consequence of this situation is that often there is no adequacy at all between the user's real needs and the system's answers (for an outstanding detailed description of a realistic scenario, see: [29]).

We may synthetically define the informative process described above as a process where Information is offered as a product while the Information needed is a service. Typically, in most realistic non trivial situations, one needs to express his/her intentions, desires, constraints and investigate the system's available Information before being able to formulate correctly a query. The classical run time behavior of an Information system requires as a prerequisite for the user's satisfaction to support a complex conversational phase in order the subsequently formulated query to be adequate with the user's need.

In the case that the user's needs do not fit with just one Information system (e.g.: I wish to organize my holidays next summer) each partial information (about available flights, trains, ... and about hotels ... and about cultural events, climate, ... and so on) in order to acquire a meaning for the user has to be integrated with other information coming from other information sources (hence the need for interoperability of information sources). Eventually, a combination of choices will emerge from a sequence of conversations between the user and several information sources, and among information sources themselves (what justifies XML typing and Ontologies). A user wishing a "service for holidays" has currently to compose his/her own chosen "products".

Such a scenario of dynamic generation of services is the major challenge for ICTs in the next years. It is as well described as being the major challenge of the OGSA: Open Grid Service Architecture.

4.3. The dynamic generation of services for human learning

In order for Grids associated to OGSAs to be successful, one needs first a well founded definition of services that eventually may be required by users of OGSA-based Grid applications. The problem is to identify those services in order to construct the software applications necessary to generate them on the fly.

Let us jump back to the anthropomorphic metaphors. It is perhaps necessary, but not sufficient for a doctor to know the anatomy and the physiology of the human body to become a good performing doctor. For a lawyer, the knowledge of the civil code and the jurisprudence is useful but insufficient in order to be a competitive lawyer at the court. One needs practice, examples, and real cases. Further, while medical knowledge is for a large part independent from the health context (a doctor, say, in France may cure a patient in Morocco, considering that most of its citizens speak French), legal knowledge is highly culture, context dependent. Even Codes are fundamentally different: a process in a Country submitted to the Roman law is quite different from the analogous one submitted to the Anglo-Saxon tradition. Certainly, the degree of context dependency is much higher in services as it is in products.

The case of Educational services is perhaps the most extreme. The service has to stimulate, evaluate and credit human learning, knowledge and skills. Nothing is more context dependent as human knowledge and skills, as well as the associated emotional aspects (motivation, cultural awareness, ...). It is evident that no educational model will ever be successful for human learning if not highly linked to the socio-economic and cultural context of human users.

If we wish to build on Grids this kind of services, we have to identify them in an accurately context dependent way. In analogy with the lawyer and the doctor's examples above, the most secure way to identify them is to practice them concretely in well controlled experimental situations and integrate the lessons learned into new requirements and better services.

The first time, for each context, we may conceive to operate like a junior doctor or lawyer: accompanying and helping seniors, better experienced, operating exactly those services to those users[24]. However, in our case – Education – one more difficulty emerges: there are no seniors, as the classical behavior of parents and teachers – the two major educators known – does not at all include ICTs.

Therefore, we will have to use a quite traditional method for introducing innovation, perhaps to be called a "Trojan horse", hereafter indicated in steps:

a) Distribute among communities of future users (learners) the infrastructures necessary for accessing the Web in the simplest and most supportive way (by accessing a Grid portal) and rely on their motivation and enthusiasm for a quite

[24] The system described in [34,37] operated in this way.

popular, accepted activity: bidirectional access to Web Information (collaborative reading and writing). We have identified three of those communities (also to be identified as scenarios supporting complementary aspects of informal learning):
    - the VIAD: Virtual Institute for Alphabetization for Development scenario, currently ongoing in Pays Coeur d'Hérault, as well as in other remote and less developed areas of the world [38,39,40];
    - the ENCORE scenario, on the construction of an encyclopaedia for Organic Chemistry [41,42];
    - The e-Qualification scenario, focusing on monitoring and qualifying human learning services as well as their effects across ELeGI applications [43,44];

b) introduce scenario-specific "champions" able to animate the human users in virtual communities, allow collaborative activities to be developed initially in order to establish mutual confidence and interests and progressively mutate towards structured Virtual Organizations;
c) offer support to developments that are selected, identified and described by the communities themselves, coordinated by the "champions";
d) highlight, underline and make explicit the relations between any development of the community and the associated human learning; develop human learning strategies and practices as a support to higher priority goals, such as economic, cultural and scientific success of each member of the community thanks to the collaboration;
e) study the communicative processes in order to identify the technological and human requirements of services adapted to each community, then finally
f) formulate the requirements as functional specifications for the next generation of Grid's services.

Hereafter, as a consequence of the above consideration, what we believe to be an innovative definition of service developments for Grid applications, i.e.: the different function of scenarios versus more classical test beds accompanying OGSA developments for e-Learning.

4.4. SEES: Service Elicitation and Exploitation / Evaluation Scenarios

In classical software engineering, the major phases were approximately:

6. software functional (informal) specification;
7. software technical (formal) specification;
8. software design;
9. software development (coding);
10. software testing and evaluation (within test beds);
11. generation of new guidelines in order to loop to 1. and 2. until satisfied.

Testing and evaluation occurs at the end of the process by means of carefully planned and controlled experiences with real potential customers. This life cycle reflects a "product" view of software applications.

When services have to be supported by software, as it is our case, we envision a different life cycle for successful service generation and use, briefly outlined in the following. We will call the two classes of scenarios for each class of actors involved in this new life cycle: SDS (Service Developer's Scenarios) and SUS (Service User's Scenarios).

Each scenario is timed by / belongs to a "phase". Each new "phase" adds up the previous ones as a new task cumulating for a holistic integrated approach. Notice that the distinction between SUS and SDS reflects the wide spectrum of meanings the word "service" adopts: from a quite high level, domain dependent meaning (e.g.: the learning service for a minimal competence on business accounting), to a low granularity, domain independent, technical meaning (e.g.: the authentication service for a Peer to access to another Peer, both being software processes).

1 Service motivation for SUS. In this phase, one has to make sure that the potential users are aware of the value added by the service and wish to be able to use it, once it will be available. Motivation in e-Learning in our case comes from locally empowered virtual communities that experience in their practice the interest for collaborating on the Web.

2 Service definition by SUS. During this phase, potential users, coordinated by seniors – the "champions" that are aware of the opportunities potentially offered by technological innovations - formulate and discuss among themselves and with other peers initially vague, yet more and more precise functional specifications of the services they might need for their own purposes. Scenarios are generated. From scenarios, drafts of collaborative protocols are extracted. These functional specifications are then used as an input to Grid's technologists working in different work packages on OGSA for Learning (SDS).

3 Service use by SUS. While SDS are specifying, designing and developing innovative services, SUS use state of the art (Web + Grid) technologies for their goals, including progressively e-Learning, generating new experimentally founded considerations, guidelines, observations to be fed back to SDS.

4 Service evaluation by SUS. During this phase, we wish the services to be evaluated, as well as their e-Learning effects, by submitting SUS to the evaluation (e-qualification) procedures suggested by the corresponding scenario.

5 Service abstraction and generalization by SUS and SDS. This task allows one to propose and realize a significant upgrade of the "old" Service Elicitation and Evaluation/Exploitation Scenarios and the identification and implementation of completely new Scenarios. For instance, from the ENCORE scenario, one may propose biologists to use the services for their own construction of ontology's.

4.5. OGHSA: Open Grid Human Service Architecture

The role of standard architectures, such as OGSA, is to propose guidelines to the developers of Infrastructures such that the subsequent developments are cumulative and well integrated. Once the Human is considered a potential service provider and consumer in a Grid network, it becomes natural to submit human participation in Virtual Organizations to rules and conditions that regulate the correct social behavior of the VOs.

The risk in oversimplification is obvious. The advantage is as well easy to appreciate. As we have described above, Humans participate to VOs either as Users or as Developers. In both cases, they may provide or consume services. While developers are well familiar with elementary Grid services and ways of combining them into more complex ones, users reason in terms of context dependent, high level services, and their contribution is better in their decomposition into lower level ones.

The acceptance of Humans in Grid VOs seems ho bring naturally to the situation where define time and run time of software is nicely intertwined. The gap between the complexity of vaguely specified, coarse grain, but real world service demand and the formally specified, but fine grain and artificial (software) service offer, seems to be potentially bridged in a smooth way by humans playing the role of providers and consumers of services.

Finally, the OGHSA concept includes the notions of progressive enhancement of previously purely human or purely artificial services by coupling the two service sources; and smooth degradation in the sense that in case of human or software failure an alternative should remain open and feasible.

5. Conclusion

The success of the Web consists of the opportunity to access any electronic information wherever it has been produced and stored. The limits of the Web (potentially overcome by the Grid and the autonomous Agents) consist of the lack of conversational, truly collaborative tools: HTTP is a stateless protocol, and most activities on the Web consist of finding a static page somewhere. The Web is mainly a library.

The Grid may transform the source of Information into a source of Knowledge, i.e.: a set of documents, programs and humans accessible at any time from anywhere capable to proactively assist "me", a human, in my daily problems by means of conversations that indeed serve me to achieve my own goals.

If that is the new scenario for e-Learning, the success is ensured, since the major limit of traditional educational applications was due to a multimedia, passive, book-like, at best: retroactive offer while real learners - as well as teachers or humans with other roles - require one - or more - partner(s) in conversations, patient but authoritative, that keep the motivation high while offering assistance just in time, collaboratively and dialectically.

Acknowledgements

This work was partially supported by the European Community under the Information Society Technologies (IST) programme of the 6th Framework Programme for RTD - project ELeGI, contract IST-002205. This document does not represent the opinion of the European Community, and the European Community is not responsible for any use that might be made of data appearing therein.

Further support has been received by the EGIS (Environment in a Global Information Society) and SCOPE (Scientific Committee on Problems of the Environment) projects within the International Council for Science (ICSU) (Francesco Di Castri); UNESCO (DESS Montpellier) and Centre d'Ecologie Fonctionelle et Evolutive CEFE-CNRS Montpellier (Arnaud Martin), Ecole Nationale Supérieure de Chimie de Montpellier (Claude Laurenço) ; Fac. Un. Notre Dame de la Paix FUNDP-FNRS Namur (Alain Krief) and IUT de Bayonne (Guy Gouardères).

References

[1] Foster et al. The Anatomy of the Grid: Enabling Scalable Virtual Organizations , International Journal of Supercomputer Applications and High Performance Computing, 15(3), 2001.

[2] Foster et al. The Physiology of the Grid: An Open Grid Services Architecture for Distributed Systems Integration. Open Grid Service Infrastructure WG, Global Grid Forum, June 22, 2002.

[3] D. De Roure et al.: Research Agenda for the Semantic Grid: A Future e-Science Infrastructure. In: Report commissioned for EPSRC/DTI Core e-Science Programme. University of Southampton, UK, 2001.

[4] Foster, N.R. Jennings and C. Kesselman, Brain Meets Brawn: Why Grid and Agents Need Each Other. Autonomous Agents and Multi-Agent Systems AAMAS'04, July 19-23, 2004, New York, USA.

[5] S.A. Cerri, Human and Artificial Agent's Conversations on the Grid ; Proc. 1st LEGE-WG Workshop: Towards a European Learning Grid Infrastructure; Educational Models for Grid Based Services, Lausanne (2002). http://ewic.bcs.org/conferences/2002/1stlege/session3.htm

[6] S.A. Cerri, G. Gouardères and F. Paraguaçu (eds). Intelligent Tutoring Systems. Proceedings of the 6th International Conference ITS 2002, LNCS 2363, Springer Verlag: pp. XXVII-1016 , 2002. http://link.springer.de/link/service/series/0558/tocs/t2363.htm

[7] D. Maraschi and S.A. Cerri, Relations entre les technologies de l'enseignement et les agents. In: AFIA 2001 Atelier: Methodologies et Environments pour les Systèmes Multi-Agents (SMA 2001) LEIBNIZ-IMAG, Grenoble, 25-29 juin 2001; pages 61-73

[8] Newell, The Knowledge Level. Artificial Intelligence, 18 (1), 1982.

[9] G. Antoniou & F. van Harmelen. « A Semantic Web Primer ». Technical Report 03009, The MIT Press, 2005.

[10] M. Liquière and J. Sallantin. "Structural machine learning with gallois lattice and graphs". In 5th International Conference on Machine Learning, pages 305–313, Madison, Wisconsin (USA),1998. Morgan Kaufmann.

[11] S.A. Cerri and V. Loia, Knowledge Communication: motivation and foundations. Presented at ACM Workshop on Strategic Directions in Computing Research - Working group on Parallel and Distributed Computation. Cambridge, Mass. (1996). http://www-osl.cs.uiuc.edu/sdcr.html

[12] Chandrasekaran and T.R. Johnson, Generic tasks and task structures: History, critique and new directions. In D. Krivine & R. Simmons (Eds.), Second Generation Expert Systems, 232-272. Berlin: Springer Verlag. (1993)

[13] W. Clancey, Knowledge-Based Tutoring: The GUIDON-Program, MIT Press, 1987.

[14] E. Soloway, What to Do Next: Meeting the Challenge of Programming-in-the-Large. In: Soloway,E.; Iyengar,Sitharama (eds); Empirical Studies of Programmers; Ablex, 1986: 263-268 (1986)

[15] E. Soloway and K. Ehrlich. Empirical studies of programming knowledge. IEEE Transactions on Software Engineering, SE-10(5):595--609, September 1984

[16] N. Wiener, Cybernetics, or control and communication in the animal and the machine. John Wiley & Sons, New York (1948)

[17] D.A. Norman, Cognitive engineering. In: Norman, D.A. and Draper, S.W. User Centered System Design: New Perspectives on Human--Computer Interaction. pp. 31--61. Hillsdale, NJ: Lawrence Erlbaum Associates. (1986)

[18] P. Wegner, Why interaction is more powerful than algorithms. Comm. ACM 40, 5; 80-91(1997)

[19] J.R. Carbonell, AI in CAI: an artificial intelligence approach to computer-assisted instruction, IEEE Trans. On Man-Machine Systems, 11, 190-202 (1970).

[20] R. Elio and A. Haddadi, On Abstract Task Models and Conversation Policies. Autonomous Agents 99; http://www.boeing.com/special/agents99/papers.html

[21] K. Van Marcke, GTE: An Epistemological Approach to Instructional Modeling. Special issue of Instructional Science, vol 26, nrs 3-4, pp147-191. P. Goodyear (ed) and K. Van Marcke (guest ed). (1998)

[22] R. Pilkington, Analysing educational dialogue interaction: towards models that support learning, Journal of Artificial Intelligence in Education 12, (2001), 1-7.

[23] K. Porayska-Pomsta, C. Mellish, and H. Pain, Aspects of speech act categorisation: towards generating teachers' language , Journal of Artificial Intelligence in Education 11 (2000), 254-272

[24] S.A. Cerri, Computational Mathetics Tool kit: architecture's for dialogues. In: Frasson, C., Gauthier, G., and Lesgold, A. (eds.): Intelligent Tutoring Systems. Lecture Notes in Computer Science , Vol. 1086. Springer-Verlag, Montréal (1996) 343-352

[25] Kafura and J.P. Briot, Actors & Agents. IEEE Concurrency 6 (1998), 24-29

[26] S.A. Cerri, Shifting the focus from control to communication: the STReams OBjects Environments model of communicating agents. In: Padget, J. A. (ed.): Collaboration between Human and Artificial Societies, Coordination and Agent-Based Distributed Computing. Lecture

Notes in Artificial Intelligence , Vol. 1624. Springer-Verlag, Berlin Heidelberg New York (1999) 71-101

[27] Z. Guessoum and J.P. Briot, From Active Objects to Autonomous Agents. IEEE Concurrency 7, 3 (1999) 68-76

[28] W.J. Clancey, The conceptual nature of knowledge, situations, and activity. In P. Feltovich, K. Ford, & R. Hoffman (Eds.), Human and Machine Expertise in Context, pp. 247-291. Menlo Park, CA: The AAAI Press. (1997)

[29] W. Clancey, Towards On-Line Services Based on a Holistic Analysis of Human Activities, In : Pierluigi Ritrovato, Colin Allison, Stefano A. Cerri, Theo Dimitrakos, Matteo Gaeta, and Saverio Salerno (eds) Towards the Learning Grid: advances in Human Learning Services. To appear in the series: Frontiers in Artificial Intelligence and Applications, IOS Press (expected January 2005).

[30] M. Crubézy, E. Motta, W. Lu and M.A. Musen, Configuring Online Problem-Solving Resources with the Internet Reasoning Service, IEEE Intelligent Systems 18, 2 (2003), 34-42

[31] M. Crubézy and M.A. Musen, Ontologies in support of Problem Solving, Handbook on Ontologies, S. Staab and R Studer (eds), Springer Verlag (2003), 321-341

[32] J. Breuker et al. « Towards a conceptual framework for conversation and services». ELeGI Technical Report D12 : Preliminary version of Grid Service Architecture for conversational and collaboration processes / 2.3., Internal Deliverable on http://portal.sema.es/ , October 2004

[33] Jonquet, M. Eisenstadt and S. A. Cerri, Learning Agents and Enhanced Presence for Generation of Services on the Grid. In : Pierluigi Ritrovato, Colin Allison, Stefano A. Cerri, Theo Dimitrakos, Matteo Gaeta, and Saverio Salerno (eds) Towards the Learning Grid: advances in Human Learning Services. To appear in the series: Frontiers in Artificial Intelligence and Applications, IOS Press (expected January 2005).

[34] G. M. da Nóbrega, S. A. Cerri and J. Sallantin. " A contradiction-driven approach to theory formation: Conceptual issues, pragmatics in human learning, potentialities." Journal of the Brazilian Computer Society n. 2, vol. 9, (2003), 37-56

[35] S. Trausan-Matu, D. Maraschi, and S.A. Cerri, Ontology-Centered Personalized Presentation of Knowledge Extracted From the Web. In Intelligent Tutoring Systems, vol. 2363, Lecture Notes in Computer Science, Cerri, S.A., Gouardères, G., Paraguaçu, F. (Eds.) Berlin Heidelberg New York: Springer-Verlag, (2002) 259-269

[36] S. A. Cerri, Open Learning Service Scenarios on Grids, Proceedings of the 3rd International Workshop on Grid Infrastructure to Support Future Technology Enhanced Learning (IST-2001-38763) December, 2003; Berlin. Published in: British Computer Society Electronic Workshops in Computing (BCS eWiC); Category: Grid computing; http://ewic.bcs.org/conferences/2003/3rdlege/index.htm

[37] G. M. da Nóbrega, S. A. Cerri, and J. Sallantin. "On the Social Rational Mirror: learning e-commerce in a Web-served Learning Environment". In S.A. Cerri, G. Gouardères, and F. Paraguaçu, editors, Intelligent Tutoring Systems, 6th International Conference - ITS 2002, Biarritz (France), June 5-8 2002. LNCS 2363, pp. 41-50. Springer-Verlag Berlin Heidelberg 2002

[38] Di Castri, Access to information and e-learning for local empowerment. The requisite for human development and environmental protection. In : Pierluigi Ritrovato, Colin Allison, Stefano A. Cerri, Theo Dimitrakos, Matteo Gaeta, and Saverio Salerno (eds) Towards the Learning Grid: advances in Human Learning Services. To appear in the series: Frontiers in Artificial Intelligence and Applications, IOS Press (expected January 2005).

[39] Chaire UNESCO CPU-DESS Aménagement Intégré des Territoires (2003) Proposition d'élements de stratégies pour le développement touristique de la communeauté de communes du Lodévois-Larzac. CNRS CEFE, Montpellier (122 pages).

[40] Paraguaçu, S.A Cerri, C. Costa, and E. Untersteller; A peer-to-peer Architecture for the Collaborative Construction of Scientific Theories by Virtual Communities, IEEE/ITRE2003, August 10-13, 2003, Newark, New Jersey, USA

[41] C. Colaux-Castillo and A. Krief, EnCOrE (Encyclopédie de Chimie Organique Electronique): an Original Way to Represent and Transfer Knowledge from Freshmen to Researchers in Organic Chemistry, Proceedings of the 3rd International Workshop on Grid Infrastructure to Support Future Technology Enhanced Learning (IST-2001-38763) December, 2003; Berlin. Published in: British Computer Society Electronic Workshops in Computing (BCS eWiC); Category: Grid computing; http://ewic.bcs.org/conferences/2003/3rdlege/session1/paper5.htm

[42] P. Lemoisson et al. , Interactive Construction of EnCOrE. In:7th Int. Conf. On Intelligent Tutoring Systems (ITS 2004)–Workshop on Grid Learning Services (GLS04), J. Mostow and P. Tedesco (eds). Summary available at http://www.info.uqam.ca/~nkambou/gls/gls04.htm

[43] R. Yatchou, G. Gouardères and R. Nkambou, Ubiquitous Knowledge Prosthesis for Grid Learning Services : the Grid-e-Card, In:7th Int. Conf. On Intelligent Tutoring Systems (ITS 2004)–Workshop on Grid Learning Services (GLS04), J. Mostow and P. Tedesco (eds). Summary available at http://www.info.uqam.ca/~nkambou/gls/gls04.htm To be submitted to : Special Issue of the Applied Artificial Intelligence Journal.(expected Sept 2005)

[44] L. Razmerita and G. Gouardères, Ontology based User Modeling for Personalization of Grid Learning Services, In:7th Int. Conf. On Intelligent Tutoring Systems (ITS 2004)–Workshop on Grid Learning Services (GLS04), J. Mostow and P. Tedesco (eds). Summary available at http://www.info.uqam.ca/~nkambou/gls/gls04.htm To be submitted to : Special Issue of the Applied Artificial Intelligence Journal.(expected Sept 2005)

[45] Abdelkader Gouaich and Stefano A. Cerri. Movement and interaction in semantic grids: dynamic service generation for agents in the MIC* deployment environment. In 4th LeGE-WG InternationalWorkshop: Towards a European Learning Grid Infrastructure: Progressing with a European Learning Grid, Stuttgart, Germany, April 2004. Electronic Workshops in Computing (eWiC). http://ewic.bcs.org/conferences/2003/4thlege/.

[46] P. Lemoisson, S. A. Cerri, J. Sallantin. " Constructive Interactions " (revised) In : Pierluigi Ritrovato, Colin Allison, Stefano A. Cerri, Theo Dimitrakos, Matteo Gaeta, and Saverio Salerno (eds) Towards the Learning Grid: advances in Human Learning Services. To appear in the series: Frontiers in Artificial Intelligence and Applications, IOS Press (expected January 2005).

[47] N.N. Binti Abdullah, M. Liquiere and S.A. Cerri, Grid Services as Learning Agents: Steps towards Induction of Communication Protocols. In:7th Int. Conf. On Intelligent Tutoring Systems (ITS 2004)–Workshop on Grid Learning Services (GLS04),), J. Mostow and P. Tedesco (eds). Summary available at http://www.info.uqam.ca/~nkambou/gls/gls04.htm To be submitted to : Special Issue of the Applied Artificial Intelligence Journal.(expected Sept 2005)

Towards the Learning Grid
P. Ritrovato et al. (Eds.)
IOS Press, 2005

Making e-Learning a Service Oriented Utility: The European Learning Grid Infrastructure Project

Matteo Gaeta [a], Pierluigi Ritrovato [b], Saverio Salerno [a]

[a] *DIIMA - University of Salerno Via Ponte Don Melillo 84084 Fisciano (SA) Italy*
{gaeta, salerno}@unisa.it
[b] *CRMPA, Via Ponte Don Melillo, 84084 Fisciano, (SA), Italy*
ritrovato@crmpa.unisa.it

Abstract: This paper describes the ELeGI (www.elegi.org) Project. ELeGI has the ambitious goal of developing software technologies for service oriented effective human learning. ELeGI will create new potential for moving from the current information transfer paradigm focused on content and on the key authoritative figure of the teacher who provides information towards learning paradigm focused on knowledge construction using experiential based and collaborative learning approaches in a contextualised, personalised and ubiquitous way. We have chosen a synergic approach, sometimes called "human centred design", to replace the classical, applicative approach to learning. With consideration of humans at the centre, learning is clearly a social, constructive phenomenon. It occurs as a side effect of interactions, conversations and enhanced presence in dynamic Virtual Communities created and deployed using Grid technologies.

Keywords: Grid technologies, service oriented architecture, semantic web, semantic and knowledge grid, Learning models, IMS Lerning Design.

Project Vision: Advancing Technology Enhanced Learning in Europe

The overall aim of the project is to radically advance the effective use of technology-enhanced learning in Europe through the design, implementation and validation of a pedagogy-driven, service-oriented software architecture based on Grid technologies for supporting ubiquitous, collaborative, experiential-based, contextualised and personalised learning. Previous projects that have set out to improve learning through novel technologies have often failed to leave any significant mark because they did not give priority to the social, economic and technical perspectives of the key human actors. So, while the development and use of appropriate technology must be pedagogically driven, at the same time those involved in the formulation and evaluation of pedagogy must be made aware of, and shown by demonstration, state-of-the-art technological possibilities. We address this pervasive learning issue by explicitly listing the roles that actors play in the learning process and illustrate with reference to future learning scenarios. This provides us with a focus for formulating requirements in terms of learning resources, services, quality of service, and usability for end-users. It also provides a clear reference for the technical context of the project – an open and flexible software architecture for creating learning environments that accommodate the roles implied by the new learning possibilities and that demonstrate state-of-the-art technology-enhanced learning.

1. Pedagogical Goals and New Learning Modes

In order to support the implementation of new learning modes [9, 15] related to ubiquitous, collaborative, experiential, contextualised and personalised learning [10, 11, 12, 13, 14, 16], it is necessary to promote a paradigm shift in the general approach to teaching and learning.

Currently, teaching and learning practices are based mainly on the information transfer paradigm. This focuses on content, and on the key authoritative figure of the teacher that provides information. Teachers' efforts are mainly devoted to find the best way for presenting content in order to transmit information to learners. This "product - teaching oriented view" finds its perfect technical mirror in the "page oriented approach to the Web" where the goal is to produce more and "better" static pages for the consumption of interested students. Learning is then considered to be an activity which helps teachers to produce, and students to consume, multimedia books on the Web. This paradigm has been popular in earlier e-Learning projects, not because it is effective, but because it is easy to implement with basic Internet facilities and it does not require any change in the traditional roles of the actors.

The information transfer paradigm is well understood and well supported by existing e-Learning practice. In order to advance effective learning we will promote another paradigm that focuses on the learner and on socio-constructivist forms of learning. In our approach the learner has an active and central role in the learning process. Learning activities are aimed at facilitating the construction of knowledge and skills in the learner [13, 15], instead of the memorisation of information. Information transfer will still obviously exist in this paradigm, but only as a simple component, not the main goal. Accordingly we can say that the proposed paradigm subsumes the old one in its displacement.

Knowledge construction occurs through forms of learning based on:

- the understanding of concepts through direct experience of their manifestation in realistic contexts (i.e. providing access to real world data) which are constructed from sophisticated software interfaces and devices, and represented as services;
- "social learning" – active collaboration with other students, teachers, tutors, experts or, in general, available human peers, by using different kinds of collaboration technologies, including enhanced presence.

In this approach collaboration [16] is considered as a complex conversational process that goes far beyond a simple information exchange. In order to support such a "ubiquitous conversational process", one must consider the social context where the learning process occurs. Accordingly we do not consider the learner's ability in an abstract way, but relate it to a specific situation (the context). In this ambit the term "ubiquitous" does not refer simply to "anytime / anywhere", but more generally to the ability to support multiple diverse learning contexts and automatically adapt to them.

As we consider human learning [2] as a social process, collaboration implies community membership, it means working together, providing added value, sharing and executing tasks in order to reach a common goal. Learning is no longer an isolated activity – it implies mutual trust, shared interests, common goals, commitments, obligations, exchanging of services, a genuinely proactive, motivated behaviour.

In order to foster these new approaches to learning [3] we will create dynamic contexts where the learner "achieves" knowledge and skills in an active way instead of simply storing information. Communities will have the right to identify their goals, in terms of knowledge and skills to be acquired, instead of just asking an authority to define a curriculum for them. Goals will therefore genuinely correspond to needs, and be highly dependent on the local culture and its priorities.

According to this learning paradigm we consider realism as the cornerstone of the learning environment. For example, highly realistic virtual scientific experiments have only recently become possible through use of advanced technology. Innovative aspects include the definition of a standard didactical model for the achievement and representation of such experiments. In this type of model a learner is immersed in a specific context, which through appropriate simulations, develops active learning processes with progressive abstraction levels, leading to the construction of their knowledge in a dynamic way. In this learning mode the student can also receive the support of the other users (collaborative aspects) and from the comparison with them; they can build a new "mediated" knowledge.

To complement this freedom in knowledge construction, we allow the definition of personalised and individualised learning paths. This means that in a specific context we need, from one side, to create learning conditions that are adequate for a learner's preferences (individualised learning) and, from the other, guarantee that the learner will reach a cognitive excellence through different learning paths according to their skills and knowledge. Accordingly, we will study and define specific models for representing knowledge that takes the learners preferred learning styles into account. A beneficial result of allowing learners the right to construct their own knowledge is that richer and more diversified learning contexts can arise, necessitating the dynamic integration of different kinds of information and communication technologies. The dynamics of intertwined, controlled and secure construction and use of subsequent versions of our systems, by skilled as well as unskilled human actors, and of the services enabling them, constitutes our methodological approach for successful adaptive technology-enhanced solutions.

2. Meeting the Technical Challenge: The Grid technology

In order to support the paradigm and the pedagogical goals described above new learning environment need to be defined. These new learning envirnoment should provide, at least, the following features in a technology neutral fashion:

- Collaboration and social interaction: group working should be routinely supported as well as the more traditional model of the solitary learner – this includes support for self-organising online communities who share common educational goals.
- Experiential (Active Learning): learning resources should be interactive, engaging, and responsive – active learning and knowledge formation should be emphasised above simple information transfer.
- Realism: real-world input should be easy to incorporate, as should simulations, ranging from simple interactive animations to immersive VR.
- Personalised: students should find themselves at the centre of their online environment, with their individual needs addressed the quality of the learning experience should be continually validated and evaluated.
- Ubiquity and accessibility:

- o wider, more flexible access to educational resources should be provided, often referred to as "anytime/anywhere" learning.
- o multiple different types of devices, interfaces, and network connection types should be supported where possible.

- Contextualised (Adaptive): appropriate learning contexts may be naturally be short-lived, as well as the more traditional static situations such as the class-room and the library – this calls for dynamicity in the creation of contexts.

These features together with the challanging pedagogical goals have highly demanding technical requirements, many of which are also the concerns of distributed systems research. According to our investigations, Grid is the most appropriate technology for supporting the proposed learning approach.

The Grid [5] was originally designed for e-Science and was primarily concerned with supercomputing applications, but the framework it engendered to realise effective sharing of distributed heterogeneous resources (OGSA: the Open Grid Services Architecture) [4]. OGSA leverages open standards including W3C, and provides an holistic view of Grid computing based on the concepts of 'Services', 'Distributed Collaboration' and 'Virtual Organisation'. It is now being applied to many other areas, especially enterprise computing and e-Commerce. Reciprocally, by progressing Grid technologies for learning, we will also contribute towards the advancement of the open Grid service model itself. We see the use of the Grid to support a paradigm shift in pedagogy to advance effective learning as a natural step in the recent historical progress of technology enhanced learning: Internet -> Web -> Grid.

2.1. The Grid added value for next generation learning

One of the first relevant aspects is that learning is inherently distributed. Using a simple analogy with computing architectures, the traditional Information-Transfer paradigm can be compared to simple "monolithic" client-server architectures. Indeed, the roles (learner and teacher) and the nature of these roles are fixed. A learner is like a client, he is only able to consume in a passive way the information provided by the teacher that, like a "monolithic" server, is able to provide these information (e.g. the functionalities provided by a server). The proposed learning paradigm is more similar to (and more suitable for) a distributed P2P architecture, in which the roles are not a-priori fixed (an expert leaner can become a tutor for another learner) and, like in the real world, knowledge is distributed among many communities and their members and, by the reverse, different members actively contribute to create the knowledge.

With respect to other distributed architectures, we aim at exploit the OGSA [4] model for several reasons. First of all, the OGSA model is based on the service's concept against the product's one. The main differences between these two concepts are underlined in [3]. Apart from the existing differences as for the conversational process, here we simply want to emphasise that, in general, a product presents a Method-based interface while a service presents a Message-based interface. In [21], G. Fox highlights that "*Method-based interfaces are most efficient but can only be run in that fashion in a single monolithic implementation*" while "*Message-based services support standards and distributed deployment with easy use of standards compliant services from different implementers*".

The message-based strategy produces lightweight loosely-coupled services that can be distributed and replicated to achieve needed performance and functionality, and it is the better strategy to build distributed systems/architectures/applications by composition of atomic components. This is clearly useful in our vision that strongly relies upon a composition paradigm allowing the creation of (personalized) learning experiences (re-)using data, units of learning, knowledge, tools virtualized as services and distributed across different organizations. Moreover, as explained in [3], the dynamic nature of services with respect to the products is an added value for our purpose.

These are the motivations that bring us to invest in a Service Oriented technology instead of more mature "traditional" distributed computing technologies.

Anyway, the question of which of the following better supports our learning process still remains: simple Web Service or Grid? According to the ELeGI project Vision, there are some reasons to prefer Grid instead of Web Service. It is clear that Web Services and Grid are not directly comparable and it isn't a case that Next Generation Grid will leverage on Web Services standards. Indeed, looking at the past the relationship existing between Web Services and Grid is the same existing between socket (for Unix Inter-process communications) and RMI (Remote Method Invocation) or between RMI and CORBA.

2.1.1. General Technologies and standards consideration

Learning is a conversational process with long time transactions, therefore the state management is a fundamental aspect. Independently from the WS-Specification used to define the semantics of an OGSA service (currently, we have two possible candidates: the WSRF [32] proposed by Global Grid Forum OGSA Working Group [24] and under the standardization process of OASIS [35] and the family of specification WS-I+ [34] as proposed by the OMII [33]), it is clear that OGSA complaint architectures will rely upon a dynamic and stateful service model and this also affects the development of learning scenarios.

Recognizing the need for the state management in learning scenarios, an underlying stateless service model would force the developer to manage the state at a higher (e.g. Application) level. From a technical point of view, this is an additional effort that adoption of Grid technologies can minimize and, in some case, eliminate.

Learning is a knowledge-based process aiming at the knowledge creation through realistic and contextualized experiences. It is evident, from several scientific reports [9, 22], the benefits coming from the integration of semantic and knowledge technologies for learning as well as for the service orientation. It is also clear that to support realistic and experiential based learning approaches involving responsive resources, 3d simulations and immersive VR, we need the scale of computational power and data storage typical of Grid technologies as well as many features of the VO paradigm (e.g. secure and transparent access to distributed and heterogeneous resources and services, including sensors and scientific instruments).

The Semantic Grid [6, 7, 22] seems to go toward this direction gluing Semantic Web [18] technologies and Grid ones. In our opinion the Grid or the Semantic Web technologies taken alone will allow a partial accomplishment of the complex ELeGI vision and, in the framework of ELeGI project, we need to exploit both Grid and Semantic Web technologies to define a domain specialisation of the Semantic Grid that we have refereed as the Semantic Grid for Human Learning [31].

This aspect highlight another relevant added value for Grid: they ability to act as a glue among different technologies like Agent, Semantic Web, Web Service that, taken alone, can provide only partial benefits. For instance, we should rely upon Agent technologies to define Pedagogical Agent [26] acting as personal tutor able to create personalized experiences or upon Semantic Web technologies to allow the creation of Knowledge Neighbourhoods, which are defined "locations in cyberspace where learners can congregate into groups or larger communities with the goal of acquiring knowledge about some topic" [23].

In ELeGI, we need both these features (and others) to achieve our goal that, it is useful to remember, is to effectively progress the e-Learning. Having this goal in mind, we don't see an advantage to use Semantic Web technologies (providing a very good support to Knowledge management, sharing and creation) and to spend our efforts to define advanced algorithm for resources reservation (to support efficient resources management allowing 3d simulations and immersive VR) or to use Agent technologies (providing a good support for contextualization and personalization) if they must be reinforced with such a mechanism to discover, acquire, federate, and manage the capabilities/resources/contents needed to create/delivery the personalized learning experiences.

From a technological viewpoint, it is clear that the big advantage of any technology is to provide all-in-box. This is the role that we expect from Grid technologies and this is the reason of aligning our research directions with the Semantic Grid and the Next Generation Grid (NGG) [27] in order to define the so-called Semantic Grid for Human Learning.

2.1.2. Virtual Organisation and Virtual Learning Community technology implication

Learning is a collaborative and community-based process and we need to support autonomous and dynamic creation of communities. The learner should be able to search and find peers having similar skills and sharing the same learning objectives, he /she should be able to organize groups with clear educational goals and to collaborate with participants to achieve these goals. To support these functionalities, we need some glue, such as an advanced mechanism for service discovery and orchestration, managing security and trust, to provide single sign on for access services, to allow different services to be aware that they work together with other services for a common objective/goal and much more. These are features typical of a Virtual Organization (VO) as described in [30].

Of course, the Grid technologies are not mandatory for the fulfilment of the VO paradigm, that is technological neutral, but there is at least one good reason to prefer Grid technologies with respect to the others, including the Web Service ones. Grid provides a well defined taxonomy [30] in order to solve many issues involved in the creation and management of VO (and of specialised virtual environment constructed upon a VO, like our Virtual Learning Communities VLC) and, in accordance with this taxonomy, it is already defined in the framework of the OGSA V1 [17] a set of capabilities useful in the context of VO for the creation of loosely coupled large scale distributed systems.

In the framework of ELeGI, we are interested in defining, formalizing and implementing the concept of Virtual Learning Community (VLC). In ELeGI the VO and VLC represent different abstractions. Through the VO we will abstract all the aspects related to the infrastructure operational management (like the IT infrastructure of modern enterprises), through the VLC we will abstract all the aspects related to the business process management (definition, enactment, etc.).

We conceive the VO as a common "base" providing methodologies, models, contracts, policies and technological assets in order to define the environment (from both the infrastructure and deployment viewpoints). Upon the defined environment we provide the "business level" in terms of services, didactic and knowledge model, social interactions, virtual laboratory and whatever needed in order to support the ELeGI learning process: namely the ?within the VLC.

The Web Services are, of course, enabling technologies for our purposes, but we need much more (i.e. a specific instance of a Service Oriented Architecture) in order to address relevant VOs (and consequently VLC) creation and management issues.

The Web Service standards are mainly aimed at obtaining interoperability among loosely coupled components/resources (virtualized as services) distributed in heterogeneous environments while the Grid is principally aimed at the creation and management of VOs for heterogeneous resource sharing and, therefore, the level of abstraction provided by these two technologies is different. The Web Services are able to provide abstractions to the lower level of the proposed learning approach (e.g. abstracting educational contents, data, computational resources) while raising the level of abstraction is a necessary task for defining and implementing the VLC. In a VLC, it is desirable to learn in a simple and more natural way, using "high level abstractions" (e.g. abstracting models, activities, experiments) that should be shared among all the participants.

According to our investigation, the Grid is the most suitable technology providing, in terms of services (e.g. all the capabilities defined in the OGSA V1), the "middle level abstractions" able to ground what a VLC requires in a distributed infrastructure.

From a technological viewpoint, instead, they are converging towards the same standards, specifications and protocols for a common building block (e.g. a Web Service) but the issues that they address remain different. Interoperability is a fundamental pillar and it is a base requirement for the creation of VOs, but VOs need more: resource management and discovery mechanisms, information and knowledge management, resource sharing based on security and trust policies and so on.

Also the Web Services have a set of WS-Specifications that, globally, define the so-called WS-Architecture [20]. But while the Grid taxonomy and capabilities are contextualized for the VO domain, and address VO specific issues, the WS-Architecture is not contextualized for a particular issue and address general issues.

This means that if we have to implement and manage a VLC (and this is a central issue in the ELeGI project) using the Web Service technologies, we have to build ad hoc and custom solutions in order to solve: first, particular issues of the VO environments (e.g. the middle level abstractions) and next, particular issues of the e-Learning domain (e.g. the high level abstractions).

2.1.3. Learning standards implication

Learning is a pedagogical-driven process. This is a key factor that distinguishes our learning approach with respect to the Information-Transfer based learning and also to other relevant learning initiatives. As explained in [31] we will not customize the ELeGI architecture for a specific pedagogical model. Instead, we have to catch all the pedagogical features we have identified including collaboration, personalization, context-awareness, realism, ubiquity, accessibility and availability. Currently, the IMS-Learning Design (IMS-LD) specifications [28] seem to be the best approach to model learning scenarios on the basis of different pedagogies and this is a good reason to investigate the adoption of these specifications in the ELeGI project. We believe that the development of IMS-LD scenarios upon a Grid based software infrastructure such as ELeGI will provide dynamicity and adaptiveness capabilities. LD takes place at two levels, learning activity and learning approach, we foresee Grid technologies can provide both of them with benefits.

The first level relates to the learning activities. A LD scenario is composed of many learning activities, that can be defined as interactions between a learner and an environment (optionally involving other learners, practitioners, resources, tools and services) to achieve a planned learning outcome [25]. We agree that in this definition, contents and context are not separable. LD specifications aim at supporting, among the others, also reuse of activities and re-purposing of units of learning. But they are difficult to obtain with traditional technologies. For instance, if we redefine the outcome of a learning activity or change the context in which the activity is performed, it implies that different contents are required. To reuse learning activities in different contexts and/or to obtain different outcomes we need a mechanism for automatic discovery and binding of new suitable contents and services as well as self-adaptive mechanisms when deploying the LD scenarios and, also, the learning activities composing a scenario. As previously described, dynamicity and adaptiveness of Grid technologies provides better benefits with respect to other technologies.

The second level concerns the learning approach. In this level we have the contextualization of the learning activities with respect to a specific pedagogical model. Even in this case, the reuse and sharing of learning activities across different pedagogical models is a desirable feature. We are convinced that the dynamicity and adaptiveness features of Grid technologies have to be investigated in order to allow a semi-automatic reconfiguration of learning activities of a LD scenario when the adopted pedagogy changes.

3. The Methodology: Test-Beds and Demonstrators

Having described the overall objectives, the pedagogical goals and how we aim to meet the technical challenge, we now outline the methodology for the realisation and validation of ELeGI project. We have selected a particular set of demonstrators and test-beds representing scientific, social, economic and cultural cognate areas that include both formal and informal learning scenarios. The key difference between test-beds and demonstrators is that demonstrators already exist in non-Grid compliant forms, as relatively mature and well understood exemplars of the types of pedagogy ELeGI wishes to support, whereas testbeds are principally new departures, designed to test the ELeGI approach from conception to implementation and evaluation.

3.1. Testbeds: Service Elicitation and Exploitation Scenarios

As we are working towards a service-oriented architecture we refer to the test-beds as Service Elicitation and Exploitation Scenarios (SEES). The purpose of the SEES is to develop and gain insight into the processes involved from formulating pedagogic requirements to the implementing environments that meet these requirements. The following SEES, which are described in detail in the RTD section, are planned:

- Informal Learning
    - Learning and Training of Researchers in Organic Chemistry;
    - e-Qualification by Open Universities;
- Formal Learning
    - Master in ICT with remote teaching and tutoring activities (in collaboration with Carnegie Mellor University);
    - Physic course in the Open University;

3.2. Demonstrators

Demonstrators differ from SEES in that they are based on the advanced prototypes which have adopted approaches congruent with the new paradigm, and where the pedagogical issues are already well understood. The purposes of the demonstrators are:

- To provide evidence of the benefit coming from the adoption of didactical models based on socio-constructivist contextualised approach and to demonstrate the effectiveness of Grid technologies for implementing these didactical models.

- to understand the engineering issues involved in implementing/porting existing solutions as OGSA-compliant software and services
- to configure and customise these environments, for demonstrating effectiveness of specific research aspects
- To prepare advanced contents for these environments
- to provide working systems to elicit feedback and provide reference points within the project
- to act as "demonstrators" in support of publicity, dissemination and training activities

The demonstrators have been selected in order to maximise the benefits of the development work in that there is already a working non-Grid version. The three demonstrators planned are:

- Virtual Scientific Experiments for teaching high level mathematical courses.
- Learning Environment for Accountancy and Business Finance
- Learning Environment for Mechanical Engineering

4. Summary of Scientific and Technical Objectives

In summary, the project has three major goals.

Goal 1. To create new potential for ubiquitous and collaborative human learning, merging experiential, personalised and contextualised approaches

Goal 2. To define and implement an advanced service-oriented Grid based software architecture for learning. This objective will be driven by the pedagogical needs and requirements elicited from Service Elicitation and Exploitation Scenarios (SEES)

Goal 3. To validate and evaluate the software architecture and the didactical approaches through the use of SEES and Demonstrators

In order to reach these goals it will pursue the following objectives:

Goal 1

- study, define and experiment with the new paradigm for formal and informal learning taking into account socio-cultural constructivist, personalised, contextualised, experiential and collaborative approaches
- study, define, experiment and validate methodologies, techniques and standards for representing and managing knowledge construction in the learner during the learning process according to different learning styles (individualised and personalised learning);
- study, define and validate methodologies for evaluating the effectiveness from both the pedagogical and usability point of view of these new learning approaches in different disciplines and contexts;
- study, define and validate didactical learning models for virtual scientific experiments which take the learner's preferences and collaborative aspects into account;

Goal 2

- design, develop and validate a Grid based software architecture for exploiting the new learning paradigm;
- monitor and contribute to standards development for learning systems, pedagogical models, Grid technologies, semantic and knowledge technologies;

- study and evaluate how the development of the semantic Web in general, and the semantic and knowledge Grid in particular, will impact on the project software architecture and new learning paradigm;
- study, define and experiment with advanced conversational processes and enhanced presence technologies for collaborative learning in the new paradigm;

Goal 3

- experiment and validate learning approaches, strategies, and technology infrastructure through different test-beds (SEES), using feedback for re-engineering and refining the context;
- study and define strategies for the adoption of these new learning approaches and related technology facilitating the paradigm shift for the learning institutions;
- demonstrate and validate how Grid technology facilitates the realisation of new learning paradigm and the implementation of Virtual Learning Communities;
- demonstrate, customise and exploit new or re-engineered learning systems and solutions for citizens and organisations;
- facilitate the exploitation of European cultural and scientific resources though the Learning Grid infrastructure.

5. Project Results and their Evaluation

The project results will be generated and evaluated through the use of the SEES and demonstrators. The SEES will evaluate the didactical approaches from cost/benefit and pedagogical points of view, and the support provided by the technology infrastructure in term of QoS, usability, scalability, interoperability and transparency of access to the distributed resources used for realising the didactical approaches. The Demonstrators will be used for stimulating the final users and the learning community in general about the potentialities offered by the realisation of a pedagogical driven service-oriented software architecture based on Grid technology (ELeGI)

In summary, the main ELeGI project results will be:

- The service oriented Grid based Software Architecture;
- Formalisation of didactical models for the new learning approaches;
- Methodologies for evaluating the effectiveness of these new learning approaches from the pedagogical and usability points of view;
- Methodologies and techniques for representing knowledge and for allowing personalised, individualised and collaborative learning;
- Strategies for leading learning organisations and actors in the learning process to actualise the paradigm shift in learning approaches;
- Prototypes for demonstrating the potentialities offered by the ELeGI technologies and methodologies;
- New digital content in different contexts to support innovative learning approaches and in particular with respect to virtual scientific experiments;
- Methodologies and techniques for making existing applications Grid-aware;
- ELeGI evaluation and experimentation feedbacks;
- Contribution to the technical standards in the Learning, semantic Web, and Grid domains;
- Workshops, Conferences, Publications, Information Web sites, and Demonstrator Web sites for disseminating project results.

6. Summary of the research activities and related innovation

The picture below shows the organisation of the RTD activities and the relations existing among the research activities.

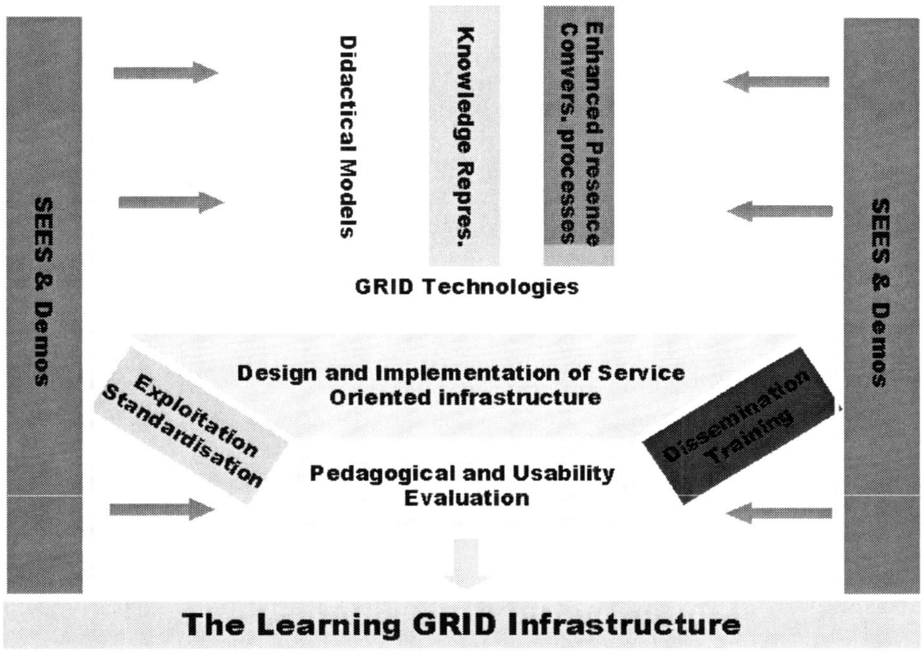

Figure 1: The EleGI integreted approach

The innovations that will be introduced with the ELeGI proposal can be classified in two different, but interrelated and objective- driven main groups. The first group is related to the pedagogical aspects the second group to the technology aspects.

The essence of innovations for pedagogical aspects is that in order to fully exploit e-learning processes we can not simply make the electronic transposition of traditional learning model. We need to investigate and define appropriate didactical models for e-learning. These models, based mainly on contextualised, experiential based and personalised approaches (socio-constructivist vision), will be defined taking into account in a synergic process both pedagogical and technological aspects fostering a learning paradigm based on socially situated, activity-based knowledge construction rather than information memorisation.

In particular, an innovative aspect is that our general model [8] is the presence of three models: Knowledge Model, Student Model and Didactic Model, which substantially interact among them to define the specific and personalised formative path. Moreover, the model will consider several characters of learning in a unitary approach. In the ELeGI proposal we will focus our attentions on the Active, Situated and Collaborative properties of learning.

- Active means that the learner is the principal actor of the process he/she takes the main decisions he/she learn choosing tools, exploring knowledge bases, accessing to virtual experiments, etc.

- Situated means contextualised with respect to activities motivated by goals, intentions, purposes, plans.
- Collaborative, means that the creation of the knowledge is a collaborative process evolving through interactions according to specific conversational processes with colleagues, teachers, tutors, experts, instruments, etc.

In this frame model for experiential based learning will be proposed, in particular with respect to Virtual Scientific Experiments.

Other innovative aspects are related to the possibility to personalise the learning process according to the learners' preferences and styles. In order to allow personalised learning processes we need to study and define methodologies for representing, through adequate knowledge structures (ontologies), and managing knowledge representing both the domain (the learning context) and the learner capabilities and skills itself including the representation of learner's attitudes, flaws as well as possible misunderstandings with respect to concepts and relations among several pieces of information related to a specific learning domain (e.g.: mathematics, physics, sociology, etc.). We are convinced we can now reach these objectives because we have already developed significant, even if quite limited, prototypes that present these features.

Exploiting these advanced knowledge representation structures, it will be possible to introduce innovative intelligent functionalities embedded into to the learning environment, namely the learning Grid infrastructure, creating a first concrete interpretation of the Ambient Intelligence vision in the learning domain.

Innovative will be the approach that we follow for implementing, experimenting and validating the learning paradigm. Indeed, each and all the research activities will be aimed at satisfying user needs and will be validated through the execution of real size test-beds in an iterative approach, thus using the results as a feed-back as well as a feed-forward for improving and changing the models defined.

It is clear that in order to reach these ambitious objectives we need to design and implement a very powerful technological infrastructure. The widest is the potential learning audience, the most sophisticated should be the technology and, at the same time, the simplest to use. From this point of view the main innovation is the use of Grid technologies for implementing a service oriented software infrastructure moving e-learning towards a service oriented utility. The use of Grid technologies implies the adoption of a framework based approach for designing our infrastructure. This means to raise the level of abstraction in the infra-structure design:

- trying to be as much as possible neutral respect to technological evolutions,
- focusing our attention on the definition of interfaces and behaviours of "learning services" in a standard way and
- implementing an infrastructure that will incrementally support the realisation and actualisation of our learning paradigm.

We are well aware, as we said in previous sections, that for actualising this new learning paradigm we need to integrate and coherently orchestrate several kinds of technologies and existing software solutions in an innovative way.

Investigating and experimenting with the use of Grid s as technology glue for implementing dynamic service oriented Virtual Learning Organisations (VLO) also introduces potential innovations fed to the technological level: the service elicitation scenarios will continuously feed the technologists with requirements for new services described at the abstraction level of the pedagogy, to be translated into combinations of services at the abstraction level of technologies. The continuous "translation" process from the one to the other abstraction level is exactly the core of the synergies declared as the innovative approach of ELeGI.

Our conversational processes research will use the methodology, models and tools successfully applied to the joint construction of shared ontologies, both in the e-Commerce and in the e-Learning domains to build semi-automatically "ontologies" of Conversations, i.e: rules for managing dynamically conversations in collaborative virtual communities.

Finally, innovations for the Grid technologies strictly connected to support dynamic Virtual Learning Organisations emerge from the study and analysis of semantic. In order to implement dynamic VLOs, we need to define mechanism for services discovery as well as to automatically "understand" the capabilities of these discovered services. In order to do that, we need to define standards for describing Grid serviced semantically. This is one of the hottest research topics in the Grid domain and we believe that with the ELeGI proposal we can contribute substantially to the progress in this field. Moreover, the exploitation of this semantic enrichment of services will be fundamental for supporting collaboration and interactivity as well as for creating the necessary awareness for implementing a Learning Ambient Intelligent vision.

Conversational processes, enhanced presence and the Semantic Grid are all activities identified in ELeGI run together: learning services, the ones needed for enabling effective learning to occur, have to be first identified by means of conversational processes by humans in virtual communities accompanied by enhanced presence in order to keep motivation and commitment to the community's goals high and performing. Identified services have then to be progressively transformed into software, i.e. the semantics of services has to be constructed in order to make an infrastructure that supports those services.

Acknowledgements

The work reported in this study was partially supported by the European Commission under the Information Society Technologies (IST) programme of the 6th Framework Programme for RTD - project ELeGI, contract IST-002205. This document does not represent the opinion of the European Community, and the European Community is not responsible for any use that might be made of data appearing therein.

References

[1] The European Learning Grid Infrastructure home page http://www.ELeGI.org/

[2] Visser, J.: Integrity, Completeness and Comprehensiveness of the Learning Environment: Meeting the Basic Learning Needs of All Throughout Life. In D. N. Aspin, J. D. Chapman, M. J. Hatton and Y. Sawano (Eds.), International Handbook of Lifelong Learning. Dordrecht, The Netherlands: Kluwer Academic Publishers, 2001.

[3] C. Allison, S. A Cerri, M. Gaeta, P. Ritrovato: "Services, Semantics and Standards: Components for a Learning Grid Infrastructure", in proceedings of the Grid Learning Service Workshop at ITS 2004 - Maceio, Brazil - August 30, 2004.

[4] Foster, I., Kesselman, C., Nick J M., and Tuecke, S. The Physiology of the Grid: An Open Grid Services Architecture for Distributed Systems Integration.

[5] Foster I. and Kesselman C.: The Grid: Blueprint for a New Computing Infrastructure, Morgan Kaufmann, 1999.

[6] De Roure D., Jennings N. R. and Shadbolt N.R.: The Semantic Grid: A Future e-Science Infrastructure, chapter in the book Grid Computing: Making The Global Infrastructure a Reality by Fran Berman, Anthony J.G. Hey and Geoffrey Fox. - John Wiley & Sons; (April 8, 2003), on pages 437-470.

[7] De Roure D., Jennings N. R. and Shadbolt N.R.: The Semantic Grid: Past, Present and Future, in the Proceeding of IEEE Volume 93, Issue 3, March 2005 Page(s):669 – 681.

[8] Albano G., D'Auria B., Gaeta M., Iovane G., Salerno S.: Education in e-learning environment: a theoretical framework and an actual proposal submitted on IEEE Transaction on Education.
[9] Anderson T., and Whitelock D.: The Educational Semantic Web: Visioning and Practicing the Future of Education. (Special Issue on) Journal of Interactive Media in Education, 2004 (1) ISSN: 1365-893X. [www-jime.open.ac.uk/2004/1].
[10] Totten, S., Sills, T., Digby, A., & Russ, P. (1991). Cooperative learning: A guide to research. New York: Garland.
[11] Bumpous D. "Constructivism and E-learning Applications" ELRN 772 - September 17, 2003.
[12] Gallagher, S. A. Problem-based learning: Where did it come from, what does it do, and where is it going? Journal for the Education of the Gifted, 20, 332-362 (1997).
[13] Hooper, Cooperative learning and computer-based instruction, in Educational Technology Research and Development, vol. 40, n. 2 (1992).
[14] Jonassen, D. H. Objectivism versus constructivism: do we need a new philosophical paradigm? Journal of Educational Research, 39 (3), 5-14 (1991).
[15] Kolb. D. A. and Fry, R. (1975) 'Toward an applied theory of experiential learning;, in C. Cooper (ed.) Theories of Group Process, London: John Wiley.
[16] Miao, Haake; Supporting Problem Based Learning by a Collaborative Virtual Environment: A Cooperative Hypermedia Approach; Proceedings of the 34th Hawaii International Conference on System Sciences – 2001.
[17] Foster I. et. al.: The Open Grid Services Architecture. Version 1.0, January, 2005.
[18] Berners-Lee T., Hendler J. and Lassila O.: The Semantic Web, Scientific American, May 2001.
[19] http://www.imsglobal.org/learningdesign/index.cfm
[20] http://www.w3.org/TR/ws-arch/
[21] Fox G.: Education and Grid Services. Talk prepared for Discussion Meeting on Education and Outreach: Developing a National Initiative (April 8, 2004, Arlington, VA), available at http://grids.ucs.indiana.edu/ptliupages/presentations/edgridapril04.ppt
[22] Final report of FP7 exploratory workshop Grid-enabled knowledge organisations and collaborative working environments, Sept. 2004, available at http://www.cordis.lu/ist/grids/pub-report.htm
[23] Stutt A. and Motta E.: Semantic Learning Webs. Journal of Interactive Media in Education. March, 2004.
[24] http://www.ggf.org/
[25] Beetham H.: JISC e-learning and Pedagogy Programme "Review: developing e-Learning Models for the JISC Practitioner Communities" Version 2.1 Helen Beetham, February 2004.
[26] Johnson, W.L.: Pedagogical agents. Proc. of ICCE '98, the Sixth Intern. Conference on Computers in Education, Beijing, China: 14–17 October.
[27] Next Generation Grids 2 Requirements and Options for European Grids Research 2005-2010 and Beyond. Expert Group Report, July 2004.
[28] IMS Global Learning Consortium, IMS Learning Design v1.0 Final Specification, http://www.imsglobal.org/learningdesign/index.cfm, 2003.
[29] Blinco K., Mason J., McLean N and Wilson S.: Trends and Issues in E-learning Infrastructure Development. A White Paper for alt-i-lab 2004 Prepared on behalf of DEST (Australia) and JISC-CETIS (UK), July, 2004.
[30] Foster I., Kesselman C. and Tuecke S.: The Anatomy of the Grid: Enabling Scalable Virtual Organizations. Intern. Journal of Supercomputer Applications, vol. 15, 2001.
[31] Gaeta A., Gaeta M., Ritrovato P. and Orciuoli F.: Enabling Technologies for future learning scenarios: The Semantic Grid for Human Learning. In the proceeding of the Second International Workshop on Collaborative and Learning Applications of Grid Technology and Grid Education CLAG + Grid.edu 2005. To be held in conjunction with the IEEE International Symposium on Cluster Computing and the Grid (CCGrid 2005) May 9 - 12, 2005, Cardiff, United Kingdom.
[32] Foster I, Frey J., Tuecke S. et al.: The WS-Resource Framework, 2004.
[33] http://www.omii.ac.uk/
[34] De Roure D., Fox G., Hey t. et al.: Web Service Grids: An Evolutionary Approach. 2004.
[35] http://www.oasis-open.org/committees/tc_home.php?wgabbrev=wsrf

Part B

Content-Centered Services

Towards the Learning Grid
P. Ritrovato et al. (Eds.)
IOS Press, 2005

Case study of virtual organization learning and knowledge testing environments

Kazys BANIULIS, Bronius TAMULYNAS, Nerijus AUKSTAKALNIS
Computer Networking Dept., Kaunas University of Technology (KTU), Assoc. prof., Rokishkio st. 7-1, 44139 Kaunas, Lithuania, e-mail: kazysba@pit.ktu.lt
Computer Networking Dept., KTU, Vytenu 65, 47482 Kaunas, Lithuania, Assoc. prof., e-mail: bronius@pit.ktu.lt
Computer Networking Dept., KTU, e-mail: nerijus.aukstakalnis@ktu.lt

Abstract. The proposed web-based knowledge assessment is based on flexible educational model and allows to implement adaptive control of learning process as well as to implement knowledge testing environment according to the requirements of student's knowledge level, his personal abilities and subject learning history. The learner knowledge model can be constructed as a subgraph of the global knowledge domain graph. The paper presents the architecture of student self-evaluation and on-line assessment system TestTool. The system is explored as an assessment engine capable to support and improve the individualized intelligent self-instructional mode of learning, grounded on the Grid distributed service architecture.

Keywords. Learning environment, knowledge testing, domain of knowledge, learning objects, data structures, Grid service architecture.

Introduction

In order to promote an effective learning process it is necessary to individuate a suitable technological infrastructure able to support such process allowing each learner to use in a transparent and shared manner all the resources already existing on-line. In the innovative vision the learning process within a learning environment can be effective only using an approach which takes into account some fundamental characteristics of learning activity and learning within a contextualized environment [1, 2].

Another fundamental and innovative aspect is the possibility of personalizing the learning process with respect to the needs of each learner. Many recent studies stress the importance of the particular learning style of each student in order to foster better learning results, so we will investigate strategies and methods to determine first the learning style preferred by the student, then, on this basis, suitable methodologies which allow performing a personalized educational process, related to the specific characteristics of the learner. So, auto adaptive systems can be defined as the capability and the intelligence of learning environments which can be increased by using suitable and innovative domain of knowledge and knowledge state of learner [1, 2 and 3].

The innovative research on the Grid goes in this direction and the Grid, at the moment, seems to be the technological infrastructure that fits such requirements best. We are trying to realize this conception by using TestTool (TT) knowledge testing environment [4, 5 and 6].

1. Virtuality of Learning Environments

When the learner enters the simulated environment, he finds himself in some initial state, and his objective is to move to some final (solution) state by performing appropriate actions, operations and moves. From the cognitive perspective, when the learner tackles a new problem, he uses a number of cognitive strategies that involve inductive and deductive reasoning, learning by trials and errors and insight. The user performs a sequence of (either mental or concrete) operations that allow him to move from one state to another until the final (solution) state of the problem is reached. So, in the simplest terms this principle may be defined as mapping from the knowledge state of a student to the domain of knowledge space of the problem [1].

Domain of knowledge is a collection of items (e.g., problems, questions, exercises, examples, and other learning objects (LO)) in a given field of knowledge. *The knowledge state of a learner* is the set of all items this student actually masters. In the domain of knowledge the items are linked by surmise relation, which allows identifying the prerequisites for each item. This relation is a partial order for representing implication relations among items in a given domain of knowledge. The knowledge state of the learner is mapped into a latent skill state, and the mapping itself is called skills map. The knowledge space is just a model of the cognitive organization of some learning material. As such, to become a valid representation with respect to some existing population of learners, it has to be tested empirically. The learner knowledge model [2, 3] can be constructed as a subgraph of the global knowledge domain graph. Such knowledge representation model belongs to a most general theory concerning multi-graphs. By decomposing information into atomic units and finding the connections among the units themselves: motivational or historical type, difficulty degrees the domain knowledge model can be based on graph paradigm. The structure, therefore, consists of both the information units and their links.

Such way of organization training environments enables tracking the improvements of the user along the whole training process. This implies a dynamic adaptation of the system to the user's skills and performance (personalization) so that his motivation and mental activity remains at a rational level during the whole training session [8]. The mechanism at the basis of this adaptation is performance and skill assessment and monitoring. The skill is the capability to perform a given sequence of operations in a purposeful way and the meta-skill is ability to combine such sequences. Such considerations suggest that the tool sharing among all the users is the key element to strengthen the effectiveness of the learning process in the situated learning framework. So all the learners, everywhere and at any time, are provided with the same equipment to know and be able actively take part in the common knowledge building.

Finally, it is important for the students to use particular resources which, due to their specific character, can be present only on remote systems. In this case the learner can invoke any application from a remote system, use the system best suited for executing that particular application, access data securely and consistently from remote sites, exploit multiple systems to complete complex tasks in an economical manner, or use multiple systems to solve large problems that exceed the capacity of a single one.

2. Case Study: Student and Data Structure Course Models

Case study is based on the use of graphical assessment system TestTool [5] in the Data structure study module.

Creation of the course model. Course model can be defined as a collection of items in a given field of knowledge. Course structure is created according to learner's needs, aims and objectives. Hierarchical principle is used to organize the learning context, i.e. the context can be enumerated or rendered as a graph by relational topics which are studied in any order. Various ways of analysis and graphical rendering are used to aggregate structure of the course. One of the many possible forms is the concept map. It should begin with the name of the key topic or concept and link it to a number of related concepts. Then, the names of concepts related to these topics as well, should be connected. A different technique for content presentation is used: hierarchical lists, chronological lists, flow charts, algorithmic schemes, content matrices, causal schemes, etc.

Case study. Teachers-experts define the three levels of knowledge (basic, intermediate and expert) the learners should be familiar with. These definitions are used to develop a course model and to form student model subsets. Creating models [2, 7] criteria of educational goals according to Bloom's taxonomy are used. Course model creation is simple:

- ✓ teacher-expert creates learning objects and describes their attributes;
- ✓ teacher-expert defines relations between one LO and several others LOs possessing some specific relationships;
- ✓ several of different relationships between two LO can existed;
- ✓ the possible relationships are defined initially or added/modified later.

According to existing e-learning standards attributes and relationships (LO metadata) are described in XML. In the same way, TestTool test-exercises (LO data) are described.

The main arguments for TestTool basis to realize the first domain of knowledge are:

- ✓ the environment is authorized and is easy modified according to the needs;
- ✓ XML files are convenient for LO presentation by adding several new features.

The domain of knowledge as data structure course and student models, as a subset of Course model are shown in Figure 1 [9]. Student model is defined according to various criteria subsets of Course Semantic Network. Graph analysis methods take into account learner possibilities and his learning progress.

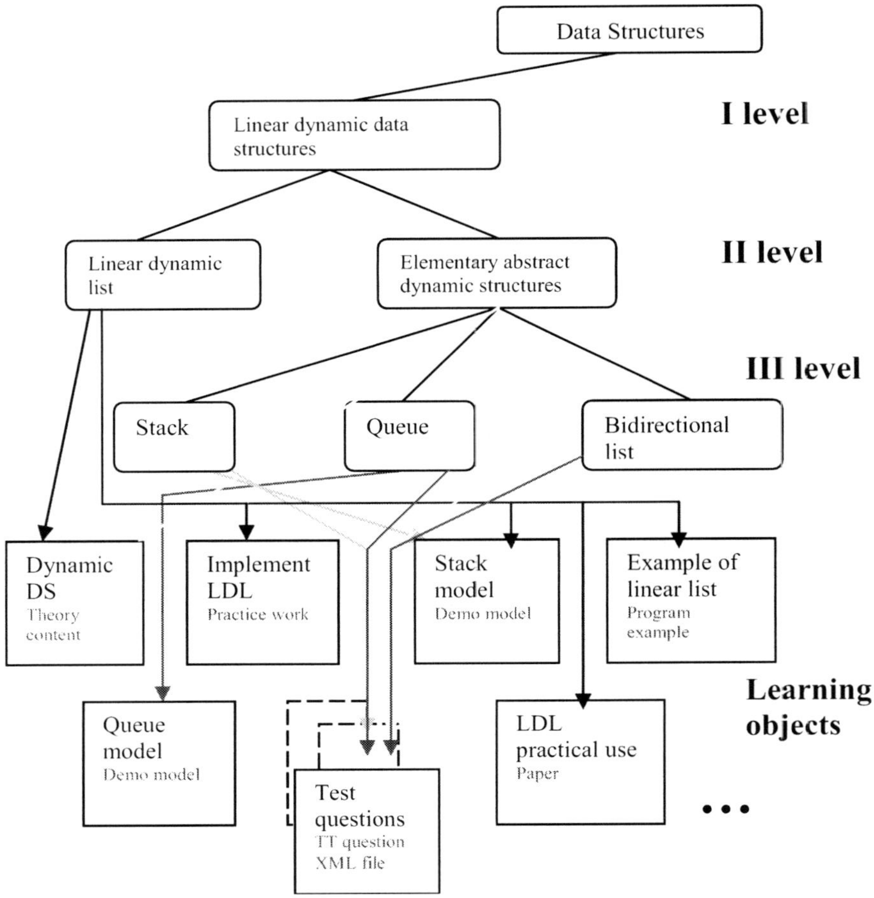

Figure 1. The Course Semantic Network

The process of knowledge acquisition according to common didactical principles is organized in two levels. Student masters only a part of knowledge $\mathbf{X} \subseteq \mathbf{Q}$ (**Q** – knowledge domain) [10] at a time by manipulating the tools for knowledge acquisition. In order to supply required content to the user the learning objects in the LO repository are divided according to common didactical principles, and multiple correspondence between sets **Q** and **P** is implemented by specific search algorithms, where **P** – known didactical ways for knowledge acquisition. The same correspondence is used to define tools and services (exercise, test, practice work and etc.) for every LO from the set **Q**. Evaluation scale will show knowledge of student by implementing the link f as realization of $f(Q) \subseteq \mathbf{X}$. This link is used as a tool for semantic splitting for the set of learning objects. Semantic splitting tool is realized via meta description of LO.

3. Grid Service Architecture and Intelligent Learning

Naturally, questions: Should the conventional web-based technologies be directly transferred onto the Grid, or should there be a more complex domain and more complex architecture, must be answered. Evidently, there is an abundance of e-learning practical and pilot cases which have been realized with conventional web-based technologies and there are no obvious reasons to transfer them directly onto the Grid. Learning subjects typical adjoined and tied to science and research, involve into more complex domains and more complex e-learning application architectures, where Grid distributed service oriented architecture prevails.

Based on the integrity and interoperability of distributed learning object systems, experimental TestTool version for Grid was implemented [6]. The following steps to transform the existing TestTool system to GridTT version are needed:

1. TestTool system based on Web services is created as a distributed system. TestTool system consists of three large subsystems of services: Client, LO Repository closely linked with LO Registry, Learner Repository. Client is a general subsystem which realizes interfaces for TT users. LO repository is the service for storage, registration and retrieval of LOs. Learners' repository is a learners' database containing individual student data records and testing results. The typical service sequence for learner is:
   - Student logs in through Learner Repository and chooses an eligible test from the list;
   - LO Registry is searched for the chosen test, LO Repository address and LO identification data are retrieved;
   - Learner Repository calls LO Factory and creates instant aggregated questions;
   - A learner communicates with the visualized LO to answer the questions;
   - LO sends the answers and the evaluations to the Learner Repository.
2. To fulfil knowledge domain requirements (Figure 2) Course model and Learner model solutions are performed.

There are a lot of additional tools in the existing integrated systems. Creation of Web service based e-learning system produce new challenges. Due to more complex architecture, course administration becomes more complicated too. Administrator has to aggregate the course from learning objects distributed in various places. Course aggregation becomes complicated to inexperienced user and possibility is high that something will be missed or mistakes will be made. One of the main goals of the distributed system (learning Grid) is to create and improve services to increase the level of automation and users utility.

High level visualization for course administration reduces interest in the structure of the course itself and administrator has to specify LO and relations between them. Graphical course aggregation tool or course visualization using tree structures in HTML file are any useful. LO is then located by the system of queries according to the attributes administrator has specified.

The installation additional software for the system to work irritates users when they have to do these themselves. To solve such problem technologies supporting standard operating system should be used. Currently, the new more intelligent version of TT based on Web services is being created. Content of LO created using earlier version of TT Author program are reusable in the new version. Reusability is achieved by using XML converter in order to transfer questions and tests into new format. The XML converter can be used to implement standardization any learning objects as well.

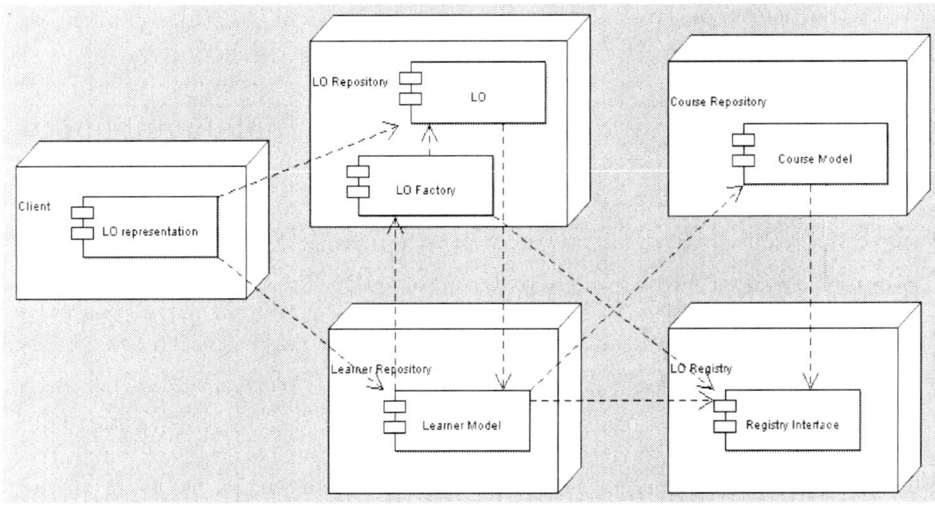

Figure 2. Conceptual learning environment using Grid service architecture

4. Meta Description of Learning Objects

Semantic network of Course model in the new version of TT is used. As learning objects are used to produce Course model thus metadata of LO is defined and its attributes are described according to the existing e-learning standards (IMS Meta-data and IEEE LOM) [11]. All standard metadata elements of LO are divided into 9 groups. At the moment most acceptable are:

1. *General* – Information Groups describing learning object as a whole;
2. *Educational* – educational or pedagogic features of the learning object;
3. *Relation* – features of the resource in relationship with other learning objects.

Most important elements in *General* group are: *Identifier* – globally unique label for learning object; *Title* – name of the learning object; *Language* – language of the learning object (or Language without Country sub code - it implies intended language of the target audience. "None" is also acceptable); *Description* – describes content of the learning object; *Keyword* – contains keyword description of the resource; *Structure* – underlying organizational structure of the resource; *Aggregation level* - the functional size of the resource. The level is from 1 to 4. Level 1 signifies the lowest level of aggregation, e.g. raw media data or fragments. Level 2 refers to a collection of atoms, e.g. an HTML document with some embedded pictures or lessons. Level 3 indicates a collection of level 1 resource, e.g. a 'web' of HTML documents, with an index page that links the pages together or a unit. Finally, level 4 refers to the highest level of granularity, e.g. a course.

Elements in *Educational* group: *Interactivity type* - type of interactivity supported by the learning object; *Learning resource type* – specific or most dominant kind of resource; *Interactivity level* – level of interactivity between the end user and the learning object; *Difficulty* – difficulty to work through the learning object for the typical target audience; *Typical learning time* – approximate or typical time it takes to work with the resource.

Elements in *Relation* group: *Kind* – nature of the relationship between the resource being described and the one identified by Resource. Types according to Dublin Core:

ispartof, haspart, isversionof, hasversion, isformatof, hasformat, referentes, isreferencedby, isbasedon, isbasisfor, requires, isrequiredby;

An example of main elements in Metadata description of learning objects in Data structure course:

Structure*. Possible values: Aggregate, Linear.*

Learning Resource type*: TestTool question XML file, practice work, paper, theory content, demo model, program example.*

Keywords*:*

Type of learning content: content, algorithm, programming.

Programming language: Java, C++, Pascal

Difficulty*: minimal, intermediate, expert.*

Relation Kind*:*

ispartof, haspart example: Stack – loop;

isbasedon, isbasisfor example: Content – Algorithm; Algorithm – Program.

Example of LO description in XML:

```
<variant>
    <lom>
            <general>
                    <Title>Stack definition</Title>
                    <Language>en</Language>
                    <Description>This question is used to evaluate what learner
                    knows about stack definition. Does he understand how stack
                    works.</Description>
                    <Keyword>Stack</Keyword>
                    <Keyword>Stack definition</Keyword>
                    <Structure>collection</Structure>
                    <Aggregationlevel>1</Aggregationlevel>
            </general>
            <Educational>
                    <Interactivitylevel>Active</Interactivitylevel>
                    <Difficulty>minimal</Difficulty>
                    <Typicallearningtime>00:20:00</Typicallearningtime>
            </Educational>
            <Relation>
                    <Kind>isbasedon</Kind>
                    <Resource>Elementary abstract dynamic structures, Data
                     Structures course</Resource>
            </Relation>
    </lom>
    <default>
<TLabel id="1" movable="false" editable="false" x="0" y="0"
background="16777215" foreground="0" opaque="false" border="default">
            <text>Which statement defines Stack?</text>
            </TLabel>
            <TRadioGroup id="3" movable="false" selectable="true" x="0"
            y="53" background="16777215" foreground="0" opaque="false"
            border="default">
                    <font size="10" style="bold"/>
                    <line id="1">Defines principle: first in, first out.</line>
```

```
                <line id="2">It's DS, when accessible only the latest
                 element.</line>
                <line id="3">It's DS, where elements are added and deleted
                no matter from which end.</line>
            </TRadioGroup>
    </default>
    <answer>
            <TRadioGroup id="3" selectable="true" x="0" y="53">
                <line id="2"/>
            </TRadioGroup>
    </answer>
</variant>
```

5. Conclusions and Discussions

Our research consists of two parts: conceptualization of virtual organization of learning and knowledge testing environments and development of web-services based knowledge assessment TestTool version. In the next stage there was created experimental service-oriented TestTool version which implements Grid environment based on *Globus toolkit* [12]. Globus tools are used for accumulation of distributed resources into one integrated system, but not for distribution of data and tasks to available computing resources. Such implementation has higher security level and usability of distributed learning resources. All web services embedded in TT Grid aware implementation are corresponding to the Grid requirements (actualizing concrete interfaces and using particular protocols of communication). While student is working with test, several of temporary LO Grid services are created and combined. These services are the most dynamical part of TestTool. When test is composed, selection of services is performed according to meantime accessible LO services (selection is performed using LO registry). All needed services according to metadata may be created on closer or less laden server. That's similar to reuse software components: at the runtime, when test execution or course content is needed. We suppose that all components already are created.

It is needed to split parts which are not closely relative in order to make TT as Grid oriented implementation in distributed E-LeGI infrastructure with multiple LO repositories. Also there should be described interfaces for communication between these parts and later suitable interfaces should be implemented using Globus distributed systems creation possibilities.

References

[1] N.Capuano, A.Gaeta, G.Laria, F.Orciuoli, P.Ritrovato, How to use technology for building next generation learning environments, Proc. of the 2-th International LeGE-WG Workshop: Towards a European Learning Grid Infrastructure, Paris, France, 2003.

[2] K. Baniulis, B. Tamulynas, Intelligent support of web-based knowledge assessment system, IEEE International Conference on Advanced Learning Technologies Proceedings, Kazan, Tatarstan, Russia, IEEE Learning Technology, 9-12 September 2002, 551-552.

[3] K. Baniulis, B. Tamulynas, Flexible Learning in an Intelligent Tutoring Environment, New Media and Telematic Technologies for Education in Eastern European Countries, Twente University Press (1997), 395-409.

[4] V. Reklaitis, K. Baniulis, T. Okamoto, Shaping e_Learning applications for a service oriented Grid. 2nd International LeGE-WG Workshop on e-Learning and Grid Technologies: A Fundamental Challenge for Europe, Paris, France. 3rd & 4th March 2003.
[5] K. Baniulis, V. Reklaitis, TestTool: Web-based Testing, Assessment, Learning, Informatics in Education, ISSN 1648-5831, 1, Vilnius, Institute of Mathematics and Informatics (2002), 17-30.
[6] V. Reklaitis, K. Baniulis, G. Paulikas, Implementation of Assessment Web-service for TestTool, Proc. of the International Conference "Advanced learning technologies and applications (ALTA'03)', Kaunas, Lithuania (2003), 39-40.
[7] L. Anderson, D. Krathwohl, A Taxonomy for Learning, Teaching and Assessing: A Revision of Bloom's Taxonomy of Educational Objectives, Longman, New York, 2001.
[8] P. Brusilovsky, H. Nijhawan, A Framework for Adaptive E-Learning Based on Distributed Re-usable Learning Activities, Proc. of World Conference on E-Learning, E-Learn 2002, Montreal, Canada, 2002.
[9] N. Aukstakalnis, Virtual learning environment development technologies on Grid network, Information Technologies 2004, Kaunas, Lithuania (2004), 181-185.
[10] L. Stefanutti, D. Albert, C. Hockemeyer, Derivation of Knowledge structures for distributed learning objects, Proc. of the 3-rd International LeGE-WG Workshop: Grid Infrastructure to support future technology enhanced learning, Berlin, Germany, 2003.
[11] IEEE LOM. (2002) Draft Standard for Learning Object Metadata, http://ltsc.ieee.org/wg12/files/LOM_1484_12_1_v1_Final_Draft.pdf.
[12] Globus Toolkit 3.2 Documentation, http://www-unix.globus.org/toolkit/docs/3.2/index.html.

Towards the Learning Grid
P. Ritrovato et al. (Eds.)
IOS Press, 2005

SCORM and the Learning Grid

Fred NEUMANN, Rüdiger GEYS
FIM-NeuesLernen, Friedrich-Alexander-Universität Erlangen-Nürnberg, Germany

Abstract. The Sharable Content Object Reference Model (SCORM) is a profile of several eLearning specifications to ensure the reusability and interoperability of eLearning content in web based Learning Management Systems (LMSs). Learning Grids - learning environments built on the technology of Grid services - are a promising new approach to enhance quality of eLearning by overcoming the page oriented structure of the web. This paper investigates how SCORM can be used in conjunction with Learning Grids. After an introduction to the relevant aspects of SCORM two major scenarios are discussed: the use of Grid enhanced content in a SCORM compliant LMS and the use of SCORM content in the context of a Learning Grid.

Keywords. eLearning Standards, ADL SCORM, Learning Grid

Motivation

Compared with the high aims of a Learning Grid infrastructure, current web based learning management systems (LMSs) like WebCT or Blackboard are sometimes described as monolithic, server-centric and content delivery oriented. However, we should not underestimate the efforts and achievements of many institutions to formulate an eLearning strategy, to select and establish an LMS, to customize and adapt it and to train their authors, tutors and lecturers in using it.

In the last years we saw a growing common sense on the functionalities and concepts of web based eLearning. This is accompanied by the development of standards and their increased acceptance by the vendors of authoring tools and learning management systems. Currently the specifications with the highest impact are:

- IEEE LOM for metadata describing learning objects (LOs), enabling the search for content,
- IMS Content Packaging to exchange LOs between authoring tools and learning environments,
- AICC for the run-time communication between the content and the learning environment,
- SCORM as a reference model to integrate the specifications above.

For a certain period it seemed that especially the content packaging and run time environment are more adopted in commercial eLearning applications for the use of commodity content modules available on the market. But meanwhile these specifications became also relevant in the academic scene, often after years of experiments with internally developed applications and contents using proprietary formats.

As a consequence, tools with scientific origin are modified to support eLearning standards. For example ILIAS, an open source LMS popular at German universities, is now being extended to handle SCORM compliant content. This is a remarkable step, because light-weight, open source solutions are especially important for smaller, non profit organisation that try to apply eLearning for new target groups and cannot afford expensive commercial servers that support the current eLearning standards.

Grid computing is a promising new technological paradigm but the concepts for a Learning Grid are at the very beginning. To get a further understanding of their potential they may be developed in an idealistic way and evaluated in dedicated test beds. But in the mean time the development of conventional web based eLearning solutions and standards will continue and the investments will increase. Therefore it is essential for the success and acceptance of a Learning Grid development to provide a smooth migration path from current web based to Grid based solutions. This can be accomplished by taking into account the current exchange and interoperability standards in the eLearning domain to enable:

- the use of Grid services in a wide range of web based LMSs,
- the use of existing standard compliant content in a Learning Grid.

In this paper we will look at SCORM [1] for that purpose, as it provides an integrated view on a set of standards and specifications that focus on single aspects.

1. SCORM Overview

In 1997 the US Department of Defense (DoD) launched the Advanced Distributed Learning (ADL) Initiative as a collaboration between government, industry and academia to specify a learning environment that permits the interoperability of learning tools and course content. ADLs major outcome is the Sharable Content Object Reference Model (SCORM), a "collection of specifications adapted from multiple sources to provide a comprehensive suite of e-learning capabilities that enable interoperability, accessibility and reusability of web-based learning content." (www.adlnet.org).

Table 1. Standard compliance of products (counted 3/2004).

Cetis standards-compliant products directory (www.cetis.ac.uk)	19 products supporting IMS Metadata 18 products supporting IMS Content Packaging 16 products supporting AICC 25 products supporting SCORM
ADL (www.adlnet.org)	40 products SCORM certified 96 vendors listed as SCORM adopters
AICC (www.aicc.org)	16 vendors certified 21 vendors self-checked
IMS (www.imsglobal.org)	40 products in product directory (with conformance information given by vendors)

SCORM is an application profile for the use of existing standards and not a specification or standard itself. The underlying specifications are slightly amended to be suitable for the DoD's education and training needs. However, the interoperability promoted by ADL became attractive to the commercial e-learning industry in general. Table 1 gives a rough impression of the current situation. It is remarkable that more software vendors are certified or declare themselves as compliant to SCORM then to its major underlying specifications.

In January 2004 ADL released SCORM 2004, formerly referred to as SCORM Version 1.3. The major change is the introduction of the IMS Simple Sequencing specification. Other changes reflect the evolution of some specifications to IEEE standards or drafts:

- IEEE Learning Object Metadata (LOM)
- IEEE Draft XML binding for LOM
- IEEE ECMAScript API Interface for Content to Runtime Services Communication
- IEEE Data Model For Content Object Communication
- IMS Content Packaging
- IMS Simple Sequencing

SCORM concentrates on the interfaces between content and an LMS and does not specify the internal structure or features of an LMS. It is concerned with the functionalities to deliver, track, report and manages learning content, learner progress and learner interactions. For this purpose it defines the basic infrastructure to use content objects but not the context in which they are used. It is often stated that SCORM is best used in web-based training for individual learners with a self-paced and self-directed approach. But SCORM claims to be pedagogically neutral and may be used in any scenario, with or without the additional use of collaborative tools.

The reference model is divided into three parts ("Books") to which we will have a further look in the next sections: the Content Aggregation Model (CAM), the Run-Time Environment (RTE) and the Sequencing and Navigation (SN) Book. SCORM defines both, requirements for an LMS and for the content. Especially in the RTE and the new SN model the minimum requirements are very much higher for an LMS to achieve than for the content.

1.1. CAM: Content Aggregation Model

The CAM defines how instructional components are described by metadata and how they are organized and packaged. A content package includes all needed physical files and an xml based file named imsmanifest.xml describing the content and its structure. The manifest is composed of the following sections:

- *Meta-data* describing the content package as a whole.
- *Organisations* describing the content structure. Multiple organisations are possible, each defining a hierarchical tree structure, optional context-specific meta data and optional definitions of sequencing and navigation behaviour.
- *Resources* defining the bundled learning resources.
- Optional *(sub)Manifest(s)* describing logically nested units of instruction.

SCORM defines two types of resources: Assets and Sharable Content Objects (SCOs). An Asset is a learning content in its most basic form, e.g. a HTML page, a picture or a video. It does not communicate with the LMS and is intended to be *completed* as soon as it is started. In contrast, an SCO can be composed of Assets. It communicates during run-time with the LMS and must not provide direct links to other SCOs, so that the possibility of repackaging is ensured.

1.2. RTE: Run-Time Environment

If we look for the applicability of SCORM in a Learning Grid, then the most interesting part is the run-time environment which specifies how an SCO is launched and how it communicates with the LMS. This section introduces the main RTE characteristics that will be discussed for a combination with Grid services later. Figure 1 shows the RTE architecture.

The LMS uses the URL of an SCO defined in the manifest to launch the SCO by HTTP in the client's web browser, either in a child window or a child frame of the LMS window. Each SCO must be able to be launched this way. After that the SCO has to search in the DOM hierarchy of its window parents for an API object provided by a run-time service of the LMS that resides in the browser. SCORM does not specify how the run-time service is implemented and how it communicates with the LMS. All it defines are the API functions, how the API is locally found and that it must be called by JavaScript.

Every communication is initiated by the SCO. The SCO is responsible for starting the communication with an Initialize() and to end it with a Terminate() before it is removed from the browser. Between these calls it is able to read and write run-time data with GetValue() and SetValue(). Written data may be cached in the client by the run-time service. The SCO cannot check whether data is cached but it may use Commit() to force the cached data being written back to the LMS. The remaining functions defined by the API are for error handling and diagnostic purposes.

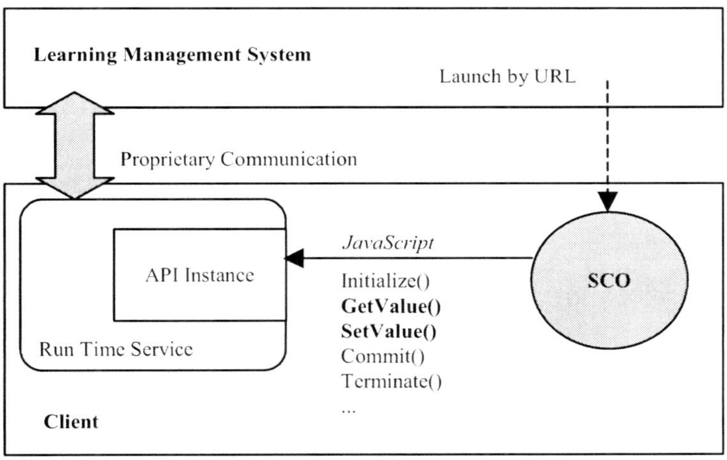

Figure 1. SCORM Run-Time Environment.

The main interaction between SCO and LMS is done by exchange of run-time data according to a data model based on the IEEE draft standard with added requirements for the run-time behaviour. All data model elements are optional to an SCO but the LMS must provide them. Their initial values may be defined in the content package, by a learner registration process or by learner profiling requirements.

The data model elements have different purposes. Some are used to track status, scores and objectives of an SCO, some provide learner specific data and others have impact on the sequencing behaviour of SCOs. The run-time data is initialised at the beginning of a *learning attempt* which may span one or more learning sessions and can be suspended while keeping the actual values stored. Additionally a content package may define that the SCOs run-time data must be kept persistent over several attempts.

1.3. SN: Sequencing and Navigation

SCORM 2004 introduces the Sequencing and Navigation (SN) Book by applying the IMS Simple Sequencing specification to define how content objects may be sequenced through learner-initiated or system-initiated navigation events. For this purpose an organisation within a content package is derived into an *activity tree* for a learner. The leaf activities of that tree have content objects associated and the sequence of launched content objects builds an actual *learning experience*. The progression through learning activities may be sequential, non-sequential, user-directed or adaptive. It follows sequencing rules defined in the activity tree and takes the current RTE data into account.

IMS Simple Sequencing 1.0 is a rather complex specification and the amount of changes done by ADL in its pseudo code indicates that there is still some flow in the specification process. Therefore it will take reasonable time until the whole SCORM 2004 will be implemented by a wide range of systems and in the mean time SCORM 1.2 will remain a state of the art that supports only a hierarchical content menu and a simple forward and backward navigation through the SCOs.

2. SCORM and Grid

Grid computing is a new technology for the flexible, secure and coordinated sharing of distributed resources and data. The Open Grid Services Architecture (OGSA) is built on web service technology and supports "transient services as named, managed entities with dynamic, managed lifetime" [2]. For eLearning this allows the creation of Learning Grids – learning environments built on OGSA-compliant software and services. Learning Grids promise to introduce a new quality of eLearning by:

- enabling collaborative learning with peer-to-peer communication,
- making computing-intensive visualisations or simulations available for the learners,
- giving access to real-world data and resources like virtual laboratories.

Do SCORM and a Learning Grid have much in common? Looking at the core aims of SCORM (accessibility, adaptability, interoperability and reusability); they seem partially similar with the aims of Grid technology. However, SCORM is focussed on the exchange and delivery of instructional content in web based LMSs, while Grid technology is concerned with sharing of any resources in a distributed environment.

First we have to clarify what a Learning Grid will look like compared to a web based LMS. Will it be an infrastructure hidden behind a "portal" with conventional web access or will the learner's device be an active resource on the Grid? Both architectures have their justifications depending on the target group of learners. In the first case the Grid functionality can be designed in any way, as long as the interaction with the user is done through HTML pages. But if a Learning Grid intends to overcome the page oriented design of the web then it must bring dynamic functionality to the learner's client. For best applicability this should be done in a transparent and system independent way, e.g. without the need for an extra installation. This requires an execution technology that is widely available in common browsers, which currently means to use Java applets.

Pankratius and Vossen propose an eLearning Grid architecture that consists of two major parts: an LMS that is internally based on web services and a core Grid middleware [3]. They also introduce the concept of a Grid-enabled learning object (GLOB) that includes conventional learning resources as well as an application layer for the use of Grid services. Figure 2 is a simplified illustration of their concept without showing the detailed internal services. At the initial login to the LMS the fabric layer of the Grid is delivered to the learners' device as a Java applet. The login service of the LMS is able to authentify the user and his device against the Grid and may also be trusted to create or delete Grid users. The LMS will request a TGT (ticket-granting-ticket) from the Grid middleware and deliver it to the client. When a GLOB is delivered to the client, it is able to use the fabric layer and the TGT initially provided by the LMS to further request session tickets and directly access the Grid services.

The proposed architecture describes a loose coupling between LMS and Grid middleware with little requirements for the LMS: the call of a few operations from a Grid login service and the delivery of a Grid enabling applet to the client at login time. Therefore it seems possible to enhance nearly every web based LMS this way, regardless of whether the LMS is already internally built on web services or not.

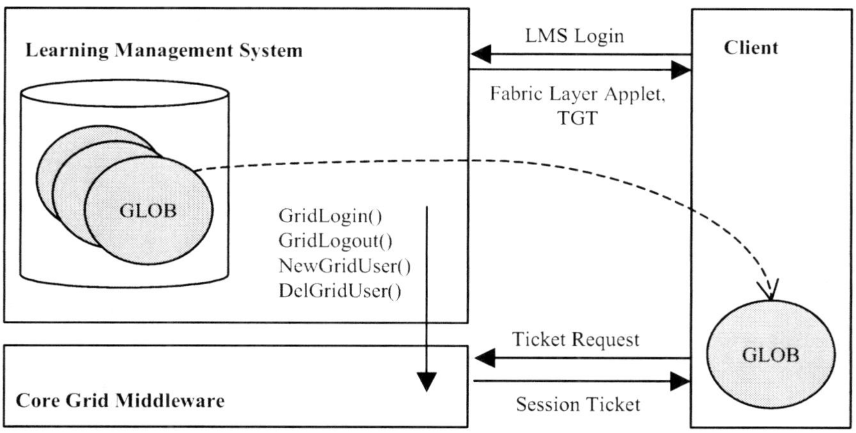

Figure 2. A proposed Learning Grid Architecture [5].

However, sometimes it will not be possible to introduce Grid support by extending an LMS, for example in the following scenarios:

- An eLearning content provider wants to offer Grid services in conjunction with his content. To not restrict possible customers he must support as many platforms as possible.
- A lecture chair wants to offer Grid based applications for a virtual course but has to use a campus-wide LMS that can't be modified.

There are many possible scenarios in which Grid services can be integrated into a learning content: database searches, exercises, simulations, virtual laboratories or visualisations. For that we could ask whether it would be possible to realize GLOBs as Grid enabled SCOs and to use them in an LMS without the need to modify it.

2.1. Grid enabled SCORM content

In the following we assume that the whole functionality needed to access the Grid is implemented by a Java applet ("Grid applet") and included in a SCORM compliant content package. Depending on the learning purpose the applet may implement the whole fabric layer of the Grid to include the learner's device as a resource on the Grid or it may be just a client to access the Grid via an ordinary web service. The most important aspect to clear is how to provide a single-sign-on from the LMS - that means how to authentify the LMS user for the desired service and how to transmit user related information between LMS and the Grid.

For this purpose we have to take a look back to what the SCORM run-time-environment specifies. The Grid applet must have access to the JavaScript API of SCORM for the exchange of data. The following data elements provided by the RTE are of special interest:

- launch_data is taken from the content package and is read-only
- learner_id is provided by the LMS and read-only
- learner_name is provided by the LMS and read-only
- interactions are used to store the results from interactive exercises
- suspend_data can be anything up to 4000 characters to be stored between sessions

Figure 3 shows a possible implementation. First the LMS launches the SCO containing the Grid applet and the normal initialisation process is done. Now the applet has to authentify with the Grid service. For this purpose it requests the launch_data from the LMS and extracts an included static key which is created by the vendor of the Learning Grid. The key is stored in the imsmanifest.xml of an SCO and may be set individually for an LMS or a course. Additionally the applet may determine its own origin with a getCodeBase() call. Due to JavaScript security restrictions in modern browsers the applet must come from the same domain as the API and so the code base helps to ensure that the applet is delivered from an LMS which is allowed to use the Grid functionality [4]. The learner is identified by ID and the Grid login is done with a combination of static key, code base and learner ID. The Grid may log this data e.g. for billing purposes. A session ticket provided by the Grid can be stored in the suspend_data element of the SCO's run-time-data.

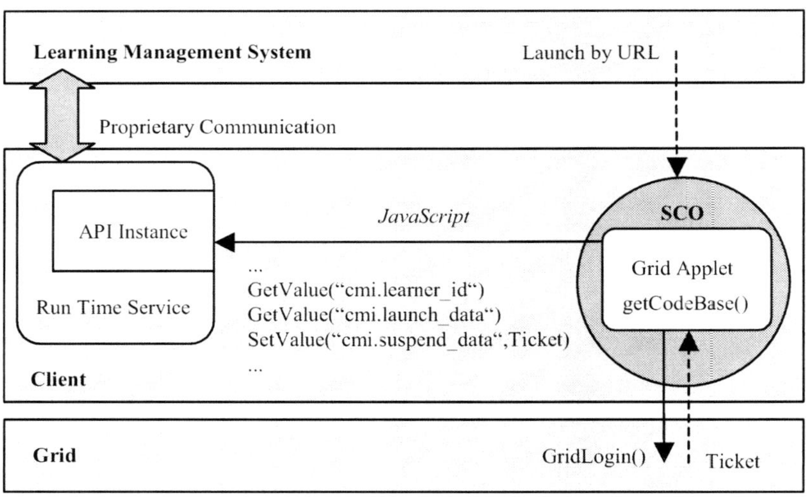

Figure 3. Using Grid enhanced SCOs.

How secure is the proposed implementation? This questions is about preventing the Grid from being misused (e.g. for stealing computing power) and preventing user accounts from being misused (e.g. for faking their activity). The communication between LMS and run-time-service is not specified and may have lower security than the Grid provides, e.g. it may not be encrypted. Security is then determined by the weakest part - the LMS.

Theoretically it is also possible to simulate an SCO session, extract the authentication from the LMS and to store and recompile the Grid applet. Then a "cracked" standalone applet can be created for the use of a Grid service with the ID of another user. However, this will mean a reasonable effort and will leave traces if both LMS and Grid service log their accesses, so we can assume a medium security level. The problem comes from the fact that the authentication is based on static information (key and learner_id) delivered from the LMS to the client. Solutions to overcome this weakness may be applicable in special scenarios:

- The LMS is able to create session-tickets and deliver them to the SCO, e.g. in an extended run-time data model element. However, this would require the inclusion of a Grid client on the LMS server and a modification of the LMS.
- In an Intranet the learners' device may already be a resource on the Grid. Then the Grid applet in the SCO can use the local host and user for an authentication.
- The learner has to manually authentify for the Grid at least once and receives a ticket that is stored in the suspend_data. Subsequent authentication may be necessary after time-out of the ticket.

A Grid enhanced SCO may be designed to support all scenarios with priority for the most advanced authentication method but a cascading fallback mechanism to the others.

Aside from security issues, a content oriented solution will not be appropriate for all purposes of Grid enhanced eLearning. A learner will work on content, but also use content-independent communication and collaboration facilities, e.g. for getting tutorial support or working in groups. A Grid solution for general supporting tools shouldn't be embedded in an SCO that is only accessible on a table of contents. SCORM can't be a help for this purpose and therefore the LMS has to be extended. An introduction of Grid support may follow the architecture described in [3] but with the Grid applets being directly embedded in the user interface of the LMS.

2.2. SCORM Content in Learning Grids

The obvious requirement for a SCORM compliant Learning Grid solution is to handle existing SCORM content, at least to import it as content packages and to launch and track the SCOs for the learner. The question is how this content can be seamlessly integrated in a highly collaborative, Grid-enabled environment. At present the reusability of SCOs prohibits a tight coupling of content with additional functionalities provided by an LMS like forums, conferences, or advanced tele-presence tools available in a Grid infrastructure. The IMS Simple Sequencing provides minimal hooks for the invocation of so called "Auxiliary Resources", however SCORM does not yet define their further behaviour and ADL recommends content developers and LMS vendors to use them with extreme care to ensure future interoperability [1] (SM-5-11). The other direction is of equal interest: how may content objects easily be referred by the learners as in their communication messages? SCORM requires that each SCO must be launched by its URL, but it may not be possible to simply copy it from the browser location into a message because it is hidden or includes user-specific parameters.

The conceptual relationship between content and collaboration is intensively addressed by the IMS Learning Design [5] which specifies an XML based language to describe complete learning scenarios including group work or collaborative learning. It formalizes the definition of actors and their roles in a learning scenario, its activities and the use of learning objects or services in an activity. IMS Learning Design is not included in SCORM and it is open whether it will be in the future. But a learning design may be integrated in a content package and SCOs may be used in a Learning Design. A Learning Grid designed to support both may enable pedagogically well defined collaborative learning with the use of widely available content. Learning Design is a conceptual model and does not define the technical implementation and the process of instantiating the activities. IMS provides a best practice guide with suggestions for developing a runtime environment but these are not normative. This gives freedom for the design of a service oriented Learning Grid architecture, especially in the decision which services should run locally on the learner's device or will be called remotely and whether the collaborative actions will behave in a peer-to-peer or server mediated manner.

On the other hand, if it is intended to include SCORM content in a Learning Grid, the architecture must take care of the requirements for a SCORM run-time environment. SCORM proposes that an LMS has a service based architecture, but it doesn't define anything of it, even not whether the services are real or just internal functionalities of a monolithic system. If we look at the run-time architecture in figure 1, a first step towards an integration of SCORM and Grid technology would be to specify the proprietary communication between LMS and the run-time service as a web or Grid service. The API functions defined by SCORM must be translated to service operations. An SCO should have the choice whether to use the JavaScript API or whether to directly communicate with the service, for example, if it is launched from a different content server. In this context the following statement from the SCORM specification is of special interest:

> *"There are ongoing research and development efforts investigating alternative methods (e.g., as a Web Service) for LMS vendors to provide SCOs access to the API Instance. (...) Future versions of SCORM may introduce other communication protocols that support the fundamental requirements defined by the IEEE standard." [1] (RTE-3-26)*

The current SCORM API service may be one of a set of services for content to LMS communication and we could imagine a suite of conformance levels with the SCORM API as the lowest common denominator and other services as extensions. Once the communication between LMS server and run-time service is specified, generic run-time services can be implemented as a bridge between service oriented LMSs and API oriented content. The JavaScript API may also wrap the extended services so that content developers can use them in a familiar way. This may be done by the introduction of new API functions or by extensions to the run-time data model, e.g. with information on user groups and shared data for collaborative work.

To give a practical example, one extension could be the support for collaborative annotations. The editing and storage of annotations would be implemented by the LMS but their appearance must be rendered by content specific functions. The content must be adaptive to enable or disable this feature depending on what conformance the LMS provides and it must be able to invoke the editing function. We could also imagine that the annotations may be extended with presence indicators showing whether the originator is currently online (or logged in to the LMS) and allowing to start a synchronous communication. Again, this information is provided by the LMS, but rendered in the content, if possible.

3. Conclusion and Discussions

Using Grid services in a SCORM compliant LMS may be possible without modification as long as the Grid functionality can be wrapped by learning object in a didactically reasonable way and as long as a medium security is acceptable. Otherwise the LMS has to be extended with Grid functionality. Using SCORM in a Learning Grid may not just mean to "simple implement it" but will lead to extensions of the run-time-environment defined by SCORM if a real integration of content and communication facilities is intended.

We see that many aspects need a further investigation and many issues are still open, both in the SCORM and the Grid world. However, the main open question is: how relevant will SCORM be in the future? Will it be the dominating model for content sharing at the time when a Learning Grid infrastructure is ready to use? Critic voices argue that SCORM is pedagogically poor while at the same time being too complex and too difficult to implement. How high is the value of having access to existing SCORM compliant content and how large will this pool be? Should a Learning Grid have its own reference model with a different set of supported specifications, e.g. with IMS Learning Design instead of Simple Sequencing? It would be a considerable effort to repeat the integration and profiling work already done by ADL.

A strategy may be not to rely on SCORM for the core architecture of a Learning Grid but to check for each concept how it harmonizes with SCORM content. In parallel, providing pluggable SCORM compliant, Grid-enhanced content packages and creating small and smart Learning Grid applications with guidelines on how to integrate them in any LMS will raise the attention of the eLearning world. This may create the "critical mass" for a broad acceptance of a Learning Grid architecture leading to its inclusion in the main standardisation processes in the eLearning domain.

References

[1] Advanced Distributed Learning (ADL). "Sharable Content Object Reference Model (SCORM®) 2004". Available at http://www.adlnet.org

[2] Foster, I. C. Kesselman, J. Nick, S. Tuecke. "The Physiology of the Grid: Open Grid Services Architecture for Distributed Systems Integration". Proc. 4th Global Grid Forum (GGF4) Workshop 2002. Available at http://www.globus.org/research/papers/ogsa.pdf

[3] Pankratius, V., G. Vossen. "Towards E-Learning Grids: Using Grid Computing in Electronic Learning". Proc. IEEE Workshop on Knowledge Grid and Grid Intelligence, Halifax, Canada, Oct 2003, pp. 4-15

[4] Advanced Distributed Learning (ADL). "Cross-Domain Scripting Issue". Paper, October 2003. Available at http://www.adlnet.org

[5] IMS Global Learning Consortium, Inc. "IMS Learning Design Version 1.0 Final Specification". Available at http://www.imsglobal.org/learningdesign

Towards the Learning Grid
P. Ritrovato et al. (Eds.)
IOS Press, 2005

Shaping e-Learning Applications for a Service-Oriented Grid

Vytautas REKLAITIS [a], Kazys BANIULIS [b], Toshio OKAMOTO [a]
[a] *Graduate School of Information Systems, University of Electro-Communications, Japan*
[b] *Computer Networks Department, Kaunas University of Technology, Lithuania*

Abstract. This paper discusses technical issues related to establishing e-learning services on a Grid. The XML based technology for implementing e-learning applications in web service form is analyzed from the standpoint of making an application Grid-aware. A special e-learning repository service is proposed as a technique for coordinated use of distributed e-learning resources through the access and invocation of web services.

Keywords. e-learning, web service, Grid technology.

Introduction

Network-based education and Grid technologies have until recently been two distinct areas, although e-learning is now increasingly addressing learning resources interoperability and various modes of interactions along with wide scale sharing and reuse. In fact, it is within these areas that Grid technology can contribute to the e-learning domain.

Actually, Grid technology including appropriate software tools is currently available, i.e., Open Grid Service Infrastructure (OGSI) specifications [1] identify mechanisms associated with Grid service creation, discovery, and management. One particular further down evolution of OGSI is the Web Service Resource Framework (WSRF) [2] that makes a distinction between the service and the stateful resources backing up that service.

There is a great deal of enthusiasm around Grid technology as it enables us to interconnect and interoperate diverse distributed resources and thereby provides services. Following well-known iterative and incremental methodology being used by software engineers, the e-earning community should also address technical issues and move actively into an e-learning Grid service design and implementation phase. The viability and applicability of technology for e-learning areas has to be proven by building instructionally meaningful and practically usable e-learning services, though simple enough at the beginning. Testbeds for large-scale coordination and deployment of distributed learning resources on a Grid could then be built further such that new innovative e-learning approaches are more likely to be realized.

1. Background

When considering learning services through coordinated use of learning resources distributed on a Grid, there arise many complex problems related to Grid technology.

Any service establishment on the Grid is a multi-faced problem that includes a wide range of problems ranging from policy issues related to legal usage of resources to communication protocols and programming interfaces aimed at access and invocation of a particular service. Looking at the taxonomy of Grid resource management, a service set-up includes a wide array of difficult tasks including the development of resource models, resource name space and store organization, resource discovery and dissemination [3].

Since web services are typically implemented using existing software components, here we assume the existence of a simple e-learning application and discuss how it can be implemented as an e-learning service on a Grid. The process used is progressively elaborated on by proposing a generic e-learning repository service that is designed to be responsible for e-learning services composition and management within a restricted Grid domain. OGSI and WSRF are taken as de facto standards for the Grid and also as the specification of techniques for configuring an extensible set of Grid services.

Our analysis and discussion is carried out by postulating a simplified and idealized e-learning application model. Let us suppose that the application consists of some portion of a learning material presentation, i.e., a few HTML pages followed by a problem-solving task or other kind of activity performed by learner. Both the Web content and activity can be logically considered as two cohesive but principally distinct learning objects that are built and described according to the IEEE-accredited Learning Object Metadata (LOM) data model standard [4].

From the perspective of the design of the application that is meant to be used on a Grid, the principal distinction is that Web pages are represented as passive content while the activity to be performed by the learner can be an interactive simulation program, assessment test, or any reality-based application [5] which is always represented in the form of an executable software component. The LOM standard fixes this distinction by describing the learning resource type and providing two interactivity types - expositive and active - under the 5th Educational category. From the standpoint of application software architecture, those two components may reside on different hosts. Moreover, the activity must be executed on the particular server on which the corresponding active learning object (LO) is stored, and to invoke it, the public interfaces must be provided that specify the functions and protocols that may be used to communicate with other components.

E-learning applications are in general significantly different from conventional computational ones focused on computing power and wide-scale resource sharing on computational Grids. In contrast, a great majority of current e-learning applications may leave high-performance computing as a secondary task such that it may appear, may be necessary in specific learning applications. Meaningful interactivity and collaboration are instead usually of greater importance for e-learning. The Greenfield Engineering Education Coalition reality-based case studies for manufacturing engineering education enhanced by Web-based simulations could be considered as learning examples adequate to e-learning Grid infrastructure [5, 6]. As such they could to be shaped as Web services driven by distributed learning objects.

2. From a Web Service to a Grid Service

Internet technology is becoming service oriented and grounded on messaging protocols and standards for XML interfaces for coordinated use of distributed resources. This approach destroys barriers between software development platforms and leads to a high level of interoperability. The basic concept and building block for Internet computing therefore becomes a Web service that in this context is viewed as a network-enabled entity providing some capability such as e-learning capability. More specifically, Web service is a software component that supports interoperable machine-to-machine interaction and has a network-addressable interface described in a machine-processible format (WSDL). Services interact in a manner prescribed by its description using Simple Object Access Protocol (SOAP) messages, typically conveyed using HTTP with an XML serialization in conjunction with other Web-related standards [7]. This definition, as an alternative to object-oriented middleware-based services [8], focuses on the description in XML format language and making use of XML binding for interprocess communication between network entities.

The core of Web service technology is the Web Service Description Language (WSDL) [9], being an XML-based language containing elements to completely define Web services. Service description in WSDL is an XML document that (i) describes SOAP message formats for communication between network resources involved in the service provision, (ii) specifies the interface to which messages are sent, and (iii) describes conventions for mapping the content of the message into and out of the software components implementing the service.

Distributed applications of Web services are centered on the design of service description using WSDL. Similar to other software analysis and design cases, there are in general two methods for creating Web service descriptions: (1) Bottom-up - takes a service implementation class, i.e., the existing application software component, and uses a conventional Web-service development toolkit to generate the appropriate WSDL automatically, and (2) Top-down - initially works out the high level design for the service by modelling client and server interrelationships, manually describing in WSDL service interfaces, messages, port types, and access protocols. The bottom-up approach is considered more effective when services are simply implemented by wrapping a readily available software product into a Web service interface. In contrast, the top-down approach initially assumes service architecture design in WSDL, then implementation of a new or adoption of existing software components. Of particular interest, the latest IMS Learning Design Best Practice and Implementation Guide suggests an identical approach in which the analysis and modelling leads to a Learning Design specification in XML, which in turn forms the basis for the development of the actual content resources for the given design [10].

Web services are typically implemented today using existing application software components. E-learning Web services can also be built using active learning objects as software components [11]. Although it somewhat doubtful whether the learning paradigm shift from a knowledge transfer model to a learner-centered learning will occur along with the invasion of Web services technology into the e-learning domain by taking such a straightforward approach. This is primarily because a service provided by software radically differs from software products [12]. Therefore, e-learning service must be modeled and designed in a such way that the service description in WSDL becomes the part of the design process before the actual code of the learning object is written, but not otherwise - a service description produced as an artifact of the learning object itself. Those interested in e-learning Web service development must understand the detailed steps involved in service-oriented modelling and architecture, particularly when composing services by writing their interfaces in WSDL.

However, there is one inherent characteristic of Web services that should be taken into consideration when designing e-learning services. Web services are stateless in that they do not retain state information from invocation to invocation. Meanwhile, it is quite likely in a series of related e-learning activities to take into consideration the results of previous invocations. WSRF extends Web service concept to a Grid and makes state management possible by making distinction between the service and the stateful resources acted upon by that service. This extension is made using existing Web service specifications and technology.

A Grid as a distributed resource and service-oriented architecture deploys the Web service, yet within a Grid the concept is being extended to cover global integrity and interoperability issues. Systems in a Grid can not only be running different operating systems, but can also represent different virtual organizations with different availability policies to their service resources to share. A Grid adds middleware services including security, authorization, accounting, and registries such that a Web service built up for a Grid can function as a Grid service. While Grid services are naturally completely based on the same set of XML based protocols, establishing Grid services raises additional questions regarding service location and access, discovery, and manageability that should be taken into account.

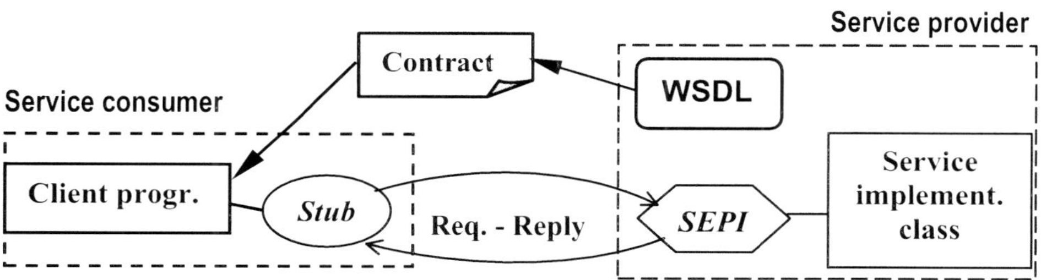

Figure 1. Web service deployment scheme

The 'WSDL first' approach leads to a Web service deployment scheme shown in Figure 1. Using a WSDL service description the server side Service End Point Interface (SEPI) and client's stub are generated by a Web service development software toolkit. A simple note 'Contract' partly represents specific Grid service attributes such as service registry and service discovery path by querying the registry, eventually they are not shown on the Figure 1 explicitly. The remainder of the paper addresses those specific Grid service attributes for the case of building e-learning Grid services.

3. e-Learning Grid Service Design Considerations

Above we looked tentatively at making a software application as a Web service. Creation of the service kernel, i.e. its description in WSDL, which contains everything needed to invoke the service, is the inevitable first step in the path of e-learning Grid service design.

Here we propose a second step, although not inevitable, but being quite reasonable and justifiable for practically realizing a service-orientation for specific e-learning domain. This involves the creation of e-learning repository Grid service whose major objective would be to collect WSDLs associated with a certain Virtual Organization (VO) into one repository as a means of providing a set of e-learning services maintenance and life cycle management services. In this case there would logically be one repository service and many associated e-learning application services under the control of the repository service. Eventually the repository service could be considered as one possible solution in determining how e-learning services in some Grid domain could be grouped and managed as a set of the same type of services.

On the other hand, such a repository service associated with e-learning services is functionally a kind of attendant service intended to implement a number of management functions. The permanent repository service should firstly maintain the repository of WSDLs within the limits of VO, e.g. a regional or national node hosting environment that is a set of resources located within a single administrative domain and comprising a necessary set of execution facilities for service provision and management. Such an internal level of resource management may include important functions closely related to a successful e-learning service provision, such as 'find-access-invoke', 'access-update-store', or 'change access status'.

Another important consideration is that Web service creation or composition as the core of Web service technology also belongs to this category of functions. If we disregard specific Web service composition issues, it seems reasonable to argue that a repository service could be considered as a compact 'region' within the e-learning Grid framework where service compositions experiments and practices could be carried out. Referring to Stefano Cerri [12] it would be the location for implementing and performing Service Developer's Services for specifying, designing and developing innovative services. The top-down 'WSDL first' approach along with LO metadata and ontology language OWL-S, which describes properties and capabilities of Web services [13], could be the principles which underlie this crucial e-learning Web service composition function.

Another external function of a repository service is the dissemination of information about hosted services beyond the VO domain. In this respect the repository service plays the role of service provider, i.e. exposing a set of services, helping to discover them, maintaining full control of access to them and being responsible for their execution. A repository service represented as a typical Grid service should be registered in the global Grid UDDI registry by name and when accessed it may expose a WS-Inspection document containing a collection of service descriptions available through this particular repository.

On the other hand, the repository service itself could maintain its local registry, which serves to discover and provide e-learning services through access to WSDL files. Let us assume that only the repository service is to be registered in the global UDDI, rather than every particular e-learning service. The repository service should also maintain its lower level registry and enable user access directly to the WSDL files of the service. This feature prevents intermixing e-learning services with other Grid services in a common Grid service registry. While the service namespace would accordingly become hierarchical, this is a common case for large scale distributed systems.

4. Discussion

The failure to properly design e-learning applications could be sometimes interpreted as a consequence of a conceptual faultline between instructional designers and distributed learning object system designers. Instructional designers think in terms of cognitive categories, learning objectives, and outcomes; treat learners as active individuals with some background knowledge (learning context); and do not think much about the interaction potential an ICT-based learning system may offer. Distributed LO systems designers, on the other hand, predominantly think hard about reuse, management, standards, and overall implementation of a workable system, placing emphasis on embedded functionalities, multimedia, and communication technology itself at the expense of proper instructional design. A question that arises is how the use of e-learning Web services may mitigate that kind of contradiction.

This paper briefly considered employing e-learning applications as a Web service deployable within a Grid environment. Web service technology involves constructing e-learning scenarios when e-learning application constituent parts are distributed on the network or globally located for other practical reasons. The predominant issue in this process is the building a service description in Web service description language. It is not a simple sequencing of content learning objects, but it is rather design and description of interfaces being used for messaging between constituent parts of the service, including both types of expositive and active learning objects. Here, instructional design and technology become closely linked due to an altered viewpoint of the way learning objects are used in a service-oriented e-learning setting.

The proposed analysis reveals another essential question to be considered in parallel with design and realization of e-learning Web services: how should WSDLs be effectively designed and built for e-learning services and to what extent should learning object metadata contribute to automated WSDL generation? Current LOM specification is designed to support reusability of learning objects, i.e. provides "a uniform way for describing learning resources so that they can be easier discovered, by different metadata aware search tools and taken for delivery or aggregation with other resources" [4]. Learning objects are indexed with metadata so that they may be identified, located, retrieved, and assembled into sharable content packages. The LOM instance accordingly does not contain appropriate elements to provide details associated with methods and data types being used by that object, which is essential data to be used for WSDL descriptions in order to automatically realize specifications for e-learning service interfaces.

Of particular interest, a question currently under discussion pertains to the revision and augmentation of LOM specification in order to better support pedagogic and economic goals when used in service-oriented architectures [14, 15]. It is also worthy to note the Java Specification Request (JSR) efforts to define metadata for Web services and integrate metadata into the Java platform to support better automatic generation of components needed for Web services [16]. Similarly the LOM specification could acquire such a responsibility to support automatic generation of descriptions for e-learning Web services based on learning objects.

Finally, construction of WSDL is not just a technical problem because it is associated with learning sessions and has direct influence on learning scenarios and objectives. Here we do not present experimental implementation results, nor illustrate a novel e-learning application functioning on the Grid, instead providing technical analysis and arguments on how e-learning applications can be built with "Grid-awareness". It is expected that this approach will be justified in the near future through experience gained in implementing real, though simple learning services based on various types of content components.

References

[1] S. Tuecke, et al (2003) Open Grid Service Infrastructure (OGSI), Version 1.0, http://www.globus.org/research/papers/Final_OGSI_Specification_V1.0.pdf

[2] I. Foster et al (2004) Modeling Stateful Resources with Web Services. Version 1.1, http://www-106.ibm.com/developerworks/library/ws-resource/ws-modelingresources.pdf

[3] K. Krauter, R. Buyya, M. Maheswaran (2002) A taxonomy and survey of Grid resource management systems for distributed computing. Software Practice and Experience, 32, No. 2 February; pp 135-164.

[4] The Final 1484.12.1 LOM Draft Standard Document, (2002) http://ltsc.ieee.org/wg12/20020612-Final-LOM-Draft.html

[5] D.M. Schuch-Miller, M.D. Lee (2002), A Dose of Reality in the Classroom. Proceedings of E-Learn 2002, World Conference on E-Learning in Corporate, Government. Healthcare, & Higher Education, October 15-19, Montreal, Canada, vol. 4, pp 2146-2149.

[6] D. Falkenburg, D.M. Schuch-Miller (2003), The Greenfield Coalition Learning Factory. Proceedings of the World Conference on Educational Multimedia, Hypermedia and Telecommunications 2003(1), 2356-2357, available at http://dl.aace.org/13245

[7] Web Service Architecture (2004), W3C Working Group Note 11 February 2004 http://www.w3.org/TR/ws-arch/

[8] W. Vogels Web Services Are Not Distributed Objects. IEEE Internet Computing, November 2003, pp 59-66, (http://weblogs.cs.cornell.edu/AllThingsDistributed/archives/000343.html, accessed Dec. 2004)

[9] Web Services Description Language (WSDL), Version 2.0, W3C Working Draft 3 August 2004, http://www.w3.org/TR/2004/WD-wsdl20-20040803/

[10] IMS Learning Design Best Practice and Implementation Guide, Version 1.0 Final Specification http://www.imsglobal.org/learningdesign/ldv1p0/imsld_bestv1p0.html

[11] V. Reklaitis, K Baniulis, N. Aukstakalnis (2004) Building Assessment Web Service from Question Type Learning Objects. 4th International LeGE-WG Workshop: Towards a European Learning Grid Infrastructure: Progressing with a European Learning Grid, Stuttgart, Germany. 27-28 April, 2004, British Computer Society, Electronic Workshops in Computing (eWiC), http://www.bcs.org/ewic/

[12] S.A.Cerri (2003) Open Learning Service Scenarios on Grids. 3rd International LeGE-WG Workshop: Grid Infrastructure to Support Future Technology Enhanced Learning, Berlin, Germany. 3 December, British Computer Society, Electronic Workshops in Computing (eWiC), http://www.bcs.org/ewic/

[13] D.Martin et al. (2003), Describing Web Services using OWL-S and WSDL, DAML-S Coalition working document, http://www.daml.org/services/owl-s/1.0/owl-s-wsdl.html

[14] K. Wulf (2003) Reusability of e-Learning Objects in the Context of Learning Grids. 3rd International LeGE-WG Workshop: Grid Infrastructure to support future technology enhanced learning, Berlin. 3 December, British Computer Society, Electronic Workshops in Computing (eWiC), http://www.bcs.org/ewic/

[15] M. A. Sicilia, E. García (2003) On the Concepts of Usability and Reusability of Learning Objects International Review of Research in Open and Distance Learning ISSN: 1492-3831, http://www.irrodl.org/content/v4.2/sicilia-garcia.html

[16] JSR 181: Web Services Metadata for the Java Platform, (2004), Java Specification Requests, http://www.jcp.org/en/jsr/detail?id=181

Towards the Learning Grid
P. Ritrovato et al. (Eds.)
IOS Press, 2005

Derivation of Knowledge Structures for Distributed Learning Objects

Luca STEFANUTTI, Dietrich ALBERT and Cord HOCKEMEYER
Cognitive Science Section – Graz University (Austria)
luca.stefanutti@unipd.it, dietrich.albert@uni-graz.at, cord.hockemeyer@uni-graz.at

Abstract. Knowledge space theory [1–3] offers a rigorous and efficient formal framework for the construction, validation, and application of e-assessment and e-learning adaptive systems. This theory is the basis for some existing e-learning and e-assessment adaptive systems in the U.S. and in Europe. Such systems are based on a fixed and local domain of knowledge, where *fixed* means that the domain does not change in time, and *local* refers to the fact that the items are stored and available locally. In this paper we present some theoretical notes on the efficient construction and application of knowledge spaces for knowledge domains that are both dynamic and distributed in space. This goes in the direction of an exploitation of new technologies like the GRID for building the next generation of learning environments.

Keywords. Knowledge structures, knowledge spaces, distributed learning objects, skill maps, knowledge assessment, GRID Technology

Introduction

Knowledge space theory [1–3] offers a rigorous and efficient formal framework for the construction, validation, and application of e-assessment and e-learning adaptive systems. It has originally been developed as a psychometric theory for the assessment of knowledge; however, as adaptivity and optimal learning paths matter, its methods and models have been fruitfully exploited for e-learning purposes as well, e.g. in the ALEKS (http://www.aleks.com) or RATH (http://css.uni-graz.at/rath) systems.

According to this theory, a *domain of knowledge* is a collection Q of items (e.g., learning objects, problems, questions, exercises, examples, etc.) in a given field of knowledge (e.g., mathematics, physics, chemistry, biology, etc.). Then, the *knowledge state* of a student is the set K of all items in Q that this student actually masters, and a *knowledge structure* for Q is a pair $(Q, \mathcal{K})$ in which $\mathcal{K}$ is the collection of all knowledge states that can be observed in a certain population of students. If $\mathcal{K}$ is closed under union (i.e., $K \cup K' \in \mathcal{K}$ whenever $K, K' \in \mathcal{K}$) then it is called a *knowledge space*. Sometimes also closure under intersection holds ($K \cap K' \in \mathcal{K}$ whenever $K, K' \in \mathcal{K}$), in which case, $\mathcal{K}$ is called a *quasi-ordinal* knowledge space.

The above-mentioned theory is the basis for some existing e-learning and e-assessment adaptive systems in the U.S. and in Europe. Two of them are the ALEKS (Adaptive LEarning with Knowledge Spaces) system developed by the research group of Irvine, CA supervised by Falmagne (http://www.aleks.com), and the RATH (Relational Adaptive Tutoring Hypertext) system of the research group of Graz, Austria [4,5].

Such systems are based on a fixed and local domain of knowledge Q, where *fixed* means that Q does not change in time, and *local* refers to the fact that the items are stored and available locally. The original theory, in fact, provides methods of construction of knowledge structures which are based on these two requirements [6–8]. Later developments of the theory provide some methods of construction for the case of dynamic domains of knowledge (see, e.g., [9,10]). However, the efficient construction and application of knowledge structures for distributed (i.e., non-local) items appears to be still an open question.

New technologies like the GRID provide a promising approach for the construction and application of e-learning systems [11]. These technologies are strongly based on the concept of distributed services. In this paper we present some theoretical notes on the efficient construction and application of knowledge spaces for knowledge domains that are both dynamic and distributed in space. This means that the learning objects may reside on different locations and that every location has access to both, local and remote learning objects. Moreover, the set (repository) of learning objects in the various locations is assumed to be dynamic in the sense that learning objects may be continuously added to (resp. removed from) the local repositories. At the basis of our approach there is the concept of a *distributed skill map*, which is the subject of next section.

1. Distributed Skill Maps

A skill map [12–14] is a triplet $A := (Q_A, S_A, \sigma_A)$ in which Q_A is a nonempty set of items (problems, learning objects, exercises, questions, etc.), S_A is a nonempty set of skills, and $\sigma_A : Q_A \to 2^S$ is a mapping such that $\sigma_A(q) \neq \varnothing$ for all $q \in Q_A$. The interpretation of σ_A is the following: for any q in Q_A, $\sigma_A(q)$ is the set of all skills that (according to A) are sufficient to solve item q.

A knowledge structure can be easily derived from a skill map A. By the conjunctive model of Doignon [2,12], a subset K of Q_A is said to be *delineated* by a subset T of S_A if and only if

$$K = \varphi_A(T) := \{ q \in Q_A : \sigma_A(q) \subseteq T \}. \quad (1)$$

In words, every item q in K is solvable by (some subset of) skills in T, and K contains all such items. It turns out that the collection $\mathcal{K}(A)$ of all subsets $K \subseteq Q_A$ fulfilling (1) for some subset T of S is a knowledge structure closed under intersection. Note that this leads to a proximity to the *formal concept analysis* developed by Wille and his group [15]. He characterizes concepts through the (sub) set of objects belonging to the concept and through the properties (in our case the skills required for the respective learning object) shared by all these objects.

While large parts of the procedures developed in the context of knowledge space theory relies on structures closed under union this does not necessarily hold for knowledge structures derived from skill maps: If we have, e.g., $Q_A = \{a, b, c\}$, $S_A = \{x, y\}$, and σ_A defined by $\sigma_A(a) = \{x\}$, $\sigma_A(b) = \{y\}$, *and* $\sigma_A(c) = \{x, y\}$, the resulting structure $\mathcal{K}(A) = \{ \varnothing, \{a\}, \{b\}, \{a, b, c\} \}$, i.e. it contains the subsets $\{a\}$ and $\{b\}$ of Q but not their union $\{a, b\}$ since no subset of S_A maps to $\{a, b\}$ under σ_A. Conditions for skill maps providing knowledge spaces, i.e. knowledge structures closed under union, have been investigated by Korossy [14].

A *distributed skill map* is a pair ($\mathcal{D}$, $\vee$), where $\mathcal{D}$ is a collection of skill maps, and "$\vee$" (read: "join") is a binary operator such that, given any three skill maps $A := (Q_A, S_A, \sigma_A)$, $B := (Q_B, S_B, \sigma_B)$ and $C := (Q_C, S_C, \sigma_C)$ in $\mathcal{D}$, $C = A \vee B$ if and only if

1. $Q_C = Q_A \cup Q_B$,
2. $S_C = S_A \cup S_B$,
3. $\sigma_C(q) = \sigma_A(q) \cup \sigma_B(q)$ for all $q \in Q_C$.

It is a simple fact that the join of two skill maps is still a skill map. A distributed skill map (D^*,$\vee$), is said to be *complete* if $A \vee B \in D^*$ whenever $A, B \in D^*$. Thus, every complete distributed skill map has a *top* element $T = (Q_T, S_T, \sigma_T)$ which is determined by

$$T = \vee \{A : A \in D^*\}$$

[Note that, from a mathematical point of view, a complete distributed skill map is a complete join semi-lattice in which the join operation is "$\vee$".] It follows that the knowledge structure delineated by a complete distributed skill map ($\mathcal{D}^*$, $\vee$) having top element T, is $\mathcal{K}(T)$ where, for any $A \in D^*$,

$$\mathcal{K}(A) := \{K \subseteq Q_A : K = \varphi_A(T) \text{ for some } T \subseteq S_A\}.$$

The fact that $\mathcal{K}(T)$ is a knowledge structure closed under intersection immediately follows from the fact that T is, indeed, a skill map. Moreover, since the join-closure of any distributed skill map ($\mathcal{D}$, $\vee$) is a complete distributed skill map, the knowledge structure delineated by $\mathcal{D}$ is

$$\mathcal{K} = \varphi(\vee\{A : A \in D\})$$

Thus, a distributed skill map can be seen as a distributed representation of a knowledge structure closed under intersection.

2. Construction and Retrieval of Distributed Skill Maps

Physically, the elements of a distributed skill map ($\mathcal{D}$, $\vee$) reside in locations that are separate in space, or they can be produced at different time points. The subset $\mathcal{D}'$ of all elements in $\mathcal{D}$ that are accessible to a given user in a specific location is the distributed skill map accessible to that user.

Locally, a skill map $A := (Q_A, S_A, \sigma_A)$, is represented as a collection R of pairs (q, P), where $q \in Q_A$ is an item, $P \subseteq S_A$ is a set of skills such that $\sigma_A(q) = P$, and R is called a *local repository* of the skill map A. To create a local repository one needs to specify the pairs (q, P), each of which is a single item (problem, learning object, etc.) with a set of skills 'attached' to it. The only requirement is that the items in a local repository have to be unique (to assure consistency of the mapping σ_A), i.e., for all $q \in Q_A$,

$$(q, P) \in \mathrm{R} \quad and \quad (q, P') \in \mathrm{R} \Rightarrow P = P'$$

Technically, appropriate metadata schemas have to be defined for the representation of the elements of a local repository (i.e., the pairs (q, P)). Such a schema definition may be based, e.g., on the *generic adaptive element* proposed by Conlan et al. [16] as an extension to the IMS Learning Resource Metadata and IEEE Learning Object metadata definitions.

The user is allowed to perform three kinds of operations with local and remote repositories:

1. insert/delete/edit items (q, P) in the local repository;
2. retrieve items from the local repository;
3. retrieve items from a remote repository.

Through these three operations the user derives, in fact, a local skill map and – implicitly – a local knowledge space which can then be used for e-learning and/or assessment purposes. Thus, the advantage of distributed skill maps is that the corresponding knowledge structure can be derived locally for the specific subset of items collected by the user.

3. Assessment of the Knowledge State of a Student

Given a set Q of items, the knowledge state of a student is the collection K of all items that this student masters. Here we face the problem of how to determine this collection for a certain student in an efficient way. Knowledge space theory provides procedures for the efficient assessment of the knowledge state of the student provided that an explicit representation of the knowledge structure is available to these procedures (see e.g., [17,18]).

When the items in Q are distributed in space the derivation of an explicit knowledge space for Q turns out to be a rather inefficient approach. To see this, imagine that a user collects a set of elements (q, P) from different (local or remote) repositories creating, this way, a local skill map $A := (Q_A, S_A, \sigma_A)$ (see previous section). To use this skill map for assessing a student with the procedures mentioned above, the user needs to derive the explicit knowledge space corresponding to A. This turns out to be a time and space consuming task.

At least for quasi-ordinal knowledge spaces, an efficient assessment procedure can be derived which does not require the explicit construction of the knowledge space corresponding to a certain skill map A. In this section we provide a sketch of this procedure.

In a first step, we define a binary relation "$\leq_A$" on Q_A such that, for any two items p, $q \in Q_A$,

$$p \leq_A q \Leftrightarrow \sigma_A(p) \subseteq \sigma_A(q).$$

The interpretation of such a relation is the following: "the fact that a student masters item p can be *surmised* by the fact that this student masters q" or, equivalently, "the fact that this student does not master q can be surmised by the fact that s/he does not master p". The introduction of the relation "$\leq_A$" has a clear aim: it is a classical result in lattice theory that there exists a 1–1 correspondence between the quasi-ordinal knowledge spaces on a set Q and the surmise relations for Q [1,2,19].

As second step, we introduce the following notation: for a subset $X \subseteq Q_A$, we denote with

$$X^{\uparrow} := \{q \in Q_A : x \leq_A q \text{ for some } x \in X\}$$

the *up-set* of X in the partially ordered set $(Q_A, \leq_A)$, and with

$$X^{\downarrow} := \{q \in Q_A : q \leq_A x \text{ for some } x \in X\}$$

the *down-set* of X in $(Q_A, \leq_A)$.

Suppose now that the knowledge state $K^* \subseteq Q_A$ of a student has to be uncovered through the skill map A. This occurs in a stepwise assessment procedure where, in each step $n > 0$ the student is presented with a new question $q_n \in Q_A$ and a representation $K_n \subseteq Q_A$ of the knowledge state of the student is updated according to the student's answer. Under the assumption that at the outset ($n = 0$) there is no prior knowledge about K^*, the assessment algorithm is as follows:

```
n ← 0, Kn  ← ∅, Qn ← QA;
while Qn ≠ ∅ do:
   choose new item q from Qn;
   obtain answer r for q from student;
   if r = 1 (correct answer) then
         Kn+1 ← Kn ∪ {q}↓;
         Qn+1 ← Qn \ {q}↓;
   else
         Qn+1 ← Qn \ {q}↑;
   end
   n ← + 1;
end
```

The algorithm sketched above terminates in a finite number of steps $m \leq |Q_A|$ and – if no lucky guesses or careless errors occur during the assessment process (see in this connection [16,17]) – the knowledge state of the student $K^* = K_m$ is correctly uncovered by the procedure. One note on the efficiency of this procedure is that, especially when $|Q_A|$ is large, the number of steps m is expected to be much smaller than $|Q_A|$.

4. Validity of Distributed Skill Maps

A skill map is a (formal) cognitive model which specifies the skills underlying a certain set of items. As a model it is a hypothetical representation of the relation between items and skills and it needs to be validated. A first step of validity is reliability. The different skill maps in a distributed skill map are supposed to be created by different sources (human experts, teachers, educational institutions, etc.). Each source creates an item q and provides a skill assignment to that item. When the same item q is provided by two or more different sources, the problem arises of testing the agreement, among these sources. One question here is that, given a skill map $A := (Q_A, S_A, \sigma_A)$ and an item $q \in Q_A$, $\sigma_A(q)$ is the set of all skills in S_A that are sufficient to solve item q *according to* A. Thus, two different skill maps A and B, with $Q_A \cap Q_B \neq \emptyset$ may reflect different opinions on the sufficient skills of a given item. A perfect agreement arises when, for $q \in Q_A \cap Q_B$, $\sigma_A(q) = \sigma_B(q)$.

Given two sets X and Y, let $X \| Y$ denote their symmetric difference, i.e.,

$$X \| Y := (X \setminus Y) \cup (Y \setminus X)$$

Then, for any skill $s \in S_A \cup S_B$ and any item $q \in Q_A \cap Q_B$ an agreement occurs whenever $s \notin \sigma_A(q) \| \sigma_B(q)$. The ratio between the number of such agreements and the theoretical (maximum) number of agreements for all items in $Q_A \cap Q_B$, and all skills in $S_A \cup S_B$ provides a raw measure of the total agreement between the two skill maps A and B (for the calculation of raw agreement indexes and their statistical significance see, e.g., [20]).

Finally, note that reliability is a necessary but not sufficient condition of validity. This implies that even if reliable, a skill map should then be tested against empirical data. If the knowledge structure corresponding to a given skill map is considered, then various methods and probabilistic can be applied for this purpose [2,21,22]. Both, reliability and validity can be increased by combining structures obtained from different sources. The work of Dowling and her group [22–24] provides a good basis for further investigations in this direction.

5. Conclusions

Knowledge space theory provides formal models and methods for the efficient assessment of knowledge in a certain domain of knowledge. Existing methods, however, are applicable only in the case of a local domain of knowledge. An approach for the assessment of knowledge through knowledge spaces which is appropriate for distributed and dynamic learning objects was presented in this paper. The approach focuses on the construction of *distributed skill maps* (and corresponding knowledge spaces) and on the derivation of new local skill maps from the distributed ones. The concept of a distributed skill map allows exploiting the advantages of applying knowledge spaces in knowledge assessment when the learning objects are located in distributed repositories, rather then local. This would allow the exploitation of new technologies like the GRID for the construction of e-learning and e-assessment systems.

An algorithm for the efficient assessment of knowledge through distributed skill maps was sketched in Section 3. The algorithm applies in case of skill maps generating quasi-ordinal knowledge spaces. The explicit derivation of a knowledge space from a (local or distributed) skill map is time-consuming, especially when the domain of knowledge gets large. The advantage of the proposed algorithm is that its application does not require the explicit derivation of the knowledge space corresponding to a given skill map.

In a distributed skill map, new local skill maps can be obtained integrating existing ones. This integration poses the problem of the validity of local skill maps. This problem was discussed in Section 4 where some basic methods were proposed for obtaining statistical indexes of agreement among different skill maps.

Finally, we would like to point out that the approach proposed here is restricted to cases where all parts of a learning object are located on one server. If we base our structuring process on the component–attribute approach (see [3]) instead, also learning objects whose parts are distributed among different servers can be covered [26]. However, that approach involves higher efforts in the structuring process.

Acknowledgements

The work reported in this paper was supported by the European Commission through the LeGE-WG Thematic Network (Grant No. IST-2001-38763). Luca Stefanutti contributed to this research during his stay at Graz Unviersity as a Marie Curie Fellow of the European Commission (Grant No. HPMF-CT-2000-01044).

References

[1] Doignon, J.-P. & Falmagne, J.-C. (1985). Spaces for the assessment of knowledge. *International Journal of Man-Machine Studies, 23*, 175–196.

[2] Doignon, J.-P. & Falmagne, J.-C. (1999). *Knowledge spaces*. Berlin, Heidelberg: Springer–Verlag.

[3] Albert, D. & Lukas, J., editors (1999). *Knowledge spaces: theories, empirical research, applications*. Mahwah, New Jersey: Lawrence Earlbaum Associates.

[4] Albert, D. & Hockemeyer, C. (1997). Adaptive and dynamic hypertext tutoring systems based on knowledge space theory. In B. du Boulay & R. Mizoguchi, editors, *Artificial Intelligence in Education: Knowledge and Media in Learning Systems*, volume 39 of *Frontiers in Artificial Intelligence and Applications*, pp. 553–555. Amsterdam: IOS Press.

[5] Hockemeyer, C., Held, T., & Albert, D. (1998). RATH — a relational adaptive tutoring hypertext WWW–environment based on knowledge space theory. In C. Alvegård, editor, *CALISCE'98: Proceedings of the Fourth International Conference on Computer Aided Learning in Science and Engineering*, pp. 417–423. Göteborg, Sweden: Chalmers University of Technology.

[6] Dowling, C.E. (1993). Applying the basis of a knowledge space for controlling the questioning of an expert. *Journal of Mathematical Psychology, 37*, 21–48.

[7] Koppen, M. (1993). Extracting human expertise for constructing knowledge spaces: an algorithm. *Journal of Mathematical Psychology, 37*, 1–20.

[8] Koppen, M. & Doignon, J.-P. (1990). How to build a knowledge space by querying an expert. *Journal of Mathematical Psychology, 34*, 311–331.

[9] Albert, D. & Kaluscha, R. (1997). Adapting knowledge structures in dynamic domains. In C. Herzog, editor, *Beiträge zum Achten Arbeitstreffen der GI–Fachgruppe, 1.1.5./7.0.1 „Intelligente Lehr/Lernsysteme"* (pp. 89–100). München, Germany: Technische Universität München. Online available at http://css.uni-graz.at/publicdocs/publications/file1102342382.pdf.

[10] Stefanutti, L. & Koppen, M. (2003). A procedure for the incremental construction of a knowledge space. *Journal of Mathematical Psychology, 47*, 265–277.

[11] Ritrovato, P. (2003). How to use the GRID Technology for building the next generation of learning environments. In T. Dimitrakos & P. Ritrovato, editors, *4th International LeGE-WG Workshop - Towards a European Learning Grid Infrastructure: Progressing with a European Learning Grid.* Wiltshire: British Computer Society. Published electronically at http://ewic.bcs.org/conferences/2003/2ndlege/session1/paper3.htm.

[12] Doignon, J.P. (1994). Knowledge spaces and skill assignments. In G.H. Fischer and D. Laming, editors, *Contributions to Mathematical Psychology, Psychometrics, and Methodology*, pp. 111–121. New York: Springer–Verlag.

[13] Düntsch, I., & Gediga, G. (1995). Skills and knowledge structures. *British Journal of Mathematical and Statistical Psychology, 48*, 9–27.

[14] Korossy, K. (1997). Extending the theory of knowledge spaces: A competence-performance approach. *Zeitschrift für Psychologie, 205*, 53–82.
[15] Rusch, A. & Wille, R. (1996). Knowledge spaces and formal concept analysis. In Hans-Hermann Bock & Wolfgang Polasek, editors, *Data Analysis and Information Systems*, Studies in Classification, Data Analysis, and Knowledge Organization, pp. 427–436, Berlin, Germany: Springer–Verlag.
[16] Conlan, O., Hockemeyer, C., Wade, V., & Albert, D. (2002). Metadata Driven Approaches to Facilitate Adaptivity in Personalized eLearning systems. *The Journal of Information and Systems in Education, 1*, 38–44.
[17] Falmagne, J.-C. & Doignon, J.-P. (1988). A class of stochastic procedures for the assessment of knowledge. *British Journal of Mathematical and Statistical Psychology, 41*, 1–23.
[18] Falmagne, J.-C. & Doignon, J.-P. (1988). A Markovian procedure for assessing the state of a system. *Journal of Mathematical Psychology, 32*, 232–258.
[19] Birkhoff, G. (1967). *Lattice theory*. Providence, R.I.: American Mathematical Society.
[20] Übersax, J.S. (1993). Statistical Modeling of Expert Ratings on Medical Treatment Appropriateness. *Journal of the American Statistical Association, 88*, 421–427.
[21] Schrepp, M., Held, T., & Albert, D. (1999). Component-based construction of surmise relations for chess problems. In D. Albert & J. Lukas, editors, *Knowledge Spaces: Theories, Empirical Research, Applications*, pp. 41–66. Mahwah, NJ: Lawrence Erlbaum Associates.
[22] Ünlü, A. & Albert, D. (2004). The correlational agreement coefficient ca (≤, d) — a mathematical analysis of a descriptive goodness-of-fit measure. *Mathematical Social Sciences, 48*, 281–314.
[23] Baumunk, K. & Dowling, C.E. (1997). Validity of spaces for assessing knowledge about fractions. *Journal of Mathematical Psychology, 41*, 99–105.
[24] Dowling, C.E. (1994). Integrating different knowledge spaces. In G.H. Fischer & D. Laming, editors, *Contributions to Mathematical Psychology, Psychometrics, and Methodology*, pp. 149–158. New York: Springer–Verlag.
[25] Dowling, C.E. & Hockemeyer, C. (1998). Computing the intersection of knowledge spaces using only their basis. In C.E. Dowling, F.S. Roberts, & P. Theuns, editors, *Recent Progress in Mathematical Psychology*, pp. 133–141. Mahwah, NJ: Lawrence Erlbaum Associates Ltd.
[26] Stefanutti, L., Albert, D., & Hockemeyer, C. (2005). Structuring and Merging Distributed Content. In P. Ritrovato, editor, *Towards the Learning GRID: Advances in Human Learning Services*, pp. 113–118. Amsterdam: IOS Press.

Towards the Learning Grid
P. Ritrovato et al. (Eds.)
IOS Press, 2005

Structuring and Merging Distributed Content

Luca STEFANUTTI, Dietrich ALBERT and Cord HOCKEMEYER
Department of Psychology, University of Graz Universitätsplatz 2/III, 8010 Graz, AT
luca.stefanutti@unipd.it, dietrich.albert@uni-graz.at, cord.hockemeyer@uni-graz.at

Abstract. A flexible approach for structuring and merging distributed learning object is presented. At the basis of this approach there is a formal representation of a learning object, called *attribute structure*. Attribute structures are labeled directed graphs representing structured information on the learning objects. When two or more learning objects are merged, the corresponding attribute structures are unified, and the unified structure is attached to the resulting learning object.

Keywords. Distributed learning objects, knowledge structures, structuring content

Introduction

In order to decide which object comes next in presenting a collection of learning objects to a learner, one might establish some order. Given a set O of learning objects, a *surmise relation* on O is any partial order '$\leq$' on the learning objects in O. The interpretation of '$\leq$' is that, given any two learning objects o and o' in O, $o \leq o'$ holds if a learner who masters o' also masters o. The concept of a surmise relation was introduced by Doignon and Falmagne [5,6] as one of the fundamental concepts of a theoretical framework called Knowledge Space Theory. According to this theory the *knowledge state* of a learner is the subset K of all learning objects in O that (s)he masters. A subset $K \subseteq Q$ is said to be a knowledge state of the surmise relation '$\leq$' if $o \in K$ and $o' \leq o$ implies $o' \in K$ for all learning objects $o, o' \in O$. Then the collection $\mathcal{K}$ of all knowledge states of '$\leq$' is called the *knowledge space* derived from '$\leq$'. Knowledge spaces are used for representing and assessing the knowledge state of a learner (see, e.g., [1,2] in this connection).

The construction of a surmise relation may follow different approaches [3,2]. After a brief presentation of an existing approach based on vectors of components of a learning object, we extend this approach to a more flexible representation called *attribute structure* [4]. The mathematical properties of attribute structures make it possible to compare distributed learning objects in terms of how much informative and how much demanding they are.

1. The Component Approach

According to the *component* approach [5,6], every content object o in O is equipped with an ordered n-tuple $A = (a_1, a_2, \ldots, a_n)$ of *attributes* where the length n of the attribute

n-tuple A is fixed for all objects. Each attribute a_i in A comes from a corresponding attribute set C_i called the i-th *component* of the content object. In this sense, given a collection $C = \{C_1, C_2, \ldots, C_i, \ldots C_n\}$ of disjoint attribute sets (or components), each object $o \in O$ is equipped with an element of the Cartesian product $\mathcal{P} = C_1 \times C_2 \times \ldots \times C_i \times \ldots C_n$. Usually each component C_i is equipped with a partial order '$\leq_i$' so that $\langle C_i, \leq_i \rangle$ is in fact a partially ordered set of attributes. The partial order '$\leq_i$' is interpreted in the following way: for $a, b \in C_i$, if $a \leq_i b$ then a learning object characterized by attribute a is *less demanding* than a learning object characterized by attribute b. To give a simple example, it might be postulated that 'computations involving integer numbers' (attribute a) are less demanding than 'computations involving rational numbers' (attribute b). A natural order $\leq$ on the elements in $\mathcal{P}$, the so-called coordinate-wise order [7], is derived from the n partial orders '$\leq_i$' by

$$(x_1, x_2, \ldots, x_n) \leq (y_1, y_2, \ldots, y_n) \Leftrightarrow \forall_i : x_i \leq_i y_i$$

If $f : O \rightarrow \mathcal{P}$ is a mapping assigning an attribute n-tuple to each learning object, then a surmise relation '$\leq$' on the learning objects is established by

$$o \leq o' \Leftrightarrow f(o) \leq f(o')$$

for all $o, o' \in O$. The mapping f can easily be established even when the learning objects are distributed (see, e.g., [8]).

2. Attribute Structures

An *attribute structure* is used to represent structured information on a learning object or an asset and in this sense it represents an extension of the attribute n-tuple discussed in Section 1. From a mathematical standpoint attribute structures correspond to the feature structures introduced by Carpenter [9] in computational linguistics. Let C be a set of components and A a collection of attributes, with $A \cap C = \emptyset$. An attribute structure is a labelled directed graph $\mathcal{A} = (Q, r, \alpha, \eta)$ where:

- Q is a set of nodes of the graph;
- $r \in Q$ is the *root node* of the graph;
- $\alpha : Q \rightarrow A$ is a partial function assigning attributes to some of the nodes;
- $\eta : Q \times C \rightarrow Q$ is a partial function specifying the edges of the graph.

As an example, let C' = {picture, topic, subtopic, text, language} be a set of components, and let A' = {PICTURE1, TEXT1, ENGLISH, MATH, MATRIX INVERSION} be a collection of attributes. Suppose moreover that a simple learning object is described by the asset structure $\mathcal{A}_1 = (Q_1, r_1, \alpha_1, \gamma_1)$ where Q_1 is the set of nodes, r_1 is the root node, and α_1 and γ_1 are defined as follows: α_1 (0) is not defined, α_1 (1) = PICTURE1, α_1 (2) = TEXT1, α_1 (3) = MATH, α_1 (4) = ENGLISH, and α_1 (5) = MATRIX INVERSION; η_1 (0,picture) = 1, η_1 (0,text) = 2, η_1 (0,topic) = 3, η_1 (1,topic) = 3, η_1 (2,topic) = 3,

η_1 (2,language) = 4, and η_1 (3,subtopic) = 5. The digraph representing this attribute structure is displayed in Figure 1. The structure $\mathcal{A}_1$ describes a very simple learning object containing a picture along with some text explanation. Both text and picture have MATH as topic and MATRIX INVERSION as subtopic. The root node of the structure is node 0 and it can be easily checked from the figure that each node can be reached from this node following some path in the graph. The root node is the entry node in the asset structure of the learning object, and the edges departing from this node specify the main components of the learning object itself. Thus, in our example, the learning object represented by A_1 is defined by three different components: picture, text and topic. The values of these three components are the attributes given by $\alpha_1(\eta_1(0,$ picture)) = PICTURE1, $\alpha_1(\eta_1(0,$ text)) = DESCRIPTION, and $\alpha_1(\eta_1$ (0, topic)) = MATH.

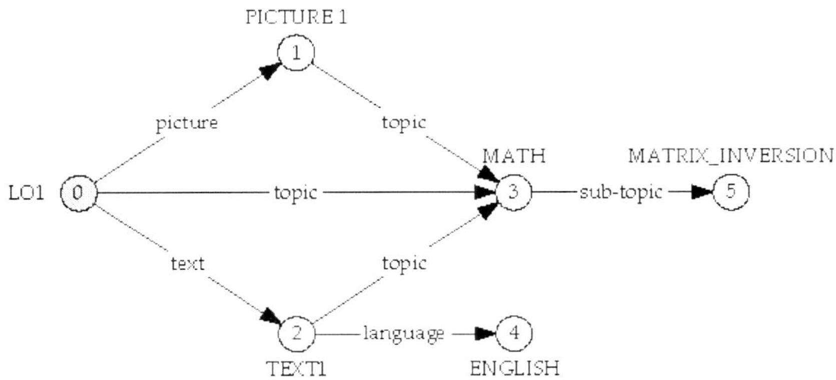

Figure 1. The attribute structure $\mathcal{A}_1$ describes a simple learning object on 'matrix algebra'.

Observe, for instance that node 5 can be reached from node 0 following the path ⟨picture, topic, subtopic⟩. The fact that, in this example, each node is reachable from the root node through some path is not a coincidence. It is explicitly required that every node in an attribute structure be reachable from the root node.

3. Comparing and Combining Attribute Structures

Attribute structures can be compared one another. Informally, an attribute structure $\mathcal{A}$ *subsumes* another attribute structure $\mathcal{A}'$ (denoted by $\mathcal{A} \sqsubseteq \mathcal{A}'$) if $\mathcal{A}'$ contains at least the same information as $\mathcal{A}$. In this sense an attribute structure can be thought as a class of learning objects (the class of all learning objects represented by that structure), and '$\sqsubseteq$' can be regarded as a partial order on such classes. Formally, an attribute structure $\mathcal{A} = (Q, r, \alpha, \eta)$ subsumes another attribute structure $\mathcal{A}' = \langle Q', r', \alpha', \eta' \rangle$ if there exists a mapping $h : Q \rightarrow Q'$ fulfilling the three conditions

(1) $h(r) = r'$;
(2) for all $q \in Q$ and all $c \in C$, if $\eta(q, c)$ is defined then $h(\eta(q, c)) = \eta'(h(q), c)$;
(3) for all $q \in Q$, if $\alpha(q)$ is defined then $\alpha(q) = \alpha'(h(q))$.

In Section 1, the attribute sets were assumed to be partially ordered according to pedagogical criteria and/or to cognitive demands. Analogously, we assume now that a partial order '$\leq$' is defined on the set A of attributes so that, given two attributes $a, b \in A$, if $a \leq b$ then a learning object defined by attribute a is less demanding than a learning object defined by attribute b. Then the subsumption relation '$\sqsubseteq$' is made consistent with '$\leq$' if condition (3) is replaced by

(4) for all $q \in Q$, if $\alpha(q)$ is defined then $\alpha(q) \leq \alpha'(h(q))$.

According to this new definition, if $\mathcal{A} \sqsubseteq \mathcal{B}$ *then* $\mathcal{A}$ is either less informative than $\mathcal{B}$ or less demanding than $\mathcal{B}$ or both.

As an example consider the three attribute structures depicted in Figure 2. Assuming that MATRIX PRODUCT $\leq$ MATRIX INVERSION, both mappings g and h fulfil conditions (1), (2) and (4). Thus both attribute structures labelled by LO2 and LO3 subsume the attribute structure labelled by LO1. However there is neither mapping from LO2 to LO3 fulfilling the subsumption conditions, nor the opposite, thus these last two structures are incomparable to each other. The derivation of a surmise relation for the learning objects parallels that established in Section 1. If $s : o \mapsto s(o)$ is a mapping assigning an attribute structure to each learning object, then a surmise relation '$\leq$' on the learning objects is derived by

$$o \leq o' \Leftrightarrow s(o) \sqsubseteq s(o')$$

for all $o, o' \in O$. Two binary operations are defined on attribute structures: *unification* and *generalization*.

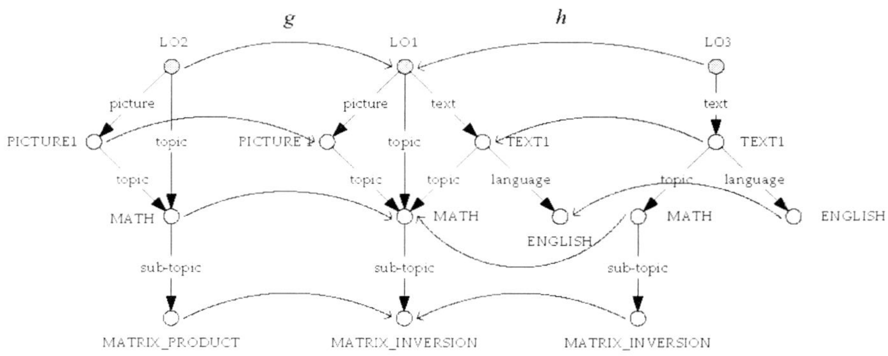

Figure 2. Both LO2 and LO3 subsume LO1. However LO2 and LO3 are incomparable.

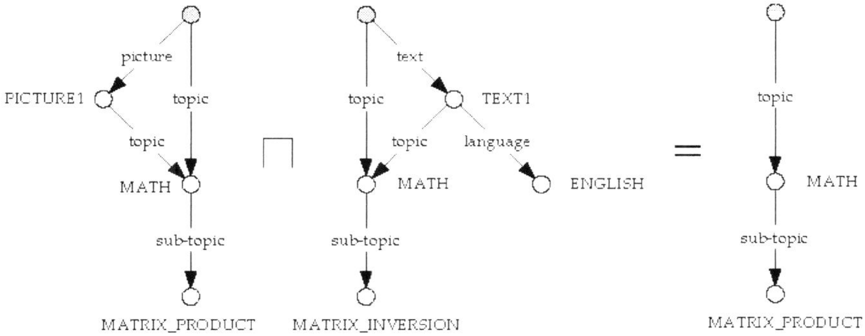

Figure 3. Generalization of two asset structures.

Mathematically, the unification of two attribute structures $\mathcal{A}$ and $\mathcal{B}$ (denoted by $\mathcal{A} \sqcup \mathcal{B}$), when exists, is the least upper bound of $\{\mathcal{A}, \mathcal{B}\}$ *with* respect to the subsumption relation. Dually, generalization (denoted by $\mathcal{A} \sqcap \mathcal{B}$) is the greatest lower bound. In particular, for any two attribute structures $\mathcal{A}$ and $\mathcal{B}$ it holds that

$$A \sqsubseteq A \sqcup B, \quad B \sqsubseteq A \sqcup B$$

$$A \sqcap B \sqsubseteq A, \quad A \sqcap B \sqsubseteq B$$

When two different learning objects are merged together, or when different assets are assembled into a single learning object, the corresponding attribute structures are unified, and the resulting attribute structure is assigned to the resulting learning object. On the other hand, the generalization operation is used to find the common structure of two or more learning objects or, stated another way, to classify learning objects. An example of the generalization operation applied to two attribute structures is shown in Figure 3. Here, the resulting structure shows that two learning objects have in common topic and subtopic. Generalized attribute structures can also be used e.g. for searching a distributed environment for all learning objects whose structure is consistent with a certain 'template' (for instance to find out all learning objects that are 'problems' involving, as cognitive operation, 'recognition' rather than 'recall').

4. Conclusions

In this paper we have discussed how adaptivity to the individual learners' current knowledge can be realised in a learning grid using a high level of distribution [10]. At first sight, the attribute structure approach may seem more difficult and more costly (in a sense of structuring efforts) than the skill map approach [8]. However, it opens a closer connection between knowledge spaces and ontological models like concept maps [11] and the semantic web [12,13]. Since these ontological models are increasingly supported by content developers, the attribute structure approach promises to lead to a derivation of prerequisite information that requires rather little additional effort from the authors of learning objects. Instead, the prerequisite information should be derivable from the already provided ontological information of the single assets.

Acknowledgements

The work reported in this paper was supported by the European Commission through the LeGE-WG Thematic Network (Grant No. IST-2001-38763) and through a Marie Curie Fellow of the European Commission (Grant No. HPMF-CT-2000-01044) given to Luca Stefanutti.

References

[1] Doignon J.P. & Falmagne J.C. (1985). Spaces for the assessment of knowledge. *International Journal of ManMachine Studies, 23*, 175–196.

[2] Doignon J.P. & Falmagne J.C. (1999). *Knowledge Spaces*. Berlin: SpringerVerlag.

[3] Albert, D. & Lukas, J., editors (1999). *Knowledge Spaces: Theories, Empirical Research, Applications*. Mahwah, NJ: Lawrence Erlbaum Associates.

[4] Albert D. & Stefanutti L. (2003). Ordering and Combining Distributed Learning Objects through Skill Maps and Asset Structures. *Proceedings of the International Conference on Computers in Education (ICCE 2003)*. Hong Kong, 25 December.

[5] Albert D. & Held T. (1999). Component based knowledge spaces in problem solving and inductive reasoning. In D. Albert and J. Lukas, editors, *Knowledge Spaces. Theories, Empirical Research, Applications*. Mahwah, NJ: Lawrence Erlbaum Associates.

[6] Schrepp M., Held T., & Albert D. (1999). Component based construction of surmise relations for chess problems. In D. Albert and J. Lukas, editors, *Knowledge Spaces. Theories, Empirical Research, Applications*. Mahwah, NJ: Lawrence Erlbaum Associates.

[7] Davey B.A. & Priestley H.A. (2002). *Introduction to lattices and order. Second edition.* Cambridge University Press.

[8] Stefanutti L., Albert D., & Hockemeyer C. (2005). Derivation of knowledge structures for distributed learning. In P. Ritrovato, editor, *Towards the Learning GRID: Advances in Human Learning Services*, pp. 105–112. Amsterdam: IOS Press.

[9] Carpenter B. (1992). The logic of typed feature structures. *Cambridge Tracts in Theoretical Computer Science.* Cambridge University Press, Cambridge.

[10] Hockemeyer, C. & Albert, D. (2003). Adaptive eLearning and the Learning GRID. In P. Ritrovato, S. Salerno & M. Gaeta (Eds.), *1st LeGE-WG International Workshop on Educational Models for GRID Based Services*. Wiltshire, UK: British Computer Society.

[11] Plotnick, E. (2001). Concept Mapping: A Graphical System for Understanding the Relationship Between Concepts. *Teacher Librarian, 28*, 42–44.

[12] World Wide Web Consortium (2004). *Semantic Web.* http://www.w3c.org/2001/sw/ (Retrieved December 3, 2004).

[13] McIlraith, S. A., Plexousakis, D., & van Harmelen, F., editors (2004). The Semantic Web - ISWC 2004. *Lecture Notes in Computer Science, 2398.* New York: Springer.

Towards the Learning Grid
P. Ritrovato et al. (Eds.)
IOS Press, 2005

Reusability of eLearning Objects in the context of Learning Grids

Konrad WULF
High Performance Computing Center Stuttgart (HLRS), Stuttgart, Germany
Email: wulf@hlrs.de

Abstract. This paper examines the requirements for eLearning Object Metadata, in order to appropriately support pedagogic and economic goals as well as service oriented architectures like the Grid. The standard IEEE LOM is being tested against these requirements. In conclusion, it can be said that while current eLearning practices are well supported by the standard, the main insufficiencies concern a) the adequate description of ELOs that are services and not downloadable, self-contained programs and b) the commercial trading of ELOs.

Keywords. Reusability, eLearning, Standards, Metadata, eLearning Objects, Learning Grid, Grid Computing, requirements analysis, IEEE LOM, IMS Metadata

Introduction

The vision of an efficient and pedagogically effective European eLearning Grid Infrastructure, in my opinion, relies heavily on the reusability and - as a prerequisite - detectability of eLearning Objects. This is why this article takes a look at the requirements on the design of Metadata for such eLearning Objects. This analysis will then compare the requirements with a widely discussed standardization effort, namely IEEE LOM which is building on IMS Metadata and on work done by Ariadne and the Dublin Core Group.

1. Definition of an eLearning Object (ELO)

There are numerous definitions out there, but most of them have similar things in mind: eLearning Objects (ELOs) are chunks of teaching material that make sense on their own. The main purpose is the reuse in several different combinations within but also across organizational boundaries. This makes it sensible to include in the definition of an ELO the fact that it is tagged with meta information about it, so that it can be found by search engines. This is in-line with the practical definition of Muzio et al. and others (see 0). The aggregation level of an ELO can range from a "learning unit" to a "set of courses that lead to some kind of certificate".

Another important question is whether an ELO should be considered as a downloadable thing or as a service. As the new generation of Grids is based on service oriented architectures (see e.g. 0), it makes sense to regard the ELO as a service as the more general case whereas the downloadable thing - that is only executed on the client machine with no interaction with servers during execution time - represents one special case of it. The more general case will be used as working definition within this paper.

2. Requirements for Reusable eLearning Objects in a Learning Grid

2.1. Pedagogic Point of View

From a pedagogical perspective, the perfect eLearning process would be 1. responsive, 2. ubiquitous, 3. collaborative, 4. experiential, 5. contextualised and personalised.

Responsiveness is a basic requirement that is valid for all Software, but especially on distributed systems like the Web, delay and also reliability are important Quality of Service (QoS) issues that need to be taken care of in order to deliver good eLearning services. Latency in delivery of requested learning resources highly influences a learner's motivation (see 0). In many occasions, among other factors, the server side limitations lead to delay (see 0). So for an ELO with service character, information about the current server performance situation and how it is influenced by the execution of another instance of the ELO is valuable for determining not only the technical, but also the motivational quality of an ELO (R_ServicePerformance). This topic is closely related to the monitoring of Service Level Agreements (SLA), which is a big issue of its own. So in terms of practicability this information will have to be concise.

Ubiquity stands for the wish for accessibility at any time and from anywhere using a variety of devices. Ubiquity is potentially a central advantage of eLearning compared to classical class room teaching, as it enables new organisational patterns of learning. This implies that interoperability of protocols and data formats is essential, stressing also the need for standardized metadata.

Collaboration and group working can be very beneficial for the motivation of the learner. The sense of community, as well as the pure possibility to discuss open questions improves the performance of the learner, may it be that there is a mentor or may it be that there are fellow learners (see 0, pp.187-206). To natively integrate a collaboration tool, it seems sensible to specify such a thing in the metadata of an ELO – perhaps not on learning unit level, but surely on course level or higher. In the simplest case a chat room could be stated, or a mailing list (R_IntegratedCollaboration).

Experiential: The learning material should be highly interactive, so that the learner can make experiences through Learning by Doing (see 0, pp. 13-26). The learner should not only read texts (=> information transfer paradigm), but also use the information in a productive way by fulfilling some task so that he really understands. Thus, this requirement asks for possibilities of direct manipulation, feedback and the possibility of making mistakes. A requirement for ELO metadata derived from this is that we need some standardized indication of interactivity of a particular ELO (R_InteractivityDegree).

Contextualization and Personalization seems to be the most challenging of the requirements. It means that the learning system needs to know about the pre-knowledge of the learner, his ways and speed of learning etc. So once the Learning Management System (LMS) knows these details about the learner, how does its search engine find suitable ELOs? The answer is that metadata should contain information on the progression pace (R_ProgressionPace) and the assumed pre-knowledge (R_AssumedPreknowledge). **Figure 2** depicts the requirements derived from pedagogic goals.

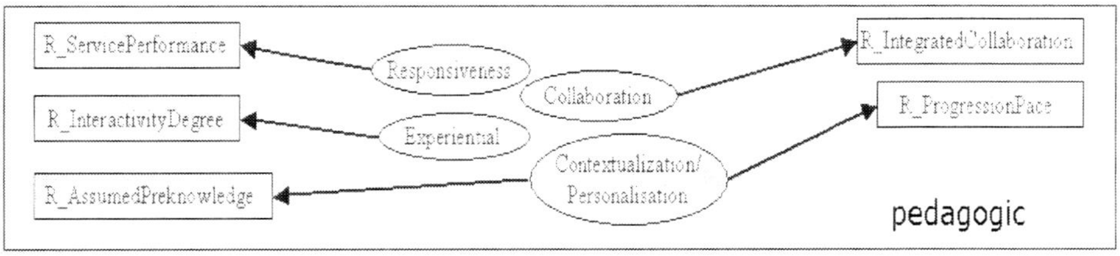

Figure 2: Requirements resulting from pedagogical goals

2.2. Economic Point of View

From an economic and enterprise point of view, the eLearning content should also be 1. cost-efficiently producible, 2. findable and 3. saleable.

Cost-efficiency: Cost-efficiency can be reached through either a) reducing the costs of production or b) through increasing the benefits. Concerning a) it can be said that up to now, the production is still very costly, as it usually implies several specialists working together: a didactical expert, a content expert and a programmer. In order for eLearning to be successful, it should be possible for a content expert to produce an ELO alone through appropriate tool support. Here, the description of the metadata of an ELO doesn't seem to influence this. But concerning b) metadata as such do increase the benefits by making reuse more probable. Depending on the design of the metadata, configurability, i.e. that the ELO can switch to different languages, different difficulty levels, allow input/ouput data etc. would additionally foster reuse (R_Configurability, see 0, pp. 8-12). Saleability, discussed below, can additionally increase the benefits that are achievable.

Findability: This requirement asks for ease of retrieving an ELO of the right quality. For Standard text formats such as ASCII, doc and PDF files searching is comparatively easy and good search engine have meanwhile been developed. The quality is thereby determined by popularity in terms of amount of referring links etc. But many pedagogically valuable ELOs are usually in a binary format, so good findability can only be achieved by standardized metatagging.

To determine the quality of an ELO, a Learning Management System might want to know the source of an ELO, as this can be an indicator. An ELO offered by MIT for example would be considered of higher quality than one offered by some unknown university (R_OriginIssuingInstitution). Different cultures also might have different understandings of particular subjects, so that another indicator for quality can be the country the ELO originates from (R_OriginCountry). Furthermore, an important factor in reality for signalling quality is certification. Also certification should be possible for ELOs (R_Certification), because we need a means of judging the overall quality of the content – whether the content is actually considered to be true, how well it is made etc. ELO meta information can be more reliable when certified by a third party authority.
Figure 3 illustrates the relations between the economic requirements as discussed in this section.

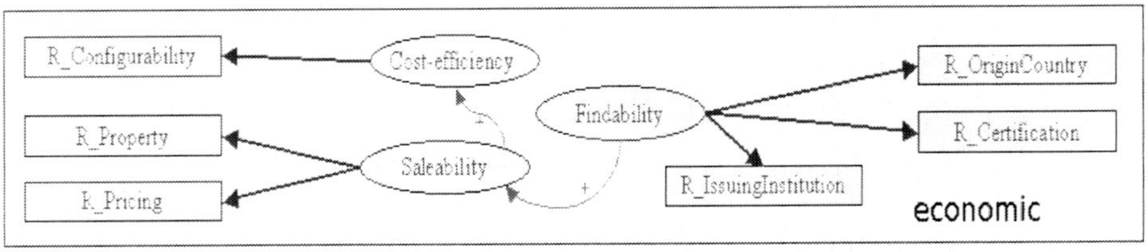

Figure 3: Economic requirements for ELO metatagging

Saleability: The requirement that an eLearning Object should be sellable in order to open up electronic market places, implies that it should be possible to protect intellectual property in the first place (R_Property, see also 0, p.7). This could be done for example by stating the copyright owner and sheltering the metadata from manipulation through e.g. encrypted checksums or watermarking. Moreover, it would be good if these eLearning Objects could already be labelled with a price, just like it can be encountered in the supermarket. Then a smooth pay by use via micro payment or similar could be used when the ELO is being requested and consumed in an open marketplace (R_pricing). It is worth noting that a free ELO is just a special case (price = 0) of the more general case (price >=0). Findability leverages saleability.

2.3. Limits to Reusability

Here, some general remarks about the limits to reusability will be made. These limits lead directly to some more requirements for the metadata.

First of all, the content that is to be delivered is nearly always tied to a language, so it is language specific and needs to be localized in order to be used in other language areas. This leads to the requirement R_Language.

Then an eLearning Object, if it is not static plain text only, has some data format that requires a complementary application, perhaps in a particular version, to access the content. This means the metadata need to specify necessary software (R_ReqSoftware). **Figure 4** depicts the limits to reusability, their origins and their relations.

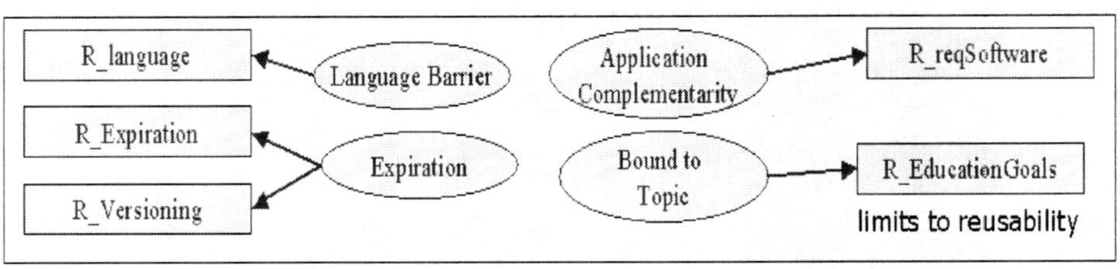

Figure 4: Limits to reusability of eLearning objects

ELOs are more or less time-bound. Sooner or later the learning material will not be "safe to use" anymore. This could be for technical reasons or because the contents simply is not valid or of interest anymore. Such expiration often cannot be forecasted. But there are some second-best indicators like the date of creation (R_Expiration) and whether a new version exists of the same ELO (R_Versioning).

At first sight trivial limit for reuse is, of course, that the topic of the ELO is only valuable if it serves a particular educational goal. But how do we know that without looking into the ELO itself? There must be some specification of the educational goals that the ELO helps to reach. A short description of the goals would help (R_EducationalGoals).

3. Analysis of the Existing Standard IEEE LOM

The IEEE Standard draft LOM is a unification effort of the US funded IMS and the EU funded ARIADNE project to merge and correlate their efforts in standardizing the metadata description of eLearning Objects (see 0 and 0). LOM is very similar to IMS Metadata. For the overall structure of IMS metadata and IEEE LOM that is being referred to, see Figure 5 in the Appendix.

Find in **Table 1** the results of the evaluation, in which IEEE LOM has been checked against the requirements that have been derived above:

Table 1: Checklist for IEEE LOM metadata format

Requirement	Judgment	Grp.
R_InteractivityDegree	☑ 5.1 Interactivity Type, 5.2 Learning Resource Type and 5.3 Interactivity Level together give a pretty good idea of the degree of interactivity of the ELO, using a closed and therefore well comparable taxonomy.	Educational Requirements
R_ProgressionPace	☑ 5.4 Semantic Density (5 points linear scale), together with 5.6- 5.8 should make it easy for search engines to find an ELO according to a learner's progression pace.	
R_AssumedPreknowledge	☑ 5.6 Context, 5.7 Typical Age Range, 5.8 Difficulty indicate the target audience using precise values out of an enumeration.	
R_ ServicePerformance	☒ In 4 Technical, no suitable entry space is designated.	
R_ IntegratedCollaboration	☒ In 4 Technical, no suitable entry space is designated.	
R_Property	☒ No answer to the difficult question as to how to protect the property from being copied and manipulated. In 6.2 and 6.3 it is possible to specify copyright and license conditions, but there are no standard license terms to choose from and a search engine will have a hard time isolating the copyright holder from the free text merged containing license conditions and the copyright holder.	Economic Requirements
R_Pricing	☒ 6.1 Cost specifies only whether the use (what kind of usage?) will be for free or not. Why not specify the price right away, with price=0 being "no cost"?	
R_IssuingInstitution	☑☒ 2.3 Contribute and 6.3 Description will give a pretty good impression about the source of an ELO, although it might not be concise enough.	
R_OriginCountry	☑☒ is NOT an extra item with enumeration values, but usually to be read (between the lines) from 2.3 Contribute	
R_Certification	☒ there is no slot for third party certification Information for indication of good quality	
R_Configurability	☒ In 4 Technical, no suitable entry space is designated.	
R_Language	☑ 1.3 Language: following ISO 639:1988 and ISO 3166-1:1997.	Requirements

R_ReqSoftware	☑☒ 4.1 Format in MIME type and 4.4 Requirement defines necessary other resources, but there is no unique taxonomy for these.	
R_Expiration	☑☒ 2.3.3 Date helps judging the "freshness", but does not help distinguishing between more or less durable ELO content.	
R_Versioning	☑ 2.1 Version allows for a check on whether you are working with the latest version	
R_educationGoals	☑ 1.4 Description: this is primarily for the user to judge, but no standard taxonomy is being used. 1.5 Keyword + 1.6 Coverage: this together with 1.4 can give indications for the search engine.	

The checklist in **Table 1** shows the results of testing LOM against the requirements. In summary, it can be said that the educational needs can be met to a wide extent using this specification. Those "educational" requirements that are not fulfilled come down to rather technical specifications that are missing and arise when ELOs are being thought of as services. The limits for reusability can also be told fairly well, although it would be desirable that the required resources (4.4) would be supplied in a more standard way (enumeration), in order to be better comparable. Also, judging the validity of content in terms of time – whether an ELO is outdated – still is an issue that is not really satisfactory solved (due to the nature of the problem). R_Configurability, here derived from economic goals, could also be seen as a limit for reusability. This limit could be widened up by allowing entries about setup choices and interfaces, which hasn't found its way into the specification, yet.

What is not adequately addressed at all, are some basic economic requirements, if the possibility of an electronic market on the level of ELOs shall be opened up through using this standard. The usual indicators for high quality can not or only insufficiently be provided. Then the problem of protection of intellectual property is not even being addressed. Finally, and this is quite simple, there is no slot allocated for specifying prices for different kinds of usages.

4. Conclusion

As this analysis has shown, the IEEE Standard LOM addresses many requirements appropriately and therefore is a good starting point for the development of eLearning Grids. But some major improvements will have to be made concerning the support of delivery of high quality ELO services. Moreover, if the ELO material is to be bought and sold, usually across organizational entities, the specification really needs some profound improvement, regarding the protection of property, pricing, definition of usage patterns / standard licenses, and signaling of certified quality.

References

[1] El Saddik, A. et al. (2001). Reusability and Adaptability of Interactive Resources In Web-Based Educational Systems. ACM Journal of Educational Resources in Computing, 1(1), Article #4, 1-19 (http://portal.acm.org/citation.cfm?id=376699).

[2] Foster, I. et al. (2002). Grid Services for Distributed System Integration. Computer, 35(6), 37-46. (http://www.globus.org/research/papers/ieee-cs-2.pdf)

[3] IMS Global Learning Consortium, Inc. (2001). IMS Learning Resource Meta-Data Information Model - Version 1.2.1 Final Specification. (http://www.imsglobal.org/metadata/)
[4] Learning Technology Standards Committee of the IEEE (2002). Draft Standard for Learning Object Metadata. (http://ltsc.ieee.org/wg12/files/LOM_1484_12_1_v1_Final_Draft.pdf)
[5] Muzio, J. et al. (2001). Experiences with Reusable eLearning Objects: From Theory to Practice. Centre for Economic Development and Applied Research (CEDAR), Royal Roads University, Victoria, BC, Canada. (http://www.cedarlearning.com/CL/elo/eLearningObjects_sml.pdf)
[6] Ramsay, J., A. Barbesi, and J. Preece, (1998) A psychological investigation of long retrieval times on the World Wide Web. Interacting with Computers, 10(10), 77-86.
[7] Ruddle, A. et al.(2002). Determining the Sources of Delay in a Distributed Learning Environment. Proceedings of 1st LEGE-WG International Workshop on Educational Models for Grid Based Services, Lausanne, CH, 16 September, eWiC (http://ewic.bcs.org/conferences/2002/1stlege/session3/paper2.htm).
[8] Schank, R. (2001). Designing World-Class E-Learning : How IBM, GE, Harvard Business School, And Columbia University Are Succeeding At E-Learning. McGraw-Hill, New York

Appendix

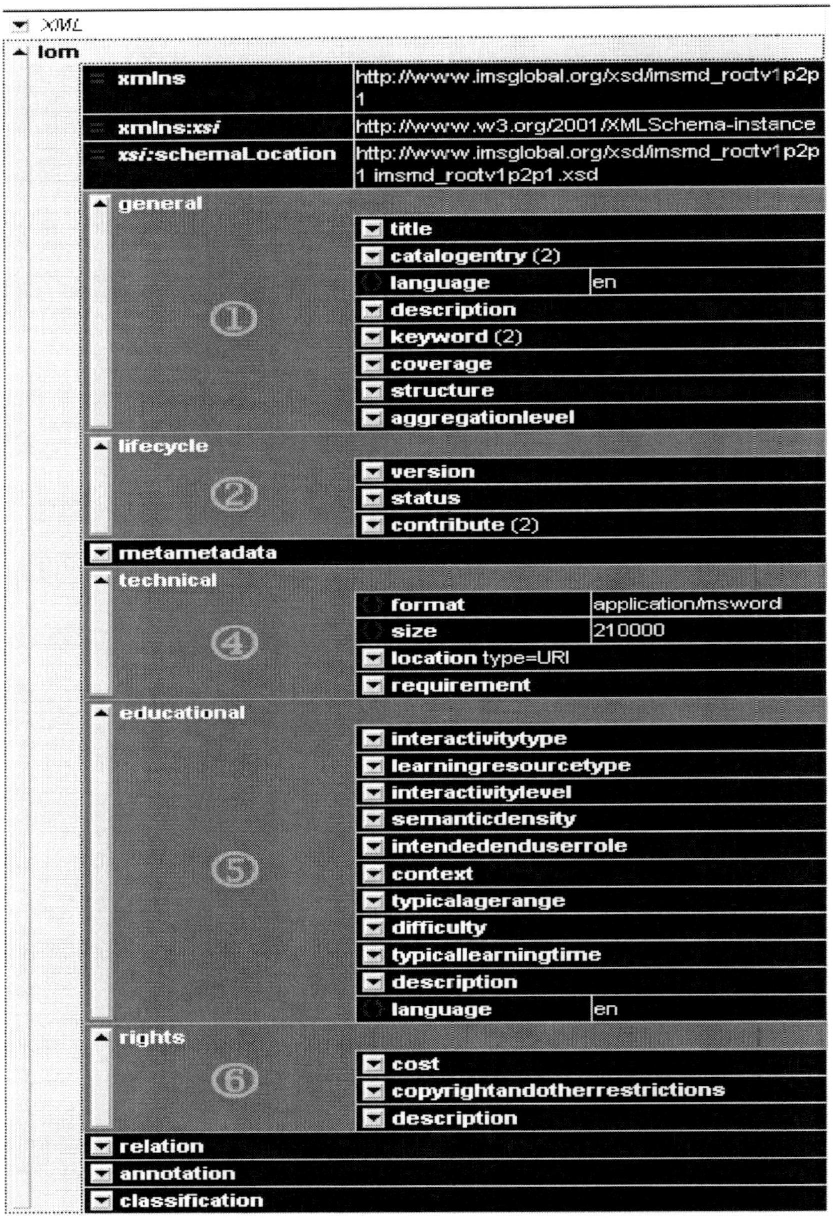

Figure 5. The overall structure of IMS metadata / IEEE LOM

Part C

Holistic Services

Towards the Learning Grid
P. Ritrovato et al. (Eds.)
IOS Press, 2005

Design Considerations for an ELeGI Portal

Colin ALLISON[a,25], Rosa MICHAELSON[b]
[a]*School of Computer Science, University of St Andrews*
[b]*Department of Accountancy and Business Finance, University of Dundee.*

Abstract. ELeGI, the European Learning Grid Infrastructure, has the ambitious goal of fostering effective learning and knowledge construction through the dynamic provision of service-based contextualised and personalised learning environments. The success of this venture will depend to a considerable extent on the usability of such environments, and their usability in turn will depend on a successful strategy for the dynamic integration and maintenance of sets of services. The concept of the portal is therefore of considerable interest, as it is often portrayed as a means whereby a user can access an integrated set of related information and services. This paper reviews the portal concept with a view to its suitability as a design basis for enabling technology that will address usability concerns. The paper proceeds by summarising the usability requirements of learning environments, reviewing some of the ideas currently associated with different types of portals (enterprise portals, institutional portals, user-centric portals, Grid portals), and concludes by deriving a taxonomy of portal characteristics against which the usability requirements of ELeGI can be assessed.

Introduction: Usability in Learning Environments

A Learning Environment (LE) in ELeGI refers to the use of a dynamically integrated set of distributed services that are used directly by learners and teachers for educational purposes. Following the holistic approach taken to Quality of Service (QoS) in [1], Fig. 1 depicts usability requirements within a broader LE architecture.

Firstly, major roles are identified with respect to a LE: institutions, teachers, learners, subject-specialists, service operators, content and service providers. Secondly, appropriate abstractions are determined by requirements analysis of each role, and groups of LE actors. Note that this approach also supports evolution of novel learning scenarios through continuous re-analysis of the principal roles and requirements, and as LEs evolve with changes in pedagogy and advances in technology. When this is done we can evaluate usability for learners from two viewpoints: i) the extent to which the LE middleware can dynamically realise usability features on top of a particular low-level infrastructure context; and ii) the extent to which the actual end-user access points can deliver these features. While the OGSA framework appears ideal for the research, development and deployment of LE middleware, it does not directly address user interface and usability issues per se. Therefore it must be complemented by a user interface management methodology and set of mechanisms, and this is exactly where the portal concept is of particular interest.

[25] Corresponding Author: Colin Allison, School of Computer Science, University of St Andrews, Scotland KY16 9SS; e-mail: ca@st-andrews.ac.uk

Usability Features	Abstractions for Learning Environment actors	**Teachers**	Users and Groups Management, Educational Resource Selection and Allocation, Activity Monitoring, Session scheduling
		Learners	Interactivity, Groupwork, High quality simulations, Real-world input, Self-Reflection Facilities, Privacy
		Content and Service Providers	Developers Application and Service Interface
		Service Operators	Manageability, Usage feedback, QoS Feedback
	Interface Accessibility	W3C Accessibility Guidelines Output formatted appropriately for interface device	
LE Middleware and QoS	Sharing, Sessions, Security, Concurrency, Availability, Replication, Distribution, Coherence, Responsiveness, Timeliness, Interoperability, Resource Management, Resource Discovery and Location, Security, Identity Management		
Low-level Infrastructure	Network Protocols, Operating Systems, Client-Server, Peer-to-Peer, Mobile Services, Authentication Authorities		
	Physical Networks, Computers, and Interface Devices		

Figure 1. Usability Features within ELeGI Learning Environment Support Architecture

1. The Portal Concept

The general purpose of a portal is to provide a single access point to a range of related information and services. It is widely used by commercial public web-based service providers in order to reduce the time that individuals spend searching, although it only promotes options that are commercially sponsored. Such portals sometimes offer facilities for personal customisation – for example, a user can specify an interest in specific types of sporting events or the local weather forecast. Examples of this approach include MyYahoo!, Lycos and MyNetscape [2-4]. However, the customisation options are very limited and, most often, these types of portal cater for anonymous users.

In contrast, the Enterprise portal is a non-public portal, which provides a type of shared corporate desktop customised for each employee. In a recent survey [5] of the US commercial sector 87% of the respondents believed that enterprise style portals would "eventually constitute the main window through which users are able to access multiple, heterogeneous software applications, along with relevant content and analysis." This type of portal is usually the front-end for an application server, which integrates various company databases and applications. While enterprise portals are customised to some extent for employees, this is mostly along the lines of which department or project they are working in/on.

In the education domain the concept of the Institutional portal is attracting attention. This is expanded and expounded in [6] where it is argued that (unlike the Enterprise portal) such a portal must be non-proprietary and under the full control of the institution it represents. The 2003 survey of the U.S. Campus Computing Project has documented the growth of institutions that have Web-based campus portals from

21.2 percent in 2002 to 28.4 percent in 2003 [7]. The institutional portal distinguishes three main content-oriented views of the institutional information base: hierarchical web pages, audience web pages and the personal web portal.

Hierarchical pages are designed for anonymous, casual visitors, and are generally read-only with limited query facilities. They may be searched and traversed according to a number of themes: studying at the University, Research at the University, and so on. Many institutions already provide this type of view.

Audience pages are targeted at specific groups such as existing students, alumni, academic staff, technical staff, and so on. Access may be restricted via an allocated password. The tenor is still predominantly read-only, but facilities such as chat and e-mail exchange may be provided. Several institutions offer this type of web service.

Personal pages are intended to go much further than the audience pages by specifically targeting each individual. This is rarely provided at present, and represents a non-trivial technical challenge.

The combination of these three views mandates a common portal reference framework. uPortal is one such framework. It is an Open Source software product sponsored by the Java in Administration Special Interest Group JA-SIG [8]. MyOneStop [9] and MyBytes [10] also claim to address this need. In the UK Higher Education sector several Universities have recently rallied round the uPortal flag [11] and abandoned efforts to create their own extensible portal technology, or to adapt proprietary commercial products.

Finally, the portal concept has been developed and exploited by Grid developers since 1997. Examples include many subject-specific portals built with the Grid Portal Developers Kit[12], and the Gridport toolkit [13]. The abundance of Grid portals is evidence of what is explicitly acknowledged in most Grid communities – that having sophisticated middleware and formidable low-level computational and network infrastructure is pointless if facilities cannot be accessed and utilised in a convenient and intuitive fashion. So, to a large extent, the take-up of Grid technologies beyond a relatively small group of users who are au fait with pseudo-cryptic job control commands and scripting languages is dependent on the development and deployment of useable interfaces, and this is what is expected from portals. Grid portals to date however have been built to support clearly identifiable communities from toolkits. They do not appear to offer the flexibility of uPortal, which can change its appearance and functionality in response to requirements without involving low-level toolkit programming.

2. Being User-Centric

As previously noted, a significant technical challenge for portal frameworks is the support of usability through relevance – that is, the production of a "personal portal" which is dynamically tailored and maintained for each individual. We refer to such portals as user-centric as they are built entirely around the identity of the user. In the traditional, institution-based, educational domain a user-centric portal should gather and present all the information and services necessary for the lecturer, based on their institutional roles. Similarly, a student should find only information that is relevant to their academic work. MMS [14] is an example of a role-based user-centric portal that has been built to operate in a traditional educational institution environment. An example MMS scenario is shown in Figure 2.

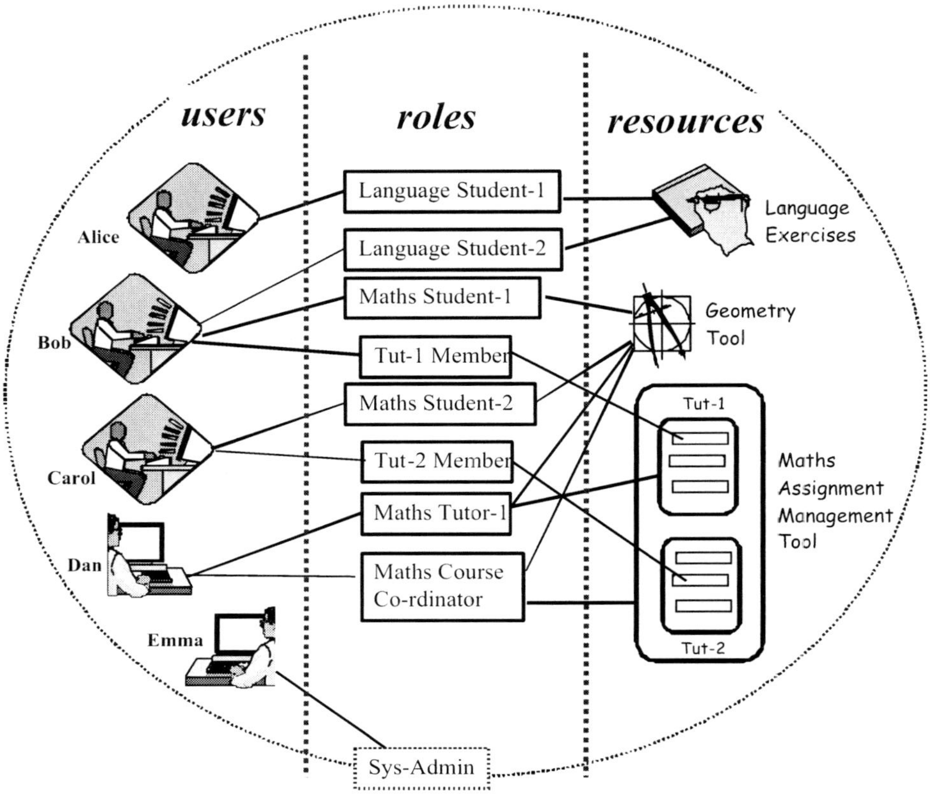

Figure 2. Role-based User-centric Views

In Fig. 2 each user has their own LE. This simple example scenario features five users: three students, an academic staff member, and a systems administrator.

- Alice is only taking a language module and only sees a set of interactive language exercises.
- Bob is taking Languages and Maths. He sees the same language exercises as Alice, a Geometry tool, and an assignment management tool for handing in work, and receiving marks.
- Carol is only taking Maths. She sees the Geometry Tool, plus her own part of the assignment manager.
- Dan is both a Course Co-ordinator and a Maths Tutor. He takes Tutorial Group Tut-1. He sees the Geometry Tool, a view of assignments limited to his own tutorial group, and also a view of the whole class, useful for a course co-ordinator.
- Emma is a systems administrator, and can, in principle see anything in the combined set of LEs. This does not preclude a resource type from providing its own privacy mechanisms.

The customised view delivered to each user in Fig.2 is based on their roles, and the qualification of the relationships between these roles and resources, based on the privileges associated with each role, and the user's identity. User-centric portal generation and maintenance is a key component of MMS, and a relatively advanced example of personalised customisation within an educational domain. MMS is based on earlier work carried out by the TAGS [15] and INSIDE [16] projects. It does not in itself fulfil the needs of ELeGI, but is an important contributing technology.

3. A Taxonomy of Portal Characteristics

The portal concept is not precise, and there are quite different approaches visible in the categories briefly reviewed in this paper – public portals, Grid portals, enterprise portals, institutional portals, user-centric portals.

Table 1 outlines a taxonomy of portal characteristics which provides a common framework for comparing different portals and portal frameworks. Space limitations preclude a complete set of comparisons, but the right hand column is used to note where a feature is likely to be of particular value to an ELeGI portal. Note that the starred items are pre-Grid features.

Table 1. Characterising a Portal

Portal Feature	**Commentary**	**ELeGI?**
Customised for the user	The portal recognises the user and accesses a profile to determine what types of services and information is relevant for them, and possibly other preferences such as presentation format.	Y
Customisable by the user	The user may: i) select from optional services and content; ii) choose a GUI look and feel; iii) organise a preferred layout.	Y
Anonymous access	Part of the portal vision is a way of evolving existing institutional web sites, so an anonymous visitor is presented with significant chunks of information, hierarchically organised, as is presently done in most public institutional web sites.	Y
Anonymous subscription	An anonymous user can request an account and create their own username and password. They may be able to subscribe to e-mail notifications of specific types of event, or partake in group activity. This is not generally supported by current institutional web sites.	Y
Single Sign-on	A user can use their institutional username and password, or certificate, to access the portal. All subsequent accesses to information and services within the portal are then trusted as the portal handles the authentication and access control issues.	Y
Application Server (Implied Read-Write)	The Enterprise portal is seen as a means of controlling access to approved corporate software, data and schemata. In contrast to most web sites, which offer basic HTML supported interaction options, portals offer genuine two-way, read-write access to services and data repositories.	Y
Content Aggregation	Content is regularly copied and updated from diverse information sources. These may be existing web sites, databases, online directories and so on. It may be copied as low-level data and then extensively formatted for presentation in the portal.	N*
Content Proxy	Rather than copying, re-organising, formatting and presenting data from external sources (as is the case with content aggregation), the portal maintains a dynamic link, as an inline frame under a tab, from an external source, typically a web site.	N
Content Referral	This is the simplest and least impressive portal capability: a standard hyperlink or URL.	N*

Support for Multiple Device Interfaces	Can the portal recognise or adapt its output to interface devices other than the standard web browser? For example, handheld computers and mobile phones.	Y
W3C Access compliant	Does the portal ensure that the organisation, formatting and presentation is consistent with W3C recommended access guidelines? Failure to do so may disadvantage users with special needs, and may contravene legislation.	Y
Sole point of access to information services	Something of a holy grail, and more than a little paradoxical. If a portal is being used as an integration mechanism, can it also expect to supplant all the other existing front-ends to diverse information services and content repositories? The problem about a portal trying to sell itself as a "one-stop-shop" is that unless it really is, it is simply another manifestation of the problem it claims to be solving.	Y
Secure	As the portal may provide access to private, or sensitive, or licensed information and services, security of access is seen as essential. Indeed, most countries have some form of legislation that places a duty of reasonable care on service provider who holds personal data.	Y

4. Conclusion

Usability without usefulness is pointless. A crucial usability feature of an LE interface is the relevance of the content and services it provides for each user. This means that the content and services delivered must be constructed, and then maintained dynamically, around the identity of each user, in their current context. ELeGI portal technology aims to combine personal profiles with middleware services to ensure that only relevant content and services are delivered to the end-user, in the appropriate format for their current interface device. This is a significant technical challenge. Fortunately, methodologies and mechanisms for building Grid portals and User-centric portals have been made extant through design and implementation experience in projects such as TAGS, INSIDE and Gridport, and this work provides a solid foundation for meeting the challenge that lies ahead.

References

[1] Allison, C., et al. (2001) An Holistic View of Quality of Service. Interactive Learning Environments. 9(1).
[2] Yahoo (2003) www.yahoo.com/.
[3] MyNetscape (2003) my.netscape.com/.
[4] Lycos (2003) www.lycos.com/.
[5] Buxbaum, P.A. (2002) "It's difficult to get a clear view of portal concept". searchebusiness.techtarget.com/originalContent/0,289142,sid19_gci779661,00.html.
[6] Gleason, B.W. (2001) Institutional Information Portal Key to Web Application Integration. crayfish.mis.udel.edu/maria/uportal/whitepaper2001.pdf. JA-SIG.
[7] CCP (2003) Campus Computing Project, National Survey of Information Technology in US Higher Education. www.campuscomputing.net/.
[8] JA-SIG (2003) http://www.ja-sig.org/.
[9] MyOneStop (2003) https://myonestop.umn.edu/mos/PortalGeneric.jsp.
[10] MyBytes (2003) www.mybytes.com.
[11] Kraan, W. (2002) Open uPortal technology gains ground in the UK, CETIS. www.cetis.ac.uk/content/20021126163827.
[12] Novotny, J. (2002) The Grid Portal Development Kit. Concurrency and Computation: Practice and Experience. 14(13-15): p. 1129-1144.
[13] Thomas, M., et al. (2001) The GridPort Toolkit Architecture for Building Grid Portals. in 10th IEEE Intl. Symposium on High Performance Distributed Computing. August 2001. IEEE.
[14] Allison, C., et al. (2003) MMS: A User Centric Portal for eLearning. in 14th Intl. Workshop on Database and Expert Systems Applications. August, 2003. Prague, Czech Republic: IEEE CS.

[15] Allison, C., et al. (2000) The TAGS Framework for Web-Based Learning Environments. in Web Based Learning Environments. June 2000. Portugal: University of Porto, FEUP Editions.
[16] Allison, C., et al. (2003) Addressing Academic Needs in Managed Learning Environments. in 4th Annual LTSN-ICS Conference. August, 2003. Galway, Ireland.

Towards the Learning Grid
P. Ritrovato et al. (Eds.)
IOS Press, 2005

An e-Learning Platform for SME Manager Upgrade and its Evolution Toward a Distributed Training Environment

Nicola Capuano, Matteo Gaeta*, Laura Pappacena

CRMPA Centro di Ricerca in Matematica Pura ed Applicata
C/O DIIMA – Università degli Studi di Salerno
Via Ponte Don Melillo – 84084 Fisciano (SA), Italia

**Dipartimento di Ingegneria dell'Informazione e Matematica Applicata*
Università degli Studi di Salerno
Via Ponte Don Melillo – 84084 Fisciano (SA), Italia

gaeta@diima.unisa.it, {capuano, pappacena}@crmpa.unisa.it

Abstract. The purpose of this paper is to describe the work related to the customisation, the trial and the evaluation of an innovative e-learning platform for manager upgrade in Small and Medium Enterprises (SME), in the framework of the EC funded project named InTraServ and its re-engineering process, aimed at adopting distributed services in the framework of another EC funded project named Diogene. The presented e-learning environment includes several state-of-the-art technologies and methodologies such as: metadata and ontologies for knowledge manipulation, fuzzy learner modelling, intelligent course tailoring, case based reasoning, business games and simulation tools. The proposed evolution is based on the distribution of working tasks among content provider services, content discovery services, content brokering services, training services, curriculum vitae searching services and collaboration services.

Keywords. e-Learning, Web Services, Distributed Environments

Introduction

The managerial capacity paradigm argues that a firm's growth is limited by the speed at which it can expand its managerial capacity. This is generally true and it is truer for Small and Medium Enterprises (SME) that often do not have a well defined managerial structure causing, in many cases, strategic and decisional lacks that obstruct the enterprise's growth.

The learning task for managers is thus a critical element for the survival and the success of the SME in the global competitive scenery. As quoted in [1] the key challenges to be addressed to satisfy SME training needs concern: distance, time and location (training must serve a dispersed group of learners where and when they require it), flexibility (training can be undertaken between work tasks), availability (training material can be easily located), immediacy (user can obtain quickly solutions to daily working problems).

Starting from these considerations, the EC funded project InTraServ [2] arranged a completely innovative e-learning platform purposed to face and solve these and further issues. The InTraServ project was concluded in May 2003 after an experimentation phase carried out in several SMEs from Italy, UK and Spain.

A further EC funded project named Diogene [3] ended in October 2004 was purposed to completely re-engineer the architecture of the InTraServ e-learning platform by applying a distributed computing paradigm based on Web Services. This allowed the distribution of training content on different servers, the integration with the forthcoming Semantic Web, the cooperation of different installations of the system, the possibility to create a training offer by combining resources offered by different providers, etc. In this sense it was a step toward Grid architecture.

The paper is organised as follows: the InTraServ project will be briefly described and its main features introduced (section 2). A sketch of the system architecture will be also presented (section 3) and the new service oriented architecture realised in Diogene will be introduced (section 4). Some conclusions (section 5) and references will follow.

1. What's InTraServ

InTraServ [2] is an EC "Trial" project funded within the 5th Framework Programme, whose purpose was to customise, try and evaluate an innovative Web-based intelligent e-learning solution for manager upgrading in real SME environments operating in different fields.

Using the InTraServ solution, it is possible for a manager to take personalised training between working tasks (on-the-job), to evaluate the acquired formal knowledge and to transform it into practical knowledge by experimenting what already learnt in simulated situations. When, finally, the manager masters such knowledge, he can apply it inside the organisation. Moreover, using InTraServ, a manager can be supported during his decision making process (just-in-time) by exploiting the CBR-based real case solver component.

The InTraServ e-learning platform is ready and accessible through the InTraServ portal [2]. It includes four courses (Business Decision, Marketing Management, Marketing Research and Management Control) available in three languages (Italian, English and Spanish) and several Business Games (BGs). The following paragraphs briefly describe its innovative features with respect to commercial e-learning platforms currently on the scene.

1.1. Metadata and Ontologies for Knowledge Management

All InTraServ learning material is organised in learning objects (LO) indexed through IMS compliant metadata [4] in order to let the system know what each of them is about and how it can be used during the learning process.

Also, to provide information about LO relations and interdependency, InTraServ applies ontologies [5] allowing to design abstract and simplified views of training domains. Within InTraServ, the ontologies are used to define and relate concepts of a training domain to four kinds of relations: (is_part_of, requires, suggested order and explains) and, also, to link concepts to LOs [6], [7].

1.2. Fuzzy Learner Modelling

InTraServ infers and maintains a learner model compliant with the IMS-LIP standard [8] composed by a cognitive state and a set learning preferences. The cognitive state stores, for each concept of a specified training domain, the knowledge degree reached by the learner, represented as a set of fuzzy numbers [9] (allowing, in this way, to manage uncertainty in the evaluation process).

Learning preferences, instead, include all information about learner cognitive abilities and perceptive capabilities i.e. to which typology of resources a specified learner is more receptive [6], [7].

1.3. Intelligent Course Tailoring

An InTraServ course is composed of a user's selected set of learning goals (key concepts that the learner has to learn) and of a learning path (a sequence of learning objects that has to be used to provide a specific learner with all necessary knowledge to fully understand the chosen goals).

Different learners can require different paths to learn the same goals depending on their learner models. For this reason, InTraServ provides an automatic curriculum generation procedure: the learner can choose what to learn (goals) and let the system organise a suitable personalised learning path to him. Such path can change dynamically during the learning process, adapting to the learner's needs in relation to the learner's performed activities [6], [7].

1.4. Case Based Reasoning

InTraServ gives learners the possibility to solve daily working problems by exploiting a CBR methodology [10] i.e. through a sub-system able to solve new cases comparing the current problem with similar solved problems in a case base and ranking found solutions.

Moreover, the system is able to extend its knowledge by interpreting a new solution in the light of similar situations and abstracting generalisations out from experiences. The strength of this approach to the problem solving is that the knowledge base is maintained as concrete problem descriptions. In this way the system maintenance could be made by a domain expert rather than a system expert.

1.5. Business Games and Simulation Tools

An important InTraServ feature is the possibility to use a set of advanced simulation tools addressing the business decision process through a "what…if" approach. They refer to a particular learning process phase called "interactive phase": after a learner studies the theory related to a specific topic, he/she can use such tools to exercise about the learned topics.

Nevertheless a simulation exercise is quite different from a classical exercise: it is based on simulation models that allow a concrete experience to be built up by the experimentation and modification of hypotheses that play a role inside the system under examination [11].

2. InTraServ Architecture: the monoITH

The main idea behind the InTraServ architecture is that any e-learning application should be supported by a general infrastructure that would put a set of common resources at everyone's disposal and, according to the specific needs of each training domain and application, by a set of further specific resources.

For this reason, the InTraServ architecture, despite customised for the management training domain, is totally adaptable and extensible and can be the ground for the realisation of a virtually infinite set of specific e-learning platforms suitable for any needs, context and domain.

Moreover, the InTraServ architecture (see sketch in figure 1), thanks to a strong separation of tasks between different components, was an ideal starting point to realise a distributed architecture as depicted in the next section.

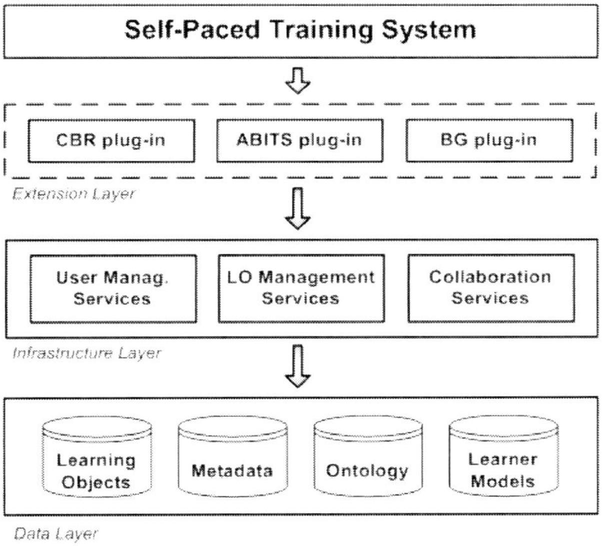

Figure 1. The InTraServ Architecture.

As seen, the InTraServ e-learning platform architecture is divided into four layers: Data, Infrastructure, Extension and Self-Paced Training System.

The Data layer stores all persistent information related to used data structures: Learning Objects, Metadata, Ontologies and Learner Models (see section 2).

The Infrastructure layer contains, instead, all general-purpose e-learning services as described below.

- **User Management Services**: allow registration and logging and provide all user and groups management functions including profiles handling;
- **Learning Objects Management Services**: provide all functions to manage LOs, Metadata and related Ontologies (including access rights handling) and to index and retrieve LOs basing on associated Metadata and Ontologies.
- **Collaboration Services**: include synchronous (text and visual chat) and asynchronous (messaging system and threaded discussion forum) tools for collaboration between users.

The Extension layer, moreover, allows adding at any time new specific domain or context dependent services through the implementation of plug-ins compliant to the system specifications. Three plug-ins have been included in the InTraServ Extension layer:

- the Case Based Reasoning (CBR) plug-in that is responsible for case bases reasoning functions (see 2.4);

- the Agent Based Intelligent Tutoring System (ABITS) plug-in that is responsible for "intelligent" training functions (see 2.1, 2.2, 2.3 and [7]);
- the Business Games (BG) plug-in that allows exploiting business games as a particular type of LOs (see 2.5).

Finally, the Self-Paced Training System layer includes the front-end related to an instance of the e-learning system (geared toward manager upgrading in SME in the case of the InTraServ project) and allows a filtered access to resources and services provided by the layers below. This layer is obtained via the customisation of a general Web Portal: a dynamic container of panels that give access to underlying services and resources.

The InTraServ e-learning platform has been entirely realised in the Microsoft .NET environment [12], using the ASP.NET language (for the front-end) and the C# language (for the back-end). Main functions have been wrapped in Web Services in order to allow a standard invocation on the Web from external applications.

3. Diogene Architecture: the Virtual Organisation for Learning

The InTraServ architecture is well structured and suitable for extensions with new services, and easily customisable for new training contexts and domains. Nevertheless, it is quite monolithic: it doesn't allow the distribution of training content on different servers, the cooperation of different installations of the system, the possibility to combine training resources offered by different providers, etc.

For this and more reasons, in the framework of another project named Diogene, we completely re-thought the InTraServ architecture in order to allow the distribution of training resources based on Web Services.

Diogene [3] is an EC funded project aimed at design, implementing and evaluating with real users an e-learning Web brokering environment for ICT individual training, able to support learners during the whole cycle of the training, from the definition of objectives to the assessment of results through the construction of custom courses.

The e-learning system that was realised under Diogene uses some InTraServ state-of-the-art technologies like metadata and ontologies for knowledge manipulation, fuzzy learner modelling, intelligent course tailoring but, also, includes a set of innovative features such as dynamic learning strategies, Semantic Web openness, Web services for Learning Object handling and IPR management, Curriculum Vitae generation, maintenance and searching facilities, free-lance teachers support and assisted Learning Objectives definition.

The architecture of Diogene is sketched in figure 2. As it can be seen, it partially derives from the InTraServ architecture in the distribution of tasks among component/services.

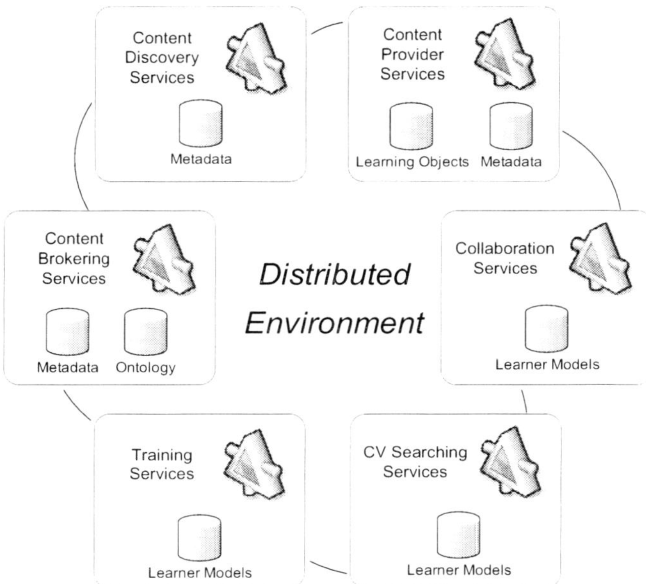

Figure 2 – The Diogene Architecture.

The meaning of the mentioned Diogene training services is described below.

- **Content Provider Services**. They are installed in content provider organisations and are used to host training content and provide a standard SOAP-based interface [12] to allow remote access to it. They provide search and retrieval functions on the local repository via metadata-based queries and are able to perform e-commerce transactions between users requesting content and the provider organisation itself to buy the access to content for limited periods of time. They are an extended version of the InTraServ Learning Objects Management Services.
- **Content Discovery Services**. They are able to extract training content directly from the Web of the present and future generation (Semantic Web). Through a keyword-based text categorisation algorithm they are able, where absent, to automatically extract metadata from textual learning objects and to link them to ontology concepts. Through a mixed approach based on keyword and ontologies, moreover, they are able to bypass compatibility problems between different ontological representations of the same domain.
- **Content Brokering Services**. They are broker of training content. They maintain indexes of learning objects of registered Content Provider and Discovery Services and allow users to use metadata- and ontology-based queries to find the right provider with the right content. They include, also, some course tailoring capabilities (see 2.3) to generate ad-hoc courses by assembling the content from registered Content Provider and Discovery Services.
- **Training Services**. They are responsible for the courses delivery and for the provision of course management and execution functions. Moreover, they deal with "intelligent" training functions such as learner modelling, course tailoring, assisted objective definition and learning strategies upgrading. They do not

maintain any local training content but strictly interact with Content Brokering Services or directly with Content Discovery and Provider Services to obtain and combine learning objects. They include and extend the InTraServ Self Paced Training System plus the User management Services and the ABITS plug-in.

- **CV Searching Services**. They provide search engine capabilities on Learner Models Databases of registered Training Services in order to let third parties interested to hire certified staff to find qualified professional (with respect to privacy requirements). They maintain, moreover, statistics of received requests in order to rank required competencies.
- **Collaboration Services**. They support social interactions, mentoring and information exchange by providing users with a set of collaborative synchronous and asynchronous facilities. They are able to automatically arrange groups among users of registered Training Services by individuating and grouping learners with similar needs and/or profiles. They are an extension of InTraServ Collaboration Services.

The following figure depicts possible interactions between multiple instances of Diogene services hosted by different organisations. They constitute the Distributed Training Environment (DTE) of Diogene.

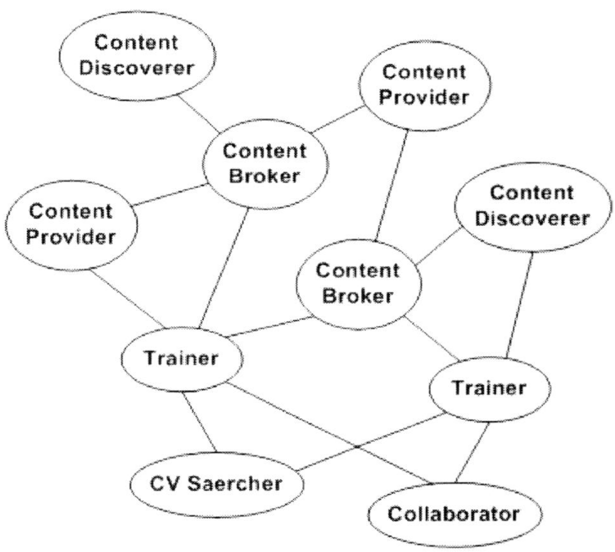

Figure 3 – Interactions Among Diogene Services.

It's obvious that the distributed architecture designed for Diogene presents several advantages with respect to the InTraServ centralised architecture.

- The maintenance of Learning Objects on content provider servers allows content provider organizations to manage and organize content locally, and, in the same time, to overcome property right related problems.
- The networking of different content provider servers filtered through content brokers allows composing training offer, aggregating content from different providers in order to best match user's needs.
- The Web is full of training content and the forthcoming Semantic Web paradigm will make it semantically understandable by machines. Content

Discovery Services exploit such power to find useful and freeware learning material and to make it available to the DTE.

- The collaboration between peers is of paramount importance to improve the training experience. Collaboration Services are able to find on the whole DTE (rather than on a single installation of the training service) learners with similar interests and to put them in contact within a co-operative environment.
- Learner models contain useful data about the know-how of students and their acquired competencies: CV Searching Services are able to find qualified professionals all over the DTE and to put them in contact with hiring companies.

4. Conclusions

In this paper we have described the e-learning platform realised within the framework of an EC funded project named InTraServ, its innovative features, its architecture and the evolution of such architecture toward a distributed services paradigm (more suitable for a Grid environment) in the context of another EC funded project named Diogene.

The InTraServ project started in December 2001 and ended in May 2003. The experimentation phase with about 20 managers of Italian, English and Spanish SMEs was carried out and gave very positive results [13]. Besides the InTraServ project, CRMPA decided to experiment the realised e-learning platform also in several Italian academic contexts (University of Salerno, University of Roma Tre and University of Molise) in four different courses about computer science and mathematics as a support for teachers in their usual didactic activities.

The Diogene project, instead, started in April 2002 and ended in October 2004. A further step of the Diogene architecture toward the Grid technology and the Virtual Organisation model is currently in progress as described in [14].

References

[1] European Commission. *Trials and Best Practice Addressing Advanced Solutions for On-the-Job Training in SMEs*. FP5 IST Action Line III.2.3 Background Paper. http://www.proacte.com.

[2] Web Site "InTraServ: Intelligent Training Service for Management Training in SMEs" FP5 IST Project (IST-2000-29377). http://www.crmpa.it/intraserv.

[3] Web Site "Diogene: a Training Web Broker for ICT Professionals" FP5 Project (IST-2001-33358).

[4] http://www.crmpa.it/diogene.

[5] IMS Learning Resource Meta-data Specification Version 1.2.2. Public Draft Specification. IMS Global Learning Consortium, 2001. http://www.imsproject.org/metadata/index.cfm.

[6] D. Fensel. Ontologies: a Silver Bullet for Knowledge Management and Electronic Commerce. Springer-Verlag, 2001.

[7] N. Capuano, M. De Santo, M. Marsella, M. Molinara, S. Salerno. Personalised Intelligent Training on the Web: A Multi Agent Approach. Electronic Business and Education, Recent Advances in Internet Infrastructures, Kluwer: Multimedia Systems And Applications Series, vol. 20, chap. 5, 2001.

[8] N. Capuano, M. Marsella, S. Salerno. ABITS: An Agent Based Intelligent Tutoring System for Distance Learning. Proceedings of the International Workshop on Adaptive and Intelligent Web-Based Education Systems. ITS 2000, Montreal, Canada, 2000.

[9] IMS Learner Information Package Specification Version 1.0. Public Draft Specification. IMS Global Learning Consortium, 2001. http://www.imsproject.org/profiles/index.cfm.

[10] D. Dubois, H, Prade. Fuzzy Sets and Systems – Theory and Applications. Academic Press, 1980.

[11] J. Kolodner. Case-Based Reasoning. Morgan Kaufmann Publishers, 1993.

[12] G. Albano, S. Miranda, S. Salerno. e-Learning e Apprendimento Manageriale. Volume Didamatica 2002 "e-Learning: metodi, strumenti ed esperienze a confronto" - pp. 253-266, 2002.

[13] M. Macdonald. Microsoft .NET Distributed Applications: Integrating Web Services and Remoting. Microsoft Press, 2003.

[14] J. Santos. InTraServ Impact Evaluation Results and Analysis. InTraServ Report (DL8), 2003. http://www.crmpa.it/intraserv/documents/DL8.pdf

[15] M. Gaeta, N. Capuano, A. Gaeta, F. Orciuoli, L. Pappacena, P. Ritrovato. DIOGENE: A Service Oriented Virtual Organisation for e-Learning. Proceedings of the 4th International LeGE-WG Workshop "Progressing with a European Learning Grid" Stuttgart, Germany, 2004.

Towards the Learning Grid
P. Ritrovato et al. (Eds.)
IOS Press, 2005

DIOGENE: A service Oriented Virtual Organisation for e-Learning

Matteo Gaeta*, Nicola Capuano, Angelo Gaeta, Francesco Orciuoli, Laura Pappacena, Pierluigi Ritrovato
**Dipartimento di Ingegneria dell'Informazione e Matematica Applicata*
Università degli Studi di Salerno
Via Ponte Don Melillo – 84084 Fisciano (SA), Italia
CRMPA Centro di Ricerca in Matematica Pura ed Applicata
C/O DIIMA – Università degli Studi di Salerno
Via Ponte Don Melillo – 84084 Fisciano (SA), Italia
gaeta@diima.unisa.it, {capuano, agaeta, pappacena, ritrovato, orciuoli}@crmpa.unisa.it

Abstract. In this paper we present the main results of the DIOGENE project where the characteristics of Virtual Organisations providing learning services have been identified and implemented using state of the art Web Services technologies. We also present a possible migration path towards the Grid emphasising the advantages stemming from the adoption of this technology.

Keywords. Virtual Organisations, Web services, Grid, Learning services

Introduction

Virtual Organizations (VOs) can be defined as a coordinated group of individuals and/or institutions who collaborate towards a common interest and share, on the basis of some policies, a set of resources (processors, instruments, data and services). The element that characterizes the participants of a VO is the common *purpose or business goal*. The participants of a VO share resources and establish sharing rules in order to obtain a common objective. Members of a VO can be geographically distributed and can access to the resources any time they are allowed.

In order to realize a VO, many problems must be resolved. Indeed, the VO is a dynamic environment, in which resources and/or individuals can join or resign in dynamic way. The resources are *heterogeneous*, d*istributed* and *shared*. The resource sharing must be controlled by a set of rules that guarantee security, through mechanisms of authentication and authorization. The resources must be monitored in real time, since their state change quickly. The VO is a highly scalable environment, so it needs mechanisms for the discovery of the single resources. In brief, for being accessible and usable any time and any place technology solutions are crucial elements.

Among the technologies available for the realization of a VO, the Web service and the Grid ones offer many advantages. They are open and provide mechanisms to address the aforementioned issues. A key factor for the realization of a VO is the adoption of technologies based on industrial standards. For example, the VO paradigm is applicable inside the boundaries of an organization structure (an intra-organization view) and across organization boundaries (an extra-organization view) but, currently, only Web Services and/or Grid technologies allow the realization of the latter view.

The following sections present the Diogene VO, which is a Web Service based VO for learning experience. We will describe the most important components of this VO and a possible deployment of the Diogene VO in a Grid infrastructure. We will end with an overview of some interesting features of the upcoming Microsoft operating system, code name Longhorn, which provides an innovative file system and communication infrastructure very useful to develop semantic and collaboration based applications.

1. THE Diogene virtual organisation

Diogene [1] is an EC funded project aimed at design, implementing and evaluating with real users an e-learning Web brokering environment for ICT individual training able to support the learners during the whole cycle of the training, from the objectives definition to the results assessment through the construction of customised courses.

The e-learning system which was developed in the framework of the Diogene project, uses state-of-the-art technologies like metadata and ontologies for knowledge representation and management, fuzzy learner modelling, intelligent course tailoring and includes a set of innovative features such as dynamic learning strategies, Semantic Web openness, Web services for Learning Objects handling and IPR management, Curriculum Vitae maintenance and searching facilities, free-lance teachers support and assisted Learning Objectives definition [2].

The Diogene scenario is modelled as a Virtual Organisation (VO) strongly based on the use of Web Services. The Diogene VO is populated by entities offering and consuming services. Such entities are grouped into four categories: **users** (human beings that provide and consume services), **organizations** (physical entities that as software components provide and consume services), **utility components** (software components embedding the technology assuring the architecture integrity) and **accessory components** (software components providing the access from outside to the Diogene VO and from the Diogene VO to outside).

1.1. Diogene Users

Diogene Users can be grouped into the following main categories (it is important to note that the same physical user can play different roles in Diogene so he/she can belong to more than one of these categories).

- Learner: is a student registered in the Diogene VO. He/she acquires knowledge through learning experiences provided by Diogene specific learning services.
- Expert Learner: is a Learner skilled about some topics. He/she can offer mentoring support to other learners about such topics, usually for free.
- Freelance Tutor: is a professional tutor offering his/her specialized mentoring support to learners about specific topics usually under the payment of some price.
- Skill Searcher is an enterprise manager interested in hiring certified staff. He/she performs queries on skill repositories.

Diogene includes further sets of users like Content Providers, Knowledge Managers and Administrators that, to improve simplicity and clearness, are not discussed in this paper.

1.2. Diogene Organisations

Organizations of different type offer services with respect to the specifications of the Diogene VO and collaborate for the realisation of their own services. The kind of organisations supported by Diogene are summarised in the following list.

- Publishing Houses (PH). They store training content and provide remote access to it. They provide search and retrieval functions on the local repository via metadata-based queries.
- Web Catcher Agencies (WA). They are able to extract training content directly from Web and Semantic Web. Through a keyword-based text categorisation algorithm they can, where absent, automatically extract metadata from textual learning objects ad link them to structures maintained by the KA.
- Tutor Agencies (TG). They work as entry point for freelance tutors; they manage the freelance tutor archive (containing tutor models) and provide searching facilities on such archive.
- Brokerage Offices (BO). They research, prepare and provide training offers for learners on demand, based on customisation information (learner model, learning strategies, price, learning goals). They collaborate with PH and WA in order to retrieve didactical material that best fit the customisation requests. They collaborate with TG to retrieve and provide freelance tutors that best fit learner needs.
- Training Agencies (TA). They provide the basic environment for learning experiences and tutoring activities. They are responsible for the delivery of courses and for the provision of course management and execution functions. They maintain learner models and are able to provide (on demand) course offers by exploiting services offered by BO.
- Knowledge Agencies (KA). They maintain and manage knowledge structures (concept dictionaries and ontologies) for the whole Diogene Network.
- Café (CA). They support social interactions, mentoring and information exchange by providing users a set of collaborative synchronous and asynchronous facilities. They automatically arrange groups among users of registered TA by individuating and grouping learners with similar needs and/or profiles.
- Skill Agencies (SA). They provide search engine capabilities on Learner Models Databases of registered TA in order to let third parties interested to hire certified staff to find qualified professional (with respect to privacy requirements). They maintain, moreover, requests statistics in order to rank the required competencies.
- Bank (BA). It's a singleton organisation that executes and logs transactions information occurred inside the Diogene VO. It interacts with an e-commerce engine to execute transactions involving real payment processes.

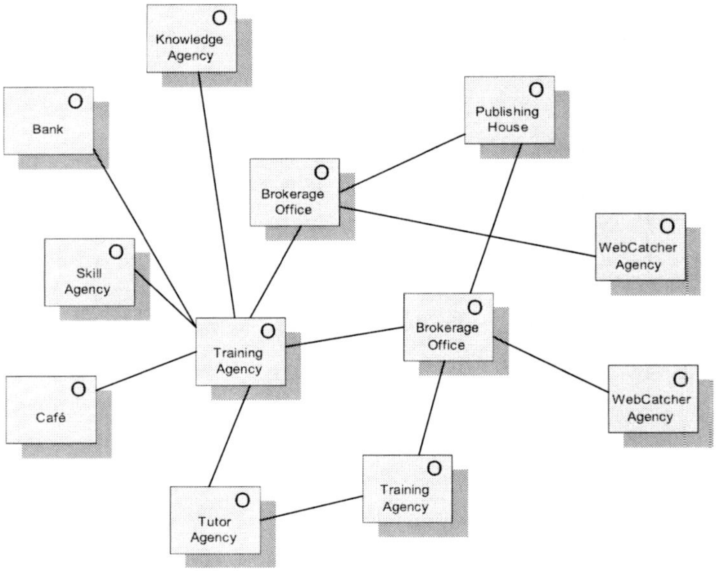

Figure 1 – Interactions among Diogene Organisations

More instances of the same Organisations live inside the VO. The various instances stand on different hosts and are managed (administered) by different users. Figure 1 depicts some interactions between Diogene organisations.

Following the principles of the Convergent Architecture [3], Diogene Organizations can manage Processes, Resources and other Organizations. *Resources* live encapsulated within the Organizations and collaborate with them to accomplish their own tasks. Resources can also be used as containers for the information exchanged between organisations. Resources can manage its own data and other Resources.

The *Processes* express and are realised by the collaboration between Organisations or between Organisations and internal Resources. The Processes can create and consume/use Resources and other Processes.

1.3. Utility and Accessor Components

Utility Components have no business-domain relevance but embed the technologies that explicitly assure the Architecture integrity. The Diogene VO includes the following two singleton components.

- Authentication Agency: it provides all services for the registration and authentication of users of the whole Diogene VO. After authentication, it releases a token that must be used as a ticket to access and be authenticated in all VO services.
- Diogene Services Registry: it includes Diogene White Pages (containing information about services offered by organisations), Yellow Pages (organizing services in categories) and Green Pages (including information about how to execute services).

Accessor Components provide the access to the Diogene VO services and also the access through the Diogene VO components to external services. The only Accessor Component of the Diogene VO is the following.

- Diogene Network Reception: the Internet entry point for all Diogene users. It provided features of user and organisation registration, it publishes characteristics and services offered by the Diogene VO, it provides administration features for the Services Registry.

1.4. Some Orchestrated Scenarios

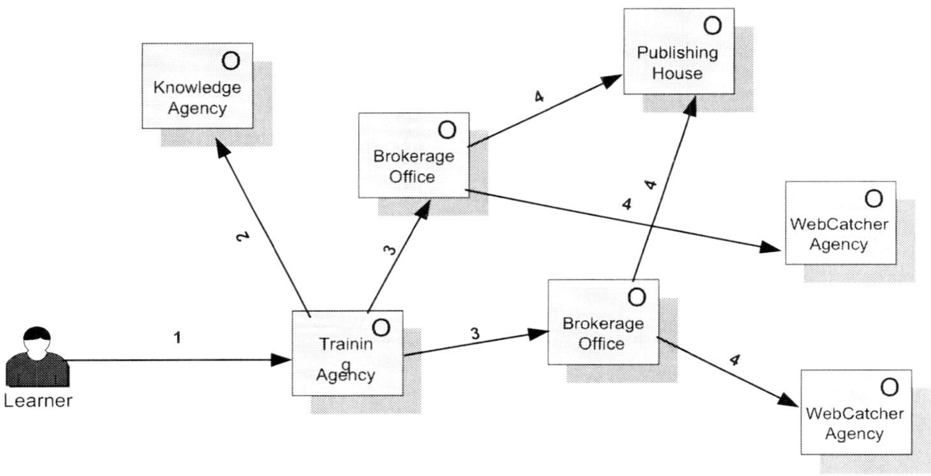

Figure 2 – Orchestrated scenario a)

In a first scenario, a **Learner** asks for a personalized training offer to his/her **Training Agency(1)** through its entry point (Training Agency web portal), starting from a concepts list that he/she wants to learn (Target Concepts). Training Agency calls the **Knowledge Agency(2)** passing to it the target concepts in order to build the learning path; it will be composed by all concepts necessaries to the learner to reach the target concepts. Knowledge Agency builds the learning path using the owned knowledge structure, ontology and concepts dictionary, and the learner acquired knowledge. Once the learning path is ready and fixed the best learning strategies for the learner the Training Agency calls the **Brokerage Office(3)** of the Diogene Virtual Organization in order to obtains the training offers to propose to the learner. Each Brokerage Office starting from the data received by Training Agency (learning path, learning strategies, learner model, etc..) will prepare a own training offer. To do this the Brokerage Office calls the **Publishing House(4)** and the **WebCatcher Agency(4)** asking them to provide the list (list entry are the metadata that describe the single Learning Object, included the price) of available material, that best fit the Training Agency requirement.

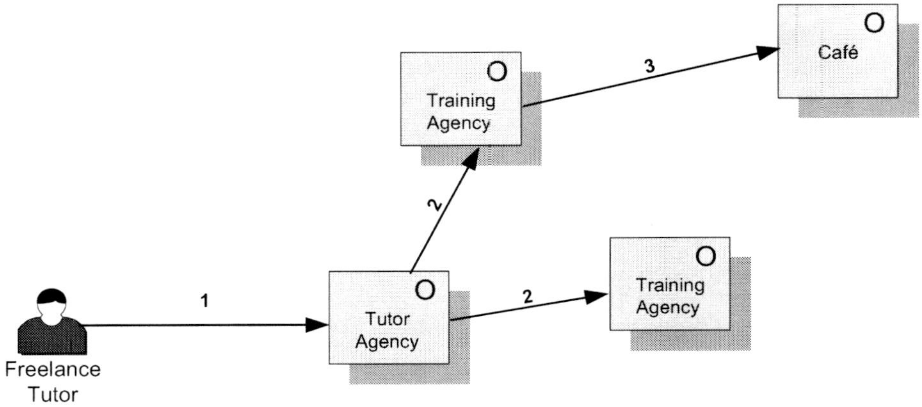

Figure 3 – Orchestrated scenario b)

In a second scenario, a **Freelance Tutor** accesses through **Tutor Agency (1)** to his/her jobs list and clicking on a specific job she/he can be redirected to a specific **Training Agency (2)**. The Training Agency offers a tutoring environment where the tutor can control learner activities, status, profile, results and progresses. Training Agency offers also an entry point for the **Café(3)** where tutor can meet his learners and collaborate and communicate with them.

2. Anatomy of the Abstract organisation

Organisations within the Diogene VO are seen as service providers. Therefore the VO is constituted by a set of cooperating services that give tangible results to the users through the available access points (web portals). Then Organizations live inside Internet and offer their services as Web-Services, they live inside a Web Server and are visible through a Web Portal.

2.1. Abstract Organisation Components

Each Organization included in Diogene VO has the same core infrastructure: the Diogene Abstract Organisation (DAO) shown in Figure 2. Main DAO elements are described below.

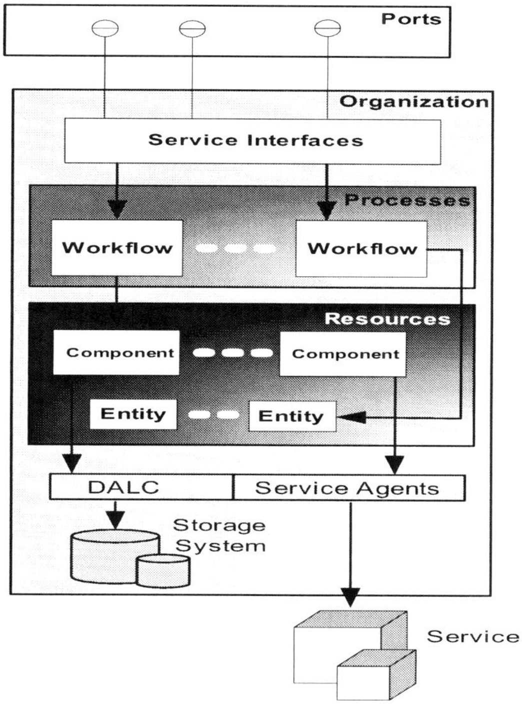

Figure 4 – Diogene Abstract Organisation.

- **Ports** are access points to particular services of an Organisation. Each service has to exhibit: a Notification Source Port (displaying an interface for those who want obtain a particular service) a Notification Sink Port (receiving the notification of the results of the required service) and a Notification Subscription Port (serving for the subscriber to manage in a source service the subscription to a particular service). Ports offer a general schema for publish and subscribe pattern.
- **Service interfaces**. To expose business logic as a service, it's necessaries create service interfaces that support the communication contracts (message-based communication, formats, protocols, security, exceptions, and so on) that different consumers require. Service interfaces are sometimes referred to as business facades. Organizations will use Façade Pattern in order to collect services invocations and dispatch calls to processes at the second layer. The business façade object authenticates and authorizes. Then façade invokes a Workflow that performs the business. The Façade Pattern provides a unified interface to a set of interfaces in a subsystem. Façade defines a higher-level interface that makes the subsystem easier to use.
- **Workflows**. Workflows define and coordinate long-running, multi-step business processes. Workflows could be wrapped in specific components that can be managed by an Application Server like COM+ in order to handle transactions.
- **Components**. Regardless of whether a business process consists of a single step or an orchestrated workflow, your application will probably require components that implement business rules and perform business tasks.

Components implement the application business logic and can be managed in an Application Server like COM+ to handle object pooling.

- **Entities**. Applications require data to be exchanged between components. The business entities that are used internally in the application are usually data structures that wrap DataSets, DataReaders, or XML streams, but they can also be implemented using custom object-oriented classes that represent the real-world entities the application has to work with.
- **Service Agents**. When a Component needs to use functionality provided in an external service, it is necessary to provide some code to manage the semantics of communicating with that particular service. Service agents isolate the idiosyncrasies of calling diverse services and can provide additional services, such as basic mapping between the format of the data exposed by the service and the format the application requires.
- **DALC** (Data Access Logic Components). Most applications and services need to access a data store at some point during a business process. DAL Components provide a standard and abstract way for accessing to the storage systems.

2.2. Some Technological Details

The Diogene Virtual Organization lives into Internet environment. Organizations expose their services as Web Services described by the WSDL standard. Actually, we think that Web Services choice is the best one for distributed environment because they are based on standards like SOAP, HTTP (protocol) and XML (meta-language for message describing) that encourage interoperability. The DAO will be implemented using Micorosft .NET technologies. Ports are Web Methods exposed as Web Services. Workflows and Components they will live in COM+ Application Server in order to take advantage from enterprise services of this environment like the Transactions management, Object Pooling management, etc… For the running and tracing of the workflows we have also used Microsoft MSMQ. Entities are simple light weight Microsoft.NET components that we have modelled using ValueObject design pattern. They are used to transport simple or complex information through the different levels of the layered architecture. DALC builds a component layer that is used to abstract from communication with storage systems.

Authentication services have been developed ex novo and have been released as a Utility Component called Authentication Agency. Services provided by Authentication Agency are: User registration, User authentication and Validity check of Security Token. Security Token is a representation of security-related information (e.g. X.509 certificate, Kerberos tickets and authenticators, mobile device security tokens from SIM cards, username, etc.).

Security Token will travel across the Diogene Network (from a service to another one) embedded in a SOAP message. In order to achieve a consistent Token passing across the Diogene Network we will use WS-Security. WS-Security is a piece of GXA specifications that describes how to attach signature and encryption headers to SOAP messages. In addition, it describes how to attach security tokens, including binary security tokens such as X.509 certificates and Kerberos tickets, to messages.

For the implementation of Diogene Services Registry we used the known UDDI (Universal Description, Discovery and Integration protocol) technology that is one of the major building blocks required for successful Web services. UDDI creates a standard interoperable platform that enables companies and applications to quickly, easily, and dynamically find and use Web services over the Internet.

UDDI also allows operational registries to be maintained for different purposes in different contexts. The UDDI project takes advantage of World Wide Web Consortium (W3C) and Internet Engineering Task Force (IETF) standards such as Extensible Markup Language (XML), and HTTP and Domain Name System (DNS) protocols.

Additionally, cross platform programming features are addressed by adopting early versions of the proposed Simple Object Access Protocol (SOAP) known as XML Protocol messaging specifications found at the W3C Web site. The UDDI protocol is the building block that will enable businesses to quickly, easily and dynamically find and transact with one another using their preferred applications.

3. Migrating toward a Grid Infrastructure

Among the technologies enabling the VO, the Grid ones are taking a leading role. The Grid computing, thought as the evolution of metacomputing, addresses issues related to access provisioning, coordinated resource sharing and problem solving in dynamic, multi institutional VO [4]. This sharing capability and support for VO implementation has been one of the main key success factors of Grid as enabling technology for e-science infrastructure. The new research directions for the development of Grid technologies are moving towards a service oriented view by the definition of the Open Grid Service Architecture (OGSA) [5] that, joining Web Service and Grid technologies, defines an open and extensible framework for distributed and highly collaborative applications.

The Diogene model can become, in simple and feasible way, a Grid-Aware model. It presents several Grid features: it is strongly based on the use of open and standard based technologies and it adopts the VO model. Furthermore, it provides, as Utility Components, a single sign on authentication mechanism to access the VO services and a Service Registry. But it has some drawbacks that, using OGSA complaint technologies instead of the web service ones, can be easily addressed in order to enhance it.

OGSA is strongly based on the service orientation and virtualization, where the first is related to definition of a uniform exposed service semantic and the identification of protocols that can be used to invoke a particular interface, and the second is related to the encapsulation behind a common interface of diverse implementation, so everything (Resources, Learning Objects and so on) in this environment is a service.

Currently, Diogene doesn't take care of (Physical) Resource Management issues. The VOs are composed by heterogeneous and distributed resources and there must be a standard way in order to manage these remote resources. Local Organizations may use a wide variety of management mechanisms (schedulers, queuing systems, reservation systems, and control interfaces), but a client need to learn how to use only one mechanism to request and use these resources.

In a Diogene VO, the Organizations are seen as service providers but there is no agreement between a provider and a client on the service level guarantee. Organizations provide services "as they can", they collaborate between them but they use only the resources of the host where their instances run. Organizations have not a full vision of all the resources of the VO, so they are not able to promise a level of QoS. Moreover, the Diogene Services Registry is a single centralized component: it maintains only static information about the services and organizes services in categories. There isn't information about the physical resources and it hasn't mechanisms to store dynamic information related to the status of the VO resources (e.g. available memory, CPU usage and so on). The VOs are dynamic, resources in a VO join and resign and their status change quickly; so it is necessary to enhance and distribute it, to avoid bottlenecks, the Diogene Service Registry.

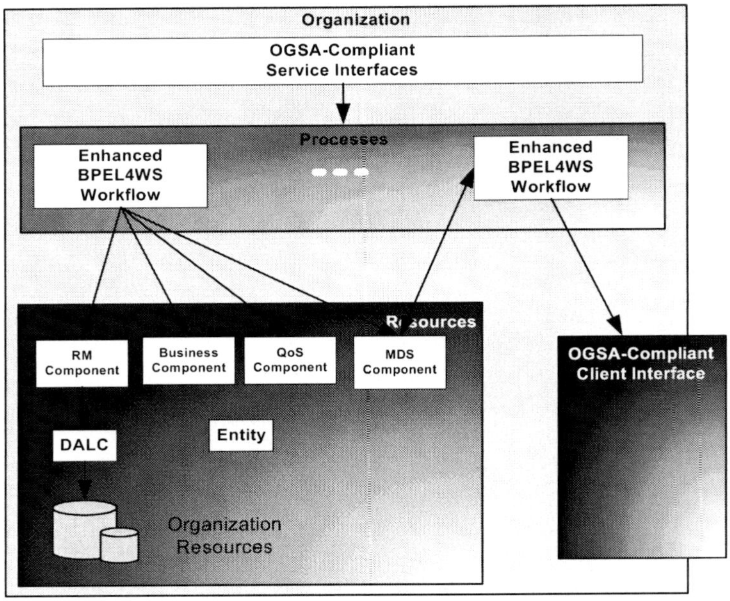

Figure 5 – DAO Grid-Aware.

In order to shift Diogene towards a Grid Service Oriented infrastructure, the Organizations should act as distributed Grid Service Providers (GSP). They should provide OGSA compliant services (e.g. Grid Services [6] or WS-Resource [7]) to clients. Organizations can share physical resources between them on the basis of VO business and security policies. They manage their own resources and they should be able to use and/or buy external resources from other Organizations.

Furthermore, the Utility Components become OGSA compliant services. They are accessible, in a standard way, from internal Organizations and external users. The Diogene Services Registry has to be modified to become an OGSA compliant Monitoring and Discovery Service (MDS) [8].

3.1. DAO Grid-Aware.

The figure 3 shows a Grid-Aware version of the Diogene Abstract Organisation. The Organizations provide OGSA compliant services. The service interface exposes the business logics and extends the notification pattern, as described in [6]. A DAO Grid-Aware does not need the Ports, as they are described in the section 3.1. Indeed, they are directly available through the OGSA Grid services.

The Organizations provide complex services obtained by composition and coordination of simple services. The Workflows, in this Grid-Aware model, are BPEL4WS [10] scripts enhanced with metadata in order to manage the Grid features (e.g. lifetime management) of the services to compose. Each organization has a BPEL enhanced engine able to parse the enhanced scripts and execute the workflow. This engine is exposed as OGSA service and accessible, by the service interface, in a standard way.

Each Organization has a Component called "MDS Component", which is functionally equivalent to a Grid Resource Information Service (GRIS) [4]. It maintains information about the service/s provided by the Organization and the resources of the Organization and has the capabilities to monitor the resources in order to obtain updated information about their status. In the Grid-Aware DAO Components, we find the Business Components that implement business rules and perform business tasks, a QoS Component that performs the mapping between high level figures of QoS (e.g. Time response) and low level figures (e.g. Required memory, Bandwidth) that can be monitored and measured and a Resource Manager (RM) Component that implements the logics to manage the local resources and exposes a standard interface.

The Organizations are GSPs but, by the other side, they take the role of clients when they negotiate or use services provided by other Organizations, so there is another interface (in figure 3 it is called "OGSA Compliant Client Interface") that allows an Organization to interact with other members of the VO. The communication with external services happens with this standard interface and the Service Agent is not required.

3.2. A simple scenario

To clarify our ideas, we explain a simple and not exhaustive scenario. In order to realize a real business scenario, the VO needs new Utility Components, besides the ones described in the sections 2.3. The first is the Resource Manager Utility (RMU), which is able to manage VO resources (virtualized as services) on demand based on the VO policies. The RMU has a complete vision of all the resources of the VO. The other Utility Components are a Negotiator (N), which provides negotiation facilities between a client (maybe a user or another Organization) and a "VO MDS". This last is equivalent to the Grid Index Information Service (GIIS) [4] and it maintains information about the services provided by the VO and information about the resources of the VO (e.g. status, access policies and so on) It interfaces itself with the "MDS Component" of the Organizations in order to obtain and index the information about resources and services.

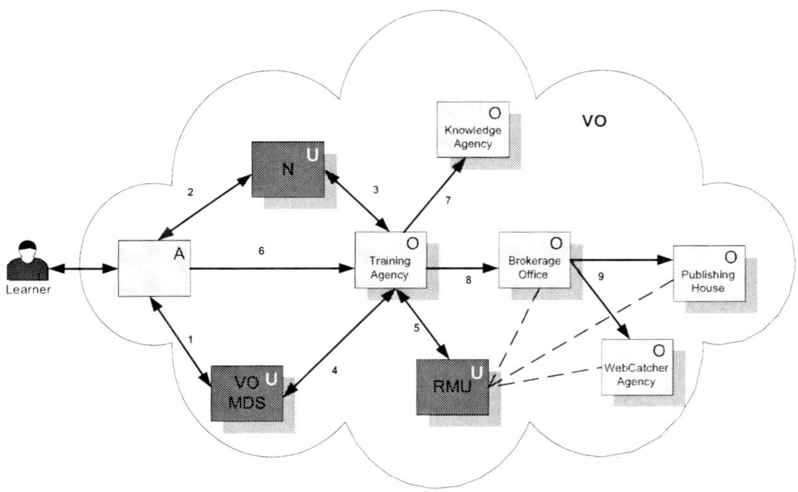

Figure 6 – Diogene VO.

Referring to Figure 4, a learner registered in the Diogene VO asks for a training session and, through the Accessor Component, performs a query against the VO MDS (1). He/she obtains a list of services provided by different Organizations inside the VO. He decides to gain experience in the business field and to play with a Business Game, but he/she provides some visualisation constrains (he/she asks for 3D representations of business game data) so he/she requires narrowing requirements on the visualisation and performance of the service. Through the Accessor Component, he/she negotiates with the Negotiator Utility (2) the QoS for the required service in a transparent way. The Negotiator interacts with TA Organization (3), which starts a simple workflow. The first operation is to map the required constrains with the resource requirements needed to satisfy it. The QoS Component performs this task. Once obtained the results, the second step is to query the VO MDS (4) to get a list of available resources and/or services of the VOs that fulfil the requirements, on the basis of the current status. Once the TA has the list of the available resources, it contacts the RMU of the VO (5). The RMU asks for the RM Components of the Organizations, which can provide the required resources, the resources reservation (in the figure, we suppose that all the necessary resources can be provided by the BO, WA and PH Organizations and this operation is shown with the dashed lines). At the end, a SLA is caught up and returned to the learner.

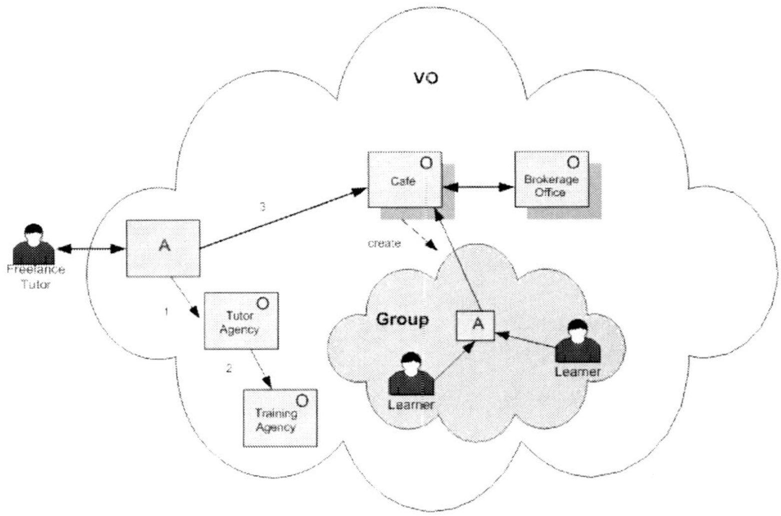

Figure 7 – Collaborative scenario.

The other steps, from (6) to (9) in figure 4, are equivalent to the first scenario presented in section 2.4 and the BO prepares and provides the business training offer for the learner based on the obtained SLA and other customised information. We suppose that the Diogene Bank Organization is able to perform a "pay per use" mechanism also on the resource usage. We haven't discussed the Accounting/Billing and SLA Monitoring issues for simplicity.

Another more complex scenario is the following, which emphasizes the features of a collaborative and experiential based learning model. Referring to Figure 5, we have a freelance tutor who wants to offer support to a group of learners. The steps (1) and (2) are the same of the second scenario described in section 2.4. Furthermore, an added value of the Grid technologies is the capability to provide collaborative features creating a group and inviting some learners, sharing needs and skills, to join a collaborative learning session. Tutor can access the **Café** organization (3) providing some target concepts and rely upon the collaborative features of the organization to provide highly realistic virtual scientific experiments. The **Café** asks **Brokerage Office** to prepare and define, interacting with other organizations, a standard didactical model for the achievement and representation of such experiments. The learners belonging to the Group can access to the virtual experiment and interact with it, using a group Accessor Component that interacts with the **Café** organization.

In this type of model, a learner is immersed in a specific context which, through appropriate simulations, develops active learning processes with progressive abstraction levels, leading to the construction of knowledge in a dynamic way. In this learning model, the student can also receive the support of other users (collaborative aspects) and, through the comparison with them; they can build a new "mediated" knowledge.

4. Conclusions and Future works

In this paper we have presented a Service oriented VO for E-Learning. We have described the Diogene model given particular emphasis on the interactions between the different members of Diogene VO in order to provide training services. Furthermore, we have shown some ideas in order to deploy the Diogene model in an OGSA complaint infrastructure, emphasising the benefits that the Diogene architecture could have from the adoption of Grid technology and in particular OGSA.

Our future work will be mainly focused on two key aspects: The implementation of Grid-aware version of DAO and the evaluation of the deployment over the new Microsoft Operating System code named Longhorn. Concerning the implementation of the Grid-aware version of the DAO we plan to use the middleware under development in the GRASP – Grid based Application Service Provision project taking into account the new development in the Grid domain concerning the WSRF (Web Services Resource Framework). Indeed, Grid community, for the motivations described in [16], is refactoring the Open Grid Service Infrastructure [6] in terms of web services specifications and technologies. The WSRF is based on the concept of WS-Resource, which is a stateful resource that participates in the *implied resource pattern* [7]. The pattern is codified using existing web service technologies, as XML, WSDL and WS-Addressing.

On the other side we will investigate how to deploy the Grid-aware version of the Diogene DAO using the new Microsoft Operating System. Longhorn, represents the first operating system built with *managed code* (i.e. .NET code completely compiled into Intermediate Language to be executed inside a CLR). Longhorn presents three key innovations for Presentation Layer, Data Layer and Communications Layer. All these layers provide their functionalities in terms of Web Services.

For the Presentation Layer, Longhorn introduced *Avalon Subsystem* [13] representing a significant evolution of the presentation technology with the goal of allowing developers to easily build rich and compelling user interfaces that can seamlessly integrate high-quality document and multimedia content.

For Data Layer, *WinFS Subsystem* [12] has been introduced. *WinFS* is the name of the new file system that provides data and storage model for "Longhorn" and has been introduced in order to simplify the process of finding and storing user data.

Indigo Subsystem has been released to fill the Communications Layer. *Indigo* is a set of technologies for developing connected applications on the Windows platform. It provides a complete and flexible messaging platform independent of network topology. With *Indigo*, developers can write applications on a simple yet powerful programming framework.

Furthermore, Longhorn exposes a set of comprehensive API, called *WinFX*, for writing Longhorn-based applications. *WinFX* APIs are entirely available in managed code.

In this frame our effort will be devoted to investigate how to extend Longhorn layers and in particular WinFS and Indigo in order to integrate the WSRF specifications. Both Indigo and WinFS provide a broad array of distributed systems capabilities in a composable and extensible architecture, spanning from data access, indexing, search and retrieval to transports, security systems, messaging patterns, encodings, network topologies and hosting models. In this way a developer can rely on an OGSA compliant infrastructure "embedded" in the operating system.

References

[1] Web Site "Diogene: a Training Web Broker for ICT Professionals" FP5 Project (IST-2001-33358). http://www.diogene.org.

[2] N. Capuano, M. Gaeta, L. Pappacena. An e-Learning Platform for SME Manager Upgrade and its Evolution Toward a Distributed Training Environment. Proceedings of the 2nd International LeGE-WG Workshop "e-Learning and Grid Technologies: a fundamental challenge for Europe" Paris, France, 2003.

[3] Richard Hubert. Convergent Architecture, Building Model-Driven J2EE Systems with UML. John Wiley & Sons.

[4] Foster, C. Kesselman and S. Tuecke, "The Anatomy Of The Grid" 2001

[5] Foster, C. Kesselman, J. Nick and S. Tuecke, "The Physiology Of The Grid" 2002

[6] Foster, C.Kesselman, S. Tuecke et al. "Open Grid Service Infrastructure V1.0" 2003

[7] Foster, Frey, Tuecke et al. "Modelling Stateful Resources With Web Services" 2004

[8] http://www.globus.org/mds/

[9] D. De Roure, N. R. Jennings, N. R. Shadbolt "The Semantic Grid: A Future e-Science Infrastructure" 2002

[10] http://www-106.ibm.com/developerworks/webservices/library/ws-bpel/

[11] http://msdn.microsoft.com/longhorn/understanding/pillars/indigo/default.aspx

[12] http://www.msdn.microsoft.com/Longhorn/understanding/pillars/WinFS/default.aspx

[13] http://www.msdn.microsoft.com/Longhorn/understanding/pillars/avalon/default.aspx

[14] http://msdn.microsoft.com/library/default.asp?url=/library/en-us/dnglobspec/html/ws-addressing.asp

[15] http://msdn.microsoft.com/library/default.asp?url=/library/en-us/dnwssecur/html/securitywhitepaper.asp

[16] Foster, Snelling, Tuecke et al. "From Open Grid Service Infrastructure to WS-Resource Framework: Refactoring & Evolution" 2004

Towards the Learning Grid
P. Ritrovato et al. (Eds.)
IOS Press, 2005

The Model of Collaborative Learning GRID to Activate Interactivity for Knowledge Building

Toshio OKAMOTO* & Mizue KAYAMA**
**University of Electro-Communications, Graduate School of Information Systems*
***Senshu University, School of Network and Information*

Abstract. The purpose of this study is to support the learning activity in the Internet learning space. In this paper, we examine the GRID technology as the knowledge management for supporting collaborative learning (CL). RAPSODY-EX (RAPSODY-EX) is a distributed learning support environment organized as a learning infrastructure. RAPSODY-EX can effectively carry out to support CL activities in asynchronous/synchronous learning mode. The mixed distributed learning environment is utilized as a new learning ecology, where individual learning, CL and videoconference are performed on the multimedia communication network. In this mixed distributed learning environment, people can arrange, modify and integrate educational information for the purpose of investigating, decision making, planning, problem solving, building knowledge and so on. Various information in the educational context is referred and reused as knowledge which oneself and others can practically utilize. We aim at constructing the growing digital portfolio database for CL-knowledge management in Internet environment. In addition, we explore the GRID technology of activating human-interactivity for knowledge mining/discovering.

Keyword. Collaborative Learning Ecology, Knowledge Building, Collaborative Learning GRID, Collaborative Memory, Social Computing

Introduction

The society is changing along with the explosive growth of Internet. This growth is so closely, tightly, and widely that everyone even feels the power of the information evolution. Education certainly is riding on the waves. Internet is becoming the catchphrase in the world of school education, which makes the distance education possible to anybody at anytime and from anywhere. As such, a new learning style 'e-Learning' emerged under the umbrella new concept of "Learning Ecology and Pedagogy", where Internet raises the level of communications and collaborations among people via technology. Nowadays, the word/system of "e-Learning" is rapidly spreading according to popularization of Internet. As for advantages of Internet, people can communicate each other for anyone, anytime and anywhere. Moreover people can share, rebuild, stock and reuse the various kind of information. Here, it seems that the concept of "e-Learning" gets the citizenship in the society instead of CAI. Along with this stream/trend, we recognize the necessity of construction to new learning society such as learning individuals, learning organization and learning community. Above mentioned, we can say that Internet is a kind of "Treasure Island" of educational resources from the world wide stance, though it includes many harmful information.

The development of the recent information communication technology is remarkable. As an effect of this, the education environment is being modified to a new environment which differs qualitatively from the previous one [26]. The new education environment contains not only computer but also communication infrastructures such as the information communication network represented by the Internet [9] [10]. We call this learning environment the Internet learning space. Information is transmitted for the learner in this learning space from the external space. The information quantity that is available to the learner is enormous. However, there is a limit to the information quantity, which the learner can process. The imbalance of this information processing quantity is a peculiar phenomenon in postmodern ages. Secondary phenomena are also triggered by this problem. These phenomena become factors which inhibit the sound transmission of knowledge and the progress of learning [22][23]. In asynchronous learning, the transformer of knowledge and the transformee of knowledge communicate with a time lag. In such a situation, more positive support is required to realize an effective and efficient learning activity. We need to build a learning infrastructure with learning spaces with various functions.

1. The focused Purpose of This Study

Recently, the thought of GRID technology in e-Learning are introduced, which means conceptual and technical aspects of electronic learning. Furthermore, this concept is being extended toward knowledge Grid, Grid Intelligence, Distributed Artificial Intelligence for effective knowledge communication/building/management. We investigate the mechanism of transmission and management of knowledge for the development of the knowledge community in the learning space, within the educational context. In this paper, we discuss about the technology the knowledge management and the knowledge representation of the learning information for the CL support in consideration of GRID technology under the context of e-Learning. The purpose of this study is to support the learning activity in the Internet learning space. RAPSODY-EX is a distributed learning support environment organized as a learning infrastructure [27]. RAPSODY-EX can effectively carry out CL support in asynchronous/ synchronous learning mode. Distributed learning means using a wide range of information technologies to provide learning opportunities beyond the bounds of the traditional classroom. Some examples of distributed learning technologies include the World Wide Web, email, video conferencing, groupware, simulations and instructional software. A distributed learning environment facilitates a learner-centered educational paradigm and promotes active learning. Distributed learning is a learning style where individual learning and CL are carried out on the multimedia communication network. In this environment, arrangement and integration of the learning information are attempted to support the decision making of learners and mediators. Various information in the educational context is referred and reused as knowledge which oneself and others can practically utilize. We aim at the construction of an growing digital portfolio based on the agent technology. In addition, the architecture of the learning environment including such a database is researched.

2. What is Collaborative Learning

2.1. Some Definitions

In terms of Roschelle & Teasley [21], they defined "collaboration" to be ".... A coordinated, synchronous activity that is the result of a continued attempt to construct and maintain a shared conception of a problem". Dillenbourg [7] takes up the following 4 points as the features of CL, which are a situation, interactions, process(learning mechanism) and effects of CL. Cowie & Rudduck [6] defined that collaboration in leaning is the opportunity to learn through the expression and exploration of diverse ideas and experiences in cooperative company..... It is not about competing with fellow members of the group and winning, but using the diverse resources available in the group to deepen understanding, sharpen judgment and extend knowledge.

In consideration of those views, Okamoto [27] pointed out that CL should emphasize 1) process/situated context, 2) individual learning achievement such as knowledge acquisition, skill formation and concept formation, learning set, 3) versatile cognition for both of holistic and serialistic thinking schema, 4) understandings of objective relationship among self/you/he or she, and 5) effects of observation learning (reflection/self-monitoring). CL doesn't depend on place and time. Especially, In Internet environment, the type of asynchronous ecology of CL is more useful rather than the synchronous one such as a Videoconference. Moreover, in the process of CL, individual learning may be sometime embedded based on a certain curriculum in schools, and vise versa.

[Activity-cognitive level]

- Discussing
- Planning/Designing
- Data/Idea sharing
- Evaluating/Finding solution
- Building knowledge

[Activity-social level]

- Observing/Suggesting
- Role-taking/Cooperating
- Coordinating/Controlling
- Social interacting
- Facilitating/Supervising

Table 1 The dimensions on features of CL

Learning Structure	Highly structured	⇔	Non structured
Teacher Control	Highly	⇔	Low
Moderation	External	⇔	Internal
Motivation	External	⇔	Internal
Learning Content	Curriculum based	⇔	Learner based
Assessment	By teacher	⇔	By learner

Table 1 shows the dimensions on features of CL.

2.2. Technological /Functional Conditions to Encourage CL

In general, we can divide the activities on collaborative learning into two classes. Based on these activities, the resources required in CL environment are taken up as follows:

- Technologically mediated dialogue channel
- Shared workplace for a group
- Personal workplace
- Learning materials/ learning tools
- Analyzing tools of Data/Information
- Repository/Memory for data /information revealed in CL
- Reference channel for the collaborative repository
- Modeling tools for monitoring the process of CL

etc.

This system can store all leaning activities log in the digital portfolio holder and participants can review those data in order to diagnose/evaluate their achievements. Also, the participants can refer the flow/stock of knowledge for an arbitrary situation of collaborative learning. We discuss the details about this function in the following chapters from the technological aspect of data/knowledge transmission.

2.3. CL with RAPSODY-EX

A learner group that guaranties the smooth transmission of knowledge can form a community (the knowledge community) by sharing and reusing common knowledge. Learning activities that occur within this group are as follows:

- Achievement of learning objectives as a group;
- Achievement of the learning objectives of each learner;
- Achievement of the learning objectives of the learner group, which consists of multiple learners.

RAPSODY-EX supports the transmission of knowledge in the learner group and the promotion of the learning activity. It is indispensable that RAPSODY-EX has the following functions:

g) Function which controls learning information for the individual learner and the group.
h) Function, which manages learning information of the learner for mediation.

The learner and group information are produced from the learning space. This information will be stored in the collaborative memory (CM). This information is defined as learning information. We also define the method of information management of such information and the structure of the CM.

3. The Management of Learning Information

The simple mechanism of the management of learning information developed in this study is shown in Figure 1. The processing mechanism consists of two components. The first one is a module that offers the learning environment. The second one is the

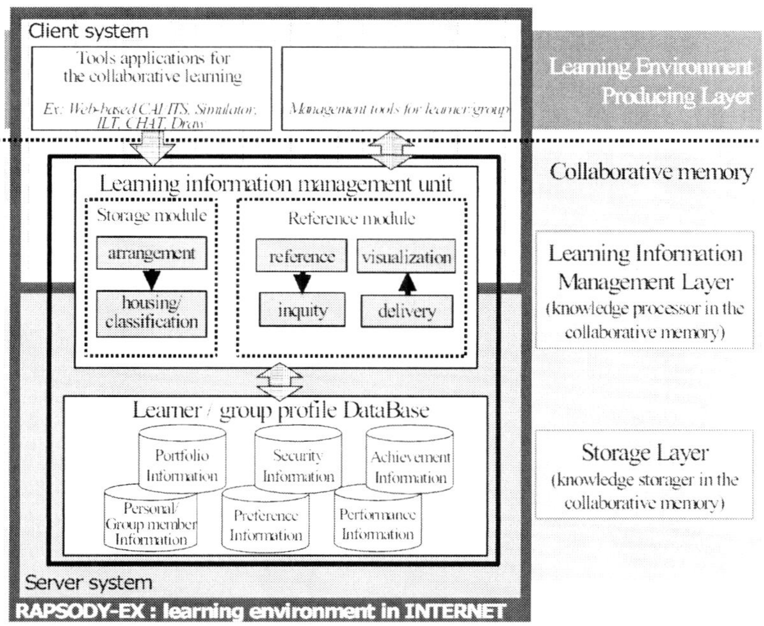

Figure 1 The mechanism schema of the RAPSODY-EX

CM that controls various information and data produced from the learning environment. In the learning environment, 2 types of functions are offered. One is the monitoring function for the learning progress. The other is the tool/application for the CL. The former function controls the learning history/record of individual learners and the progress of the collaborative group learning. The latter tool/application becomes a space/workplace for collaborative synchronous /asynchronous learning. The learning information, which emerged from such a learning environment, is handed to the CM. The CM offers 2 types of functions. One is the knowledge processing function, and the other is the knowledge storage function. In the former, input learning information is shaped to the defined form. In the latter, for the formatted information, some attributes related to content are added. The complex information processing takes place in the CM.

4. The Learning GRID Technology in RAPSODY-EX

4.1. Learning GRID as a knowledge Market

In this study, the processing described in the previous section is considered as a process of the knowledge management in the learning context. Knowledge management is defined like follows [24]. The knowledge management is "the systematic process of finding, selecting, organizing, distilling and presenting information in a way that improves an employee's comprehension in a specific area of interest."

Here, we propose the functions of Learning GRID as Knowledge Management between RAPSODY-EX and the collaborative memory in collaborative learning environment. It guarantees the mutual interactivity among learners and activate knowledge building. In some sense, GRID means the role of exchanging knowledge or artifacts in a marketplace that can stock the various kind of information. At the same time, learners need the value of sense with sharing/re-using manners. We have developed GRID technology as knowledge mining in collaborative learning process.

Figure 2 shows the meaning of Learning GRID, which plays roles of the marketplace for knowledge transmission, transformation and exchange. Moreover, the function of Learning GRID is in charge of bring about building and discover of knowledge through assimilation/accommodation, differentiating / integrating occurred in collaborative learning. We aim to realize this mechanism as social computing by active collaborative memory, which we describe its details in the chapter of Collaborative Memory.

The knowledge management in educational context is defined as follows: "the systematic process of finding, selecting, organizing, distilling and presenting information in a way that improves a learner's comprehension and/or ability to fulfill his/her current learning objectives." RAPSODY-EX aims to support participants' activities in the C (combination of knowledge) phase. Moreover, it affects not only the process of knowledge conversion from the C phase to the I (internalization of knowledge) phase, but also from the E (externalization of knowledge) phase to the C phase. The information of learning entity contains the expressed knowledge by learners. This overt knowledge can be represented by natural language as verbal information. So, we can regard this knowledge as one that would be elicited from the learner's tacit knowledge.

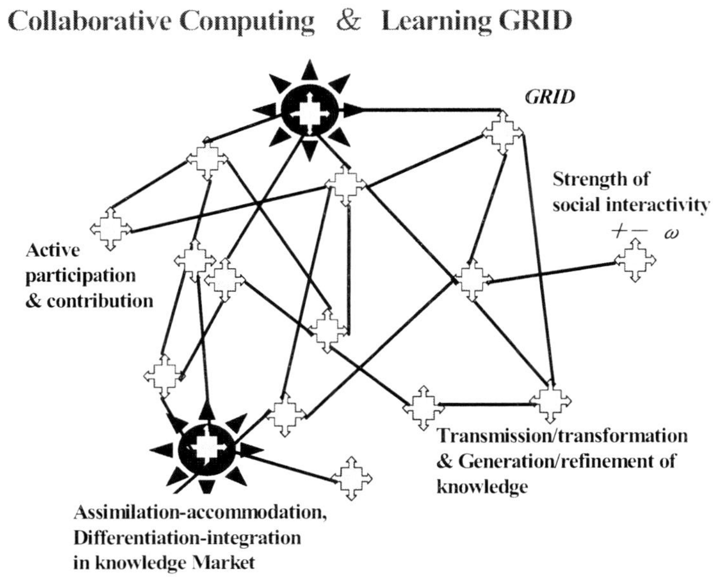

Figure 2 The Concept of Collaborative Learning & Learning GRID

In this situation, what we have to consider is as follows:

Who are the subjects of our knowledge management work?

Learners and the persons who support the learners are our subjects. Learners' task is to acquire the ability/skill for the problem solving. On the other hand, supporters' tasks are to support for acquisition of ability/skill of the learner, and to support of the problem solving by the learner. Supporter means a facilitator/tutor/coach/ organizer etc.

What are the knowledge resources in the learning group?

For learners, the knowledge for the effective and efficient problem solving is their knowledge resource. On the other hand, for the supporters, the knowledge on problem setting and activity assessment is their knowledge source.

What is the gain for the learning group?

The gains for learners are to acquire the ability in which to effectively and efficiently solve the problem, and to acquire the meta-cognition ability. For supporters, the acquisition of the ability of supporting the ability acquisition of the learner is their gain.

How are the knowledge resources controlled to guarantee the maximum gain for the learning group?

By the information processing to relate common knowledge of the CM and learning context, we try to manage the knowledge in the CL. To create the collaborative portfolio between individual and group learning, extension of acquired knowledge of learners, knowledge extraction from learning history under the problem solving and making outline of problem solving process.

4.2. The Schema and Functions of Learning GRID

Learning GRID we intend plays roles of encouraging collaborative learning. Figure 3 shows the framework of learning GRID technology. From participants' performance information and learning resource information, Learning GRID has the functions of modeling the situation of collaborative learning and perturbing a learner's behaviour for knowledge exchanging, transforming and acquiring by distributed collaborative agents in order to facilitate knowledge building. Learning GRID provides adhesive fundamentals for social computing which has also the function of collaborative filtering with recommendation function. So, we can regard this as a conductor in a marketplace and a kind of negotiation-circulation engine for knowledge management. Every agent is embedded in every Learning GRID in Internet space, each agent tries to communicate, exchange need-information among Learning GRID. In some cases, plural agents behave collaboratively or competitively for taking well knowledge negotiation along with participants' requirement. Therefore, the agent's roles become to be quite important within/ among Learning GRIDs in our system. We set up two kinds of agent who are 1) Learning GRID agent, 2) knowledge –Messenger agent for investigation, collaboration and whole watching in RAPSODY-EX.

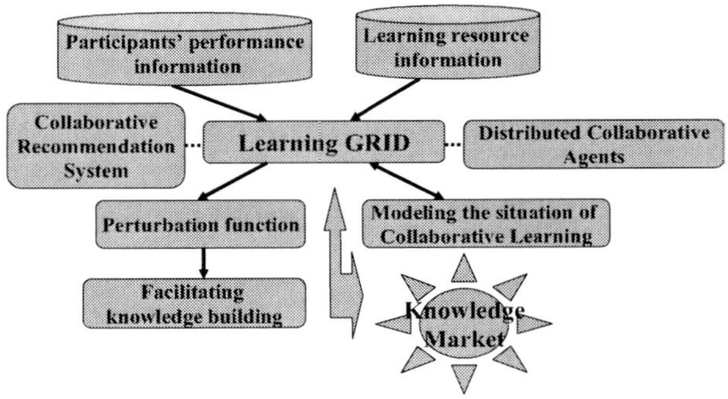

Figure 3 The Scheme and Function of Learning GRID Technology

5. The Collaborative Memory

In the CM, information generation / arrangement / housing / reference / visualization are the management processes of expressive knowledge in the learning space. RAPSODY-EX is a learning environment, which possesses a knowledge management mechanism. In this environment, 1) the review of the learning process, 2) the summarization of the problem solving process and 3) the reference of other learners' problem solving method are realized in the learning space. Learning information is expressed by an unified format. Then, that information is accumulated in the CM. This information becomes the reference object of the learner. The generation and the management of the information on the learning performance and the portfolio of the learner and group are main objects of the knowledge management. In this study, learning information is obtained from the application tools for the CL. It is necessary to control the learning record, the reference log of the others' learning information and the log of problem solving and learning progress. To realize this control not only techniques based on symbolic knowledge processing approach, but also techniques based on sub-symbolic knowledge processing approach are used.

The CM consists of two layers. One is the information storage layer and the other one is the management layer of the stored information. At the information storage layer, 4 kinds of information are mainly processes.

4. Learning information,
5. Information on the learner,
6. Information on the setting of the learning environment
7. Information on the learning result.

At the information management layer, the reference /arrangement /integration of learning information are processed. The individual learner profile information is composed of information following the IEEE Profile information guidelines [11]. The group information is expressed by the expansion of the individual learner profile information. The conversion from the learning log data to learning information is necessary to develop this profile database. The information, which should apply in learning information, is as follows:

- information and/or data on its learning context and/or learning situation
- information about the sender and the sendee of the information
- significance and/or outline in the educational context
- information on the relation structure of the learning information
- reference pointer to individual learner and group who proposed or produced the information
- relation with other material

By adding these information, the learning information is arranged into an unique form. If a learner requires some information related to his/her current learning, RAPSODY-EX shows the (estimated) desired information to the learner.

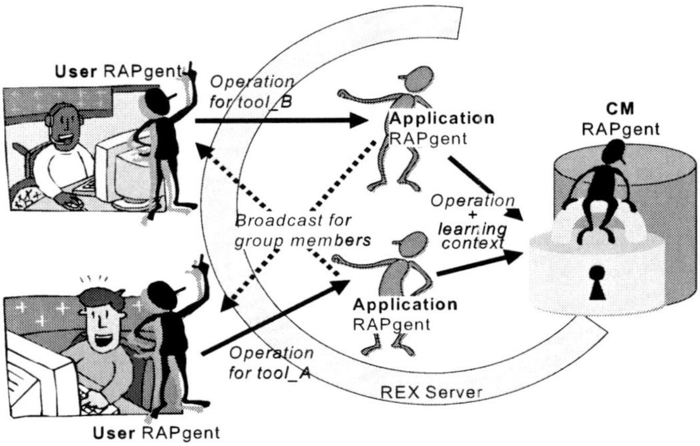

Figure 4 Communication scheme in the RAPSODY-EX

Figure 4 shows a communication scheme in the RAPSODY-EX. Three types of agents are existed in the RAPSODY-EX. These agents perform each mission with user (user-RAPgent), each CL tool (application-RAPgent) and the CM in RAPSODY-EX server (CM-RAPgent). Communication protocol between RAPgents is defined based on the FIPA ACL communicative act [8]. The missions of each RAPgent are to transform information adaptively to create group portfolio, to maintain learning contexts in the group member and to let refer information in CM. To realize the knowledge management in RAPSODY-EX, application-RAPgents develop some learning contexts by using learning information in the CM. Then they refer the suitable learning information for the collaborative tool/application.

6. Examples of the Knowledge Management in RAPSODY-EX

Figure 5 shows the window images of the collaborative applications on RAPSODY-EX. Two types of applications are loaded. One is a chat tool for the text communication among the group member. Another application is a collaborative simulator for the . Each application has each application-RAPgent. By the functions of these RAPgents, learning history data at this session is stored in the CM and formulates a set of the group portfolio.

The examples of knowledge management at this session are shown in the Figure 6. A log data of this dialog is visualized by three kinds of methods. These results are produced by three application RAPgents.

The first method is visualization of the dialog structure. The dialog layers are reasoned based on the dialog proceeding model [3] and the utterance intention information that were given to the dialog log. The result is shown as tree structure.

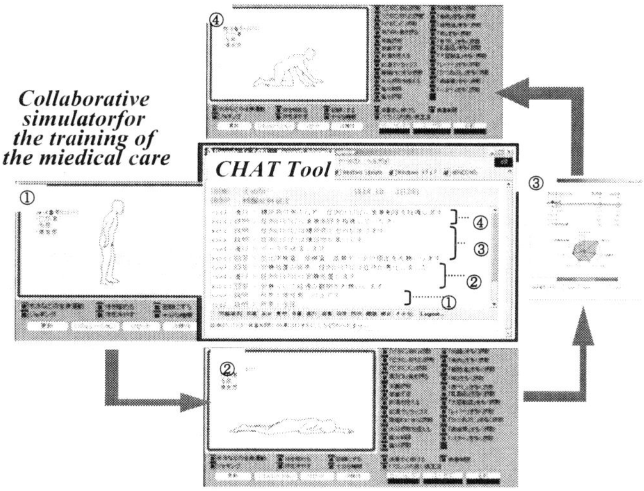

Figure 5 Two types of collaborative learning applications

<a chat tool and a collaborative simulator for the nutrition treatment>

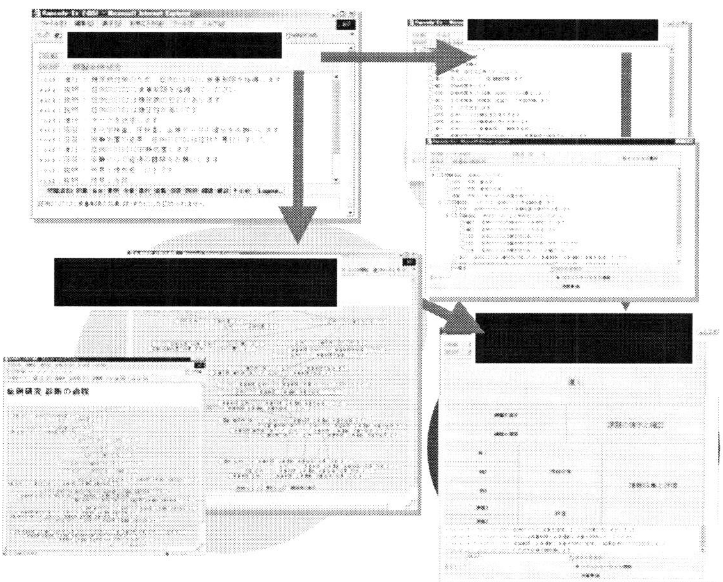

Figure 6 Examples of Knowledge Management in RAPSODY-EX

The second method is visualization of transition of the contents of a dialog. An appearance of the important term that is in a dialog is searched for using the term dictionary about the current discussion/learning domain (Chiku 2001). This result and the timing connection of each utterance are considered to detect a transition of the contents of a dialog. The result is shown as graph structure.

The third method is visualization of transition of problem solution process. One utterance can be unified as meaningless unit for the problem solving process from the first and the second processing result and an educational mentor's expertise/educational intentions. The result re-constituted as problem solution process is shown with the structure that imitated the dendrogram

Evaluation & Conclusions

The purpose of this study is to support the learning activity in the Internet learning space. We examine the knowledge management and the knowledge representation of the learning information for the CL support. RAPSODY-EX is a distributed learning support environment organized as a learning GRID technology.

In this paper, the management of learning information in RAPSODY-EX is described. RAPSODY-EX is an integrated distributed learning environment and the GRID technology for supporting tools/ applications for the CL. Also, in this paper, the knowledge management mechanism in the educational context is showed. The details of GRID technology as knowledge management and for connecting different software is exploring by using the semantic web approach, and it will be integrated with the current learning support environment.

Our Grid technology is focused in the center of connecting various information among learners' profile, log-data in learning process and learning resources as information Grid for the purpose of sharing with interoperability of applications/tools used in collaborative learning process.

References

[1] ADLNet 2000. Shareble Courseware Object Reference Model:SCORM, Ver.1.0, http://www.adlnet/org/.

[2] Agent Society, http://www.agent.org/

[3] A. Inaba and T. Okamoto 1997. Negotiation Process Model for intelligent discussion coordinating system on CSCL environment, Proceedings of the AIED 97, pp. 175-182.

[4] A. R. Kaye 1994. Computer Supported Collaborative learning in a Multi-Media Distance Education Environment, in Claire O'Malley (Ed.) Computer Supported Collaborative learning, pp.125-143, Springer-Verlag.

[5] B. Collis 1999. Design, Development and Implementation of a WWW-Based Course-Support System, Proceedings of ICCE99, pp.11-18.

[6] Cowie,H. and Ruddick,J. 1988 Co-operative Group Work; an overview, BP Educational Service, Sheffield University

[7] Dillenbourg, P. 1999 Collaborative learning, - Cognitive and Computational Approaches - , Pergamon.

[8] FIPA, http://drogo.cselt.stet.it/fipa/

[9] G. Cumming, T. Okamoto and L. Gomes 1998. Advanced Research in Computers in Education, IOS press.

[10] J. Elliott 1993. What have we Learned from Action Research in School-based Evaluation, Educational Action Research ,Vol.1, No.1, pp175-186.

[11] IEEE 2000. Draft Standard for Learning Technology -Public and Private Information (PAPI) for Learner, IEEE P1484.2/D6, http://ltsc.ieee.org/, 2000.

[12] IMS 1998. Learning Resourcde Metadata : Information Model, Best Practice and Implementation Guide, IMS Ver1.0, http://www.imsproject.org/.

[13] I. Nonoka 1995. The Knowledge-Creating Company, Oxford University Press.

[14] IPSJ Journal 1999. Special Issue on Multimedia · Distributed and Cooperative Computing, Vol.39 No.02.

[15] Journal of International Forum of Educational Technology & Society 2000. Special issue on Theme: On-line Collaborative learning Environment, Vol.3, No.3.

[16] Journal of Interactive Learning Research 1999. Special Issue on Intelligent Agents for Educational Computer-Aided Systems ,Vol.10, Nos.3-4.

[17] L. Colazzo, and A. Molinari 1996. Using Hypertext Projection to Increase Teaching Effectiveness, International Journal of Educational Multimedia and Hypermedia, AACE.

[18] M. Chiku et al. 2001. "A dialog visualization tool : Gijiroku", Proceedings of the 62th Annual Conference of the Information Processing Sciety of Japan, pp.241-244.
[19] M. Kobayashi ei al. 1998. Collaborative Customer Services Using Synchronous Web Browser Sharing, Proceedings of CSCW 98, pp.99-108, 1998.
[20] OMG, http://www.omg.org/
[21] Roschelle,J. and Teasley,S.D. 1995 The construction of shared knowledge in collaborative problem solving, In C.E. O'Malley (Ed.) Computer-Supported Collaborative learning, pp.69-97, Springer-Verlag.
[22] S. McNeil et al 1998. Technology and Teacher Education Annual, AACE.
[23] T. Chan et al. 1997. Global Education ON the Net, Springer-Verlag.
[24] T. Davenport 1997. Working Knowledge, Harvard Business School Press.
[25] The United Kingdum Government 1997. Connecting the Learning Society, The United Kingdum Government's Consultation paper.
[26] T. Kuhn 1962. The structure of scientific revolutions, University of Chicago Press.
[27] T. Okamoto, A.I.Cristea and M. Kayama 2000. Towards Intelligent Media-Oriented Distance Learning and Education Environments, Proceedings of ICCE2000.
[28] University of Phoenix Home Page: http://www. uophx.edu/
[29] Jones International University Home Page : http://www.jonesinternational.edu/
[30] V. Pankratius and G. Vossen. 2003. Towards e-Learning Grids: Using Grid Computing in Electronic Learning. Technical Report Nr. 98, Dept . of Information Systems, University of Muenster.
[31] V. Pankratius and G. Vossen. 2003. Towards the Utilization of Grid Computing in e-Learning, in Jose C. Cunha and Omer F, Rana (Eds) "Grid Computing: Software Environments and Tools", Springer Verlag.
[32] W. L. Johnson, and E. Shaw 1997. Using Agents to Overcome Deficiencies in Web-Based Courseware, Proceedings of the workshop "Intelligent Educational Systems on the World Wide Web" at the 8th World Conference of the AIED Society, IV-2.
[33] Y. Aoki and A. Nakajima 1999. User-Side Web Page Customization, Proceedings of 8th International Conference on HCI, Vol.1, pp.580-584.
[34] Y. Shimizu 1999. , Toward a New Distance Education System, Proceedings of ICCE99, pp.69-75.

Part D

New Direction in Learning Services

Towards the Learning Grid
P. Ritrovato et al. (Eds.)
IOS Press, 2005

Systems Support for Collaborative Learning

Colin ALLISON[a,26], Alan RUDDLE[a] and Rosa MICHAELSON[b]
[a]*School of Computer Science, University of St Andrews, Scotland KY16 9SS*
[b]*Accountancy & Business Finance, University of Dundee, Scotland DD1 4HN*

Abstract. One of the distinguishing features of novel network based learning environments is their capability to support group work and collaboration. TAGS, the Tutor and Groups Support Scheme, is an inter-disciplinary, inter-institutional project, which brings together software systems builders, subject-specialists and educational content developers. Collaborative Learning is central to the pedagogical goals of TAGS, and this has lead to the concept of groups being used as a fundamental organising principle. Groups form the basis of (i) privileges and access control, (ii) information dissemination and event awareness, (iii) teamwork involving shared, multi-user educational resources, (iv) online management of group learning, (v) user-centric portal generation, and (vi) replicated servers. The technical implications of this heavy reliance on the group abstraction are described.

Keywords. Group work, collaborative learning, design considerations, middleware.

Introduction

From the perspective of good educational practice an online collaborative learning environment should provide certain features for learners:

1. group-work support [1]
2. interactive, engaging, responsive
3. real-world input
4. student-centred
5. anytime/anywhere

Those pedagogical goals imply certain technical requirements.

Support for group working means that online resources may be shared and used by multiple concurrent readers and writers. This requires concurrency control and the usual associated concerns with liveness, safety and fairness. In addition, multi-user awareness is important for teamwork. Members of a group need to know what each other are doing, and have appropriate communication options to co-ordinate with each other. In particular, distributed real-time multimedia channels may be used to augment distributed resource coherence [2].

Interactivity implies that online working is much more than simply browsing lecture notes dumped on the Web. Regardless of the balance of computation between server and client the system must be geared to writers as well as readers. *Responsiveness* is essential for creating an interactive feel when working on the web. It means that the delay between a user making a request and a result being returned to

[26] Corresponding Author: Colin Allison, School of Computer Science, University of St Andrews, Scotland KY16 9SS; E-mail: ca@dcs.st-and.ac.uk

them should be no longer than some period that is considered reasonable within a particular context. For example, a user working from home over a relatively low bandwidth modem line will have lower expectations than one attached to a high-speed campus network. If a network service is perceived to be slow then it will be seen as an unproductive use of time, and may be abandoned.

Real world input is facilitated by direct Internet connection to real world data sets. For example, students of meteorology may gain access to real satellite weather image downloads within an hour of them happening and can learn from making their own weather predictions which can be later compared with established media channel predictions. The Finesse portfolio management facility [3] allows the management of a portfolio of shares by a student group. The groups maintain their portfolios by buying and selling shares chosen from a database of live data for companies quoted on the London Stock Exchange.

Student-centred means focusing on the user as an individual. It also implies strong monitoring capabilities, for manual inspection or automatic adaptation. In an interactive online environment it is of course possible to implement extensive activity logging (by careful choice of a meaningful activity), which can then be "mined" for useful feedback on a student's use of a set of educational resources. This feedback can be used to inform the resource development and adaptation process and thereby enhance the learning environment.

Anytime/anywhere implies a resilient, highly available web-based service. Availability means coping with faults. Providing a service based on multiple servers can reduce periods of non-availability caused by server crashes. These servers may be distributed across a wide area, possibly globally. If they are also used to share the load then *replication* becomes an attractive strategy as it can, in principle, also support performance by providing an appropriate ratio of users to servers. This approach is further useful as a practical means of implementing *incremental scalability*, which may be necessary to cope with a dynamically changing user population.

1. The TAGS[27] Framework for Collaborative Learning

TAGS [4] is a framework for the development, deployment and maintenance of web-based collaborative learning environments. At present TAGS is being used by tutors and students in the context of accredited degree programmes at six Scottish universities in ten departments, representing a wide range of subject areas: Physics and Astronomy; Medicine; Languages; Accountancy, Finance and Management; Information Technology; and Educational Studies. Further expansion of types of use is planned.

[27] TAGS was funded under the SHEFC Use-of-the-MANS II and ScotCIT programmes (1997-2001).

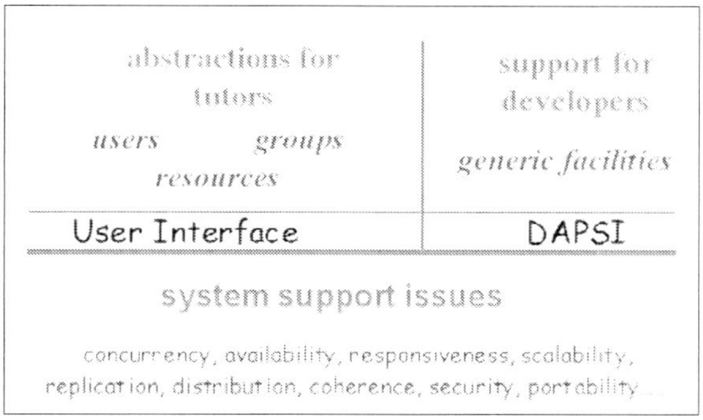

Figure 1. The TAGS Framework

The TAGS framework, see Figure 1, is concerned with supporting highly interactive multi-user, concurrent environments, accessible via standard Web browsers [5]. Requirements of the architecture include concurrency control, availability and responsiveness. When the latter two requirements are supported by replication local concurrency control mechanisms must be subsumed by global coherence. There can be a tension between strong replica synchronisation and maintaining interactive response times. TAGS accordingly provides a plug'n'play set of replication synchronisation mechanisms to support a range of resource types.

Tutors may be computer literate, but are rarely computing specialists with an understanding of distributed systems. Accordingly, a key role for TAGS is to provide useful abstractions for tutors to work with. For example, the three basic abstractions provided for tutors are users, groups, and resources. One can imagine providing tutors with further abstractions such as "course", "class", "assignment" and so on. In our experience systems, which, attempt to constrain the options of course, directors are not popular. It is more productive to provide basic building blocks. For example, the potential to group users readily supports the concept of a class, and the ability to group resources supports the notion of a course consisting of components.

TAGS also provides a developers and application programmers service interface (DAPSI), which allows educational resource developers to concentrate on content, by supplying commonly needed system services.

The project has addressed issues in usability, security, responsiveness, concurrency control, availability and infrastructure Quality of Service (QoS) that would have been unlikely to arise in a pure research environment. Much of the utility of TAGS comes from its strong support for group-based learning, which has in turn resulted in the group ethos permeating the system.

2. The Use of Groups as a Structuring Principle

The concept of the *group* is central to TAGS, where it is used to support many functions, including the following:

- privileges and access control
- information dissemination and event awareness
- teamwork involving shared, multi-user educational resources
- the management of online collaborative learning,

- user-centric portal generation
- collaborative development

In practical terms, tutors construct a collaborative learning environment by using the Users, Groups and Resources management tool. This sets up arbitrary relationships between users and resources, using groups as the basis for the mapping. Users and groups are unique by name; resources are unique by name and type. Access rights can be specified when a resource is allocated to a group. A resource may simply be distinguished as Read-only or Read-Write, or it may export a more subtle set of access methods. Figure 2 illustrates an example set of relationships between users, groups and resources.

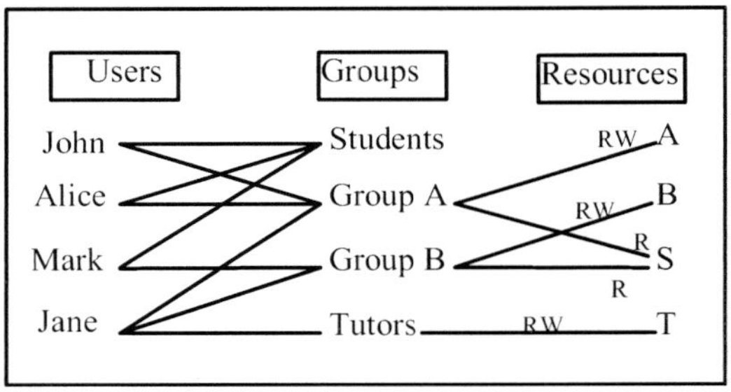

Figure 2. Basic Relations

John, Alice and Mark are members of the Students group. There are no resources shown allocated to the Students group. Jane is a Tutor and has created Groups A and B. John, Alice and Jane are in Group A and have Resources A and S allocated. S is allocated on a Read-only basis, whereas A is Read-Write. Mark and Jane are in Group B, which allows resource B as Read-Write and S as Read-only.

When a user is a member of multiple groups who have different access privileges to the same resource then they are credited with the highest level from their set of privileges.

It is hard to overstate the importance of access control and security in online environments. Privacy is essential to ensure that a student's online work is not corrupted or plagiarised (and is not in itself the result of plagiarism). Authentication is essential to the maintenance of *identity*, establishing that a user is who they say they are. Once authentication is established, authorisation needs to be performed each time a resource is accessed, to establish whether the user has the right to perform the requested operation on the resource.

The TAGS scheme for distributed authentication and authorisation is shown in Fig. 3. This allows for the secure remote access of distributed resources.

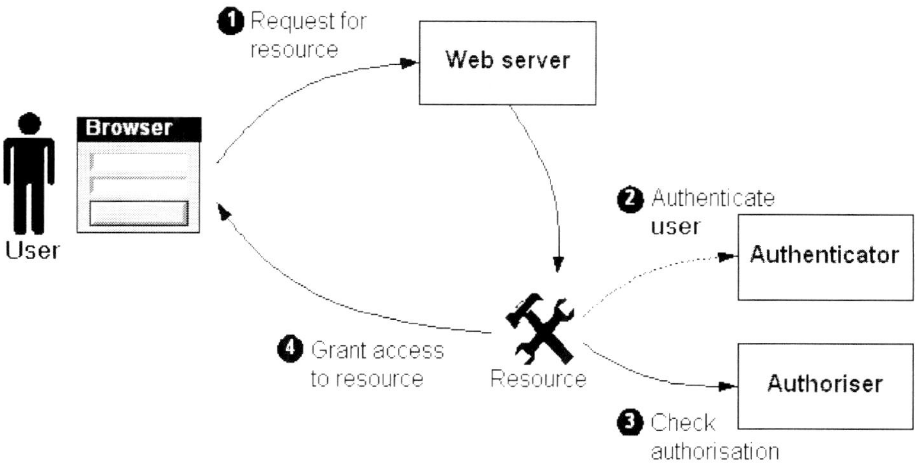

Figure 3. TAGS authentication and authorisation

When a user logs on to the system they are authenticated against a database (which may be replicated). Once a user is authenticated they may attempt to use a number of resources. Each access attempt is then authorised against the user database. Group membership allows access to resources. A simple web interface is provided to allow the allocation and revocation to groups of access rights to resources.

Note that a group does not explicitly have to be an access control group, or an information dissemination group, or any other type of group – it is the responsibility of the resource to use the groupings as it sees fit.

2.1. Support for Shared Resources

The concept of a learning resource in TAGS is deliberately loose. It can be a simple timetable, an automated assessment exercise or an interactive multi-user simulation.

In contrast to learners and tutors, developers are computing specialists. They are the people who develop and maintain resources. It is important to let people play to their strengths, and in the case of developers this means allowing them to focus on providing functionality without worrying about deployment, distribution, and management of a resource. These needs are generic and a collaborative learning environment can provide a useful set of services and interfaces for developers. Generic models for distribution allow a developer to choose the conditions, under which their resource can be made available, replicated for performance or fault tolerance, copied, re-used, and accounted for.

3. User-Centric Portal Generation

The purpose of a web portal in general is to provide a single, initial point of contact for a range of services. It is a technique widely used by web-based service providers. It reduces the time that individuals spend searching, although it only promotes options that are commercially sponsored. Portals sometimes offer facilities for personal customization; for example, an interest in specific sporting events or the local weather forecast. However, these options are very limited. They require identity and registration, which in the context of general web services must be user-driven as the service provider has little idea of who is using a portal. Any type of user may use a search engine portal for example. By and large, web portals are public and cater for anonymous users.

User portals differ from public portals in that they are built entirely around the identity of the user. Their utility in a collaborative learning environment is that they can be generated for individuals and dynamically maintained using information that is already known about an individual's roles and responsibilities. For example, if a lecturer is (i) a 1st Year Advisor of Studies for the Science Faculty, (ii) teaching modules CS3013 and CS2001 and (iii) responsible for tutorial group CS1001/5, all the links to the relevant resources associated with these responsibilities can be aggregated onto a single page. Similarly, a student who is on courses CS3020, IS 1902 and EC4221 will find all their learning resources clearly presented as on their home page.

A user's home page is updated dynamically with links to all the resources they have been allocated via their group memberships. This tends to mean that a student has a relatively clutter free, minimal home page; a tutor has more resources; and a course director may have an over-crowded view. Accordingly a view manager is being developed to help users who are members of a large number of groups to manage their home page.

4. Resource Replication on Clusters

Groups of servers are referred to as clusters. Replication and clustering can support high availability, good responsiveness and incremental scalability where appropriate middleware is provided.

A *resource* in TAGS may consist of a set of CGI programs, servlets, static HTML pages, applets, streaming media, multi-way conferencing channels and so on. The important feature of a resource in the clustering context is that it is the unit of replication management. We distinguish between resource-specific requirements and generic service needs. For example, if a resource contains continuous media then, in addition to the generic requirements of responsiveness and availability, it will also need appropriate network QoS for the satisfactory rendering of its media streams. If a resource is shared between many concurrent users then it will also require resource-specific concurrency control. If a resource is the focus of a collaborative effort then it will also need specific multi-user awareness features. Whenever a resource is replicated it will need *resource-specific replication coherence*.

The motivation for distinguishing between types of replication coherence is to avoid a "one-size-fits-all" approach. If such an approach is adopted then the synchronisation of replica updates must be able to satisfy the most stringent requirements, such as traditional atomic transactions. The undesirable consequence is that all resources, including those with relatively relaxed coherence requirements, must pay the same high price in terms of delay and protocol overhead. It can be argued that a uniform approach, such as distributed shared memory, is suitable for developers, but we believe that developers are capable of and willing to select from a range of coherence models in order to best meet the requirements of their applications. This means that the required response time can be traded off against the speed of convergence. The TAGS replicated resource architecture is more fully described in [6].

5. Conclusion

TAGS has evolved in line with the pedagogical needs of its users. The group ethos in TAGS is reflected from the application level all the way through the system design. The group mechanism provided by TAGS is part of a small and simple but powerful set of abstractions, which can be used to create a wide variety of collaborative learning environments.

References

[1] Michaelson, R. (1999) Web-based Group Work. Proceedings of the 10th Annual CTI-AFM Conference. Brighton, August, pp. 58-64. CTI-AFM Publications, East Anglia.

[2] Allison, C., Huang, F and Livesey, M.J (1999) Object Coherence in Distributed Interaction. In Correia, N., Chambel, T. and Davenport, G. (eds), Multimedia'99, pp. 123-132. Springer-Verlag: New York.

[3] Power, D.M., Michaelson R, and Allison, C. (1998) The Finesse Portfolio Management Facility. Proceedings of the 9th CTI-AFM Conference. York, October, pp. 119-125. CTI-AFM Publications, East Anglia.

[4] Allison, C., Bramley M., Michaelson R., and Serrano, J. (1999) An Integrated Framework for Distributed Learning Environments. Advances in Concurrent Engineering: the 6th ISPE International Conference on Concurrent Engineering. Bath, September, pp. 345-353. Technomic publishing.

[5] Allison, C., McKechan, D., Lawson, H. and Michaelson, R. (2000) The TAGS Framework for Web-Based Learning Environments. Web-Based Learning Environments 2000, Portugal, 5-6 June. University of Portugal: FEUP Editions.

[6] Allison, C., Bramley, M., Serrano, J., and McKechan, D. (2000) Replicating the R in URL. Proceedings of the 8th Euromicro Workshop on Parallel and Distributed Processing. Rhodos, pp. 77-83. IEEE CS Press.

Towards the Learning Grid
P. Ritrovato et al. (Eds.)
IOS Press, 2005

How To Use Grid Technology for Building the Next Generation Learning Environments

Nicola Capuano, Angelo Gaeta, Giuseppe Laria, Francesco Orciuoli, Pierluigi Ritrovato

CRMPA Centro di Ricerca in Matematica Pura ed Applicata
C/O DIIMA – Università degli Studi di Salerno
Via Ponte Don Melillo – 84084 Fisciano (SA), Italia

e-mail: {capuano, agaeta, laria, orciuoli, ritrovato}@crmpa.unisa.it

Abstract. Grid technologies promise to improve the way we think about e-learning allowing wide-scale learning resources sharing in heterogeneous and geographically distributed environments, allowing, in this way, the implementation of distributed learning spaces where different organizations and individuals are able to cooperate in pursuing similar and complementary learning and training objectives. But is the e-learning ready for this evolution? In this paper we try, starting from an existing e-learning platform named IWT, to sketch a possible migration path toward a Grid based environment. IWT was selected because it presents a flexible, service-oriented, layered architecture suitable for migration in an OGSA compliant environment. The new approach will provide more flexibility, in fact, it could leverage on the resources distributed across the Grid in order to build the learning experience that best fit student requirements. A use case scenario is also provided in order to emphasize differences between the two approaches.

Keywords: Grid Technologies, e-learning platforms, Grid aware applications, distributed learning management systems.

Introduction

Grid and learning technologies were born to solve various issues in different domains. The first, thought as the evolution of metacomputing, addresses some issues related to access provisioning, coordinated resource sharing and problem solving, towards dynamic, multi institutional virtual organization [1]. This "sharing capability" is highly controlled, with resource providers and resource consumers defining what is shared, who is allowed to share and what are the conditions allowing the sharing, based on resource management and security policies.

Learning technologies instead are tied to the binomial instruction/learning and to how it is changed after the explosive growth of the web and the web technologies. E-Learning refers to the learning that is delivered or enabled via electronic technologies such as the internet, television, videotape, intelligent tutoring system and computer-based training. This model of instruction/learning has many advantages with respect to the classical models:

- a better interaction between the learner and the learning resources he / she uses i.e. the learning is not passive;
- learning can happen anytime and anyplace i.e. there are not boundaries connected to time and place;
- a tutor or the learner himself/ herself, is able to monitor the progress and to customize the learning experience basing on learner's skills and preferences.

Nevertheless, there are some drawbacks related to current learning solutions. First of all, they are mainly focused on the content delivery, leaving in the background the collaborative view. This is also due to the implementation of distance learning platforms themselves, in which existing learning objects are platform-dependent and cannot be used outside the system. This makes more complicated the collaboration between actors of different systems. Furthermore, current learning platforms only support a specific learning-domain and are not able to support learning in different domains.

Here, but not limitedly to these issues, is where Grid technologies can help. Through the adoption of these technologies, we can have a wide-scale learning resource sharing in heterogeneous and geographically distributed environments, the implementation of learning organizations in which different actors (universities, teachers, learners), sharing a common target, are able to cooperate to achieve a result.

Grid technologies are now moving towards a service oriented view by the definition of the Open Grid Service Architecture (OGSA) [2] that, joining the Web Service and the Grid technologies, defines an open and extensible framework for distributed and highly collaborative applications. This is done through the definition of Grid Services, an extension to standard Web Services able to manage lifetime and to permit introspection of the service itself [3]. This could be the missing link in order to obtain an interactive, open and collaborative environment for distance learning built upon emerging network technologies and upcoming standards, open to the integration of third party solutions and/or services.

This paper presents a possible architecture suitable for a learning Grid accomplished by the re-engineering of an already existing traditional e-learning platform named IWT.

1. The Intelligent Web Teacher platform

The Intelligent Web Teacher (IWT) is a distance learning platform realized by CRMPA in order to fill up the lack of support for flexibility and extensibility in existing e-learning systems. IWT provides flexibility and extensibility features for low level contents and services and for higher level strategies and models. Furthermore, the IWT platform provides user-tailored didactic experiences based on the user's preferences and competences in order to offer personalized learning.

IWT arises from the consideration that every didactic/formative context requires its own specific e-learning solution. It is not thinkable to use the same application for teaching, for instance, foreign languages at primary schools and mathematical analysis at universities. It should be not only the content to vary but also its didactic model, the typology of the formative modules to be used, the application layout and, also, all the connected tools. In practice, the need to introduce the e-learning in a new didactic/formative context brings to harder work for analysts, engineers and programmers. IWT solves this problem with a really innovative solution (both at the technologies and methodologies level) modular and extensible so to become the foundation for building up a virtually infinite set of applications for either traditional or innovative e-learning.

In the next paragraph, we want to go deeper into the details of the IWT platform, showing its logical architecture.

IWT Architecture

The IWT logical architecture is divided into four main layers as presented in figure 1. The first layer at the bottom of the stack is the ***Data Layer*** that provides a way to store persistent objects as learning resources, user account information, resource indexes, etc. This layer is composed of two storage mechanisms, the first, named *Object Repository*, provides each accounted user a space for storing information and data (i.e. a Web file system). Single users can create folders and upload or download files in their folders, can create learning resources (formed by a content and a metadata [4]) directly in his/her piece of repository. The second storage mechanism, named *IWT DB*, is a relational database that maintains data related to user account; user groups and indexing structures (metadata) used for efficiently retrieve learning material stored in the *Object Repository*.

The second layer of the stack is the ***Infrastructure Layer*** that provides *Base Services* towards higher layers and also the capability to extend the services set with *Other Services*. The *Base Services* are exposed as API (Application Program Interface) instead; we can add new services installing some modules called plug-ins and plug-in drivers. Typical *Base Services* provided by the Infrastructure Layer include, but they are not limited to, *Account & Group Services*; *File System Services* providing an high level view of the *Object Repository*; *Resource & Permission Services* handling permissions over objects stored in the IWT data layer; *Knowledge & Metadata Services* providing a metadata-based searching and indexing engine for learning material in *Object Repository*; *Driver Services* providing a set of functionalities for driver handling.

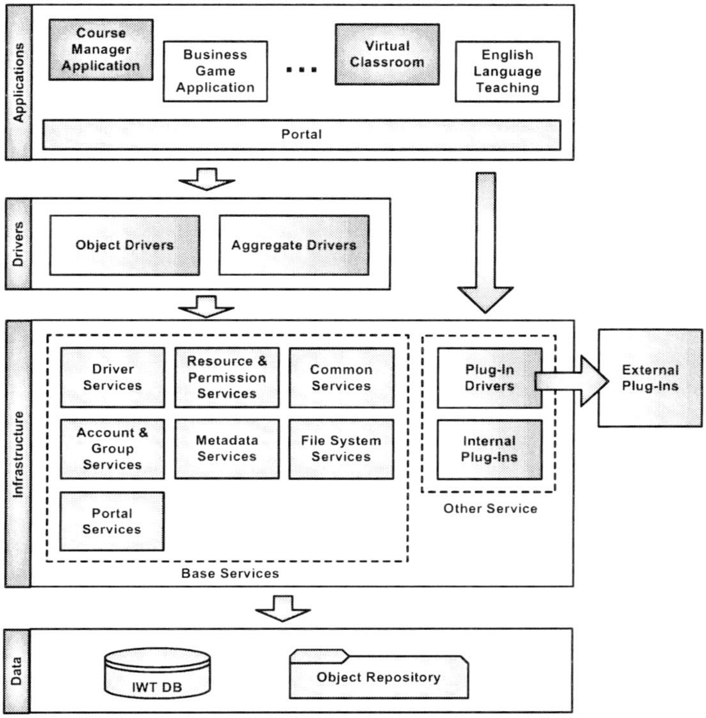

Figure 1 – IWT Logical Architecture.

The *Other Services* in IWT are represented by plug-ins. A Plug-In is an additional module installed in the IWT platform in order to provide new services (domain independent or domain specific) to the IWT architecture higher layer. There are *internal plug-ins* and *external plug-ins*, the latter need a standard interface called *plug-in driver* for their integration with IWT. As examples of plug-ins the following worth mentioning:

- Student Model Plug-In (internal plug-in) is a module that allows the earner profile handling;
- Ontology Plug-In (internal plug-in) is a module that allows to structure the knowledge about a specific domain using ontologies [5] [7];
- LIA (Learner Intelligent Advisor, external plug-in) provides the customisation of didactic experiences based on target objectives given by the teacher, the knowledge model chosen by the teacher and the student's preferences and competences; manages the student models [6] [9].

The third layer of the stack is the ***Driver Layer***. *Drivers* are pluggable components used to extend IWT services and IWT content types. There are three types of *Drivers*:

- Object Drivers, each of them manages, in a transparent way, a specific type of content (examples of contents are lesson pages, multiple choice tests, etc.);
- Aggregate Drivers, that manage complex objects (simulations, virtual experiments, etc.) arising from the aggregation of simpler objects.
- Plug-In Drivers are required to adapt to IWT the work of external Plug-Ins.

A *Driver* realizes the IWT extensibility, in fact, *Object* and *Aggregate Drivers* can dynamically extend the set of IWT managed contents, instead *Plug-In Drivers* extend the set of IWT managed services.

The highest layer in the stack is the ***Application Layer*** in which we find the specific applications we want to realize on the IWT platform.

As said before, IWT has a highly modular platform. Due to its features of flexibility and extensibility, it is fit for migrating towards a Grid environment and, in our vision, it could represent the core middleware enabling the creation of the learning Grid. Before describing how to modify the IWT platform to make it Grid-aware, we want to illustrate a typical IWT scenario.

Delivery of a Didactic Course Scenario

In this paragraph we describe and analyse the main execution flow of a typical application developed using the IWT environment, namely the "Delivery of a Didactic Course".

For a better understanding of this scenario, of fundamental importance is the introduction of the following *key abstractions*:

- Concept is a significant property in a particular domain i.e. "limit" is a concept in the domain of "mathematical analysis";
- Ontology represents a way to structure a specific domain knowledge, it can be thought as graphs in which nodes are concepts and arcs are relations between concepts;
- Target Concept is an objective fixed by a teacher for a didactic experience;
- Learning Object is a minimal unit of didactic material, the rendering of one or more learning objects represent a didactic experience, a learning object has to be described by a metadata;
- Metadata is a standard set of data used in order to describe in a consistent way a resource, metadata links learning objects to concepts covered by them;
- Student Model is a profile composed by account information, learner preferences and competences;
- Didactic Course Specification is the set of specifications required to assembly a didactic experience and is composed of a reference to ontology and a set of target concepts.
- Didactic Course Presentation is the list of learning objects that realize the didactic course described in a Didactic Course Specification.

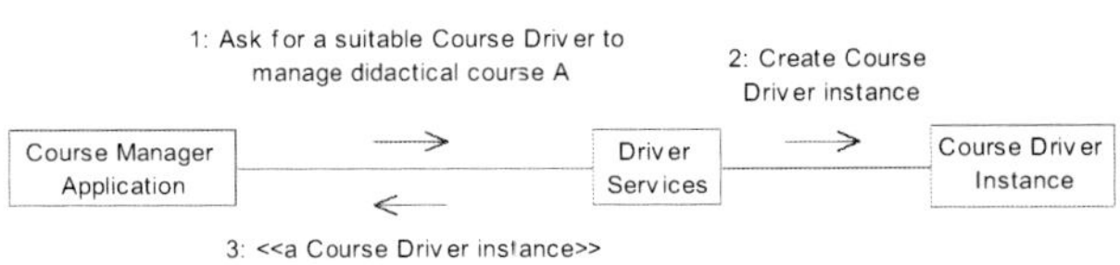

Figure 2 – Step 1.

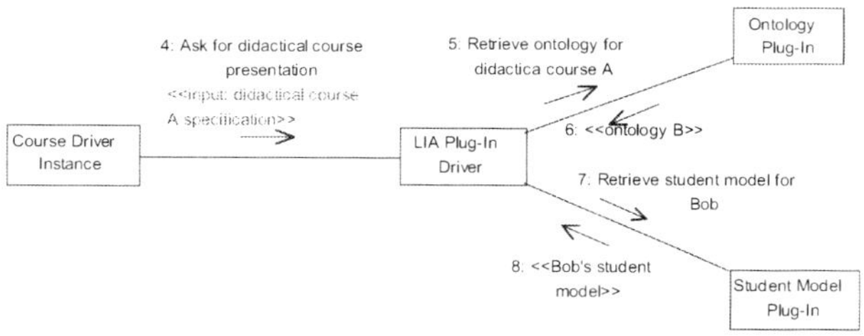

Figure 3 – Step 2.

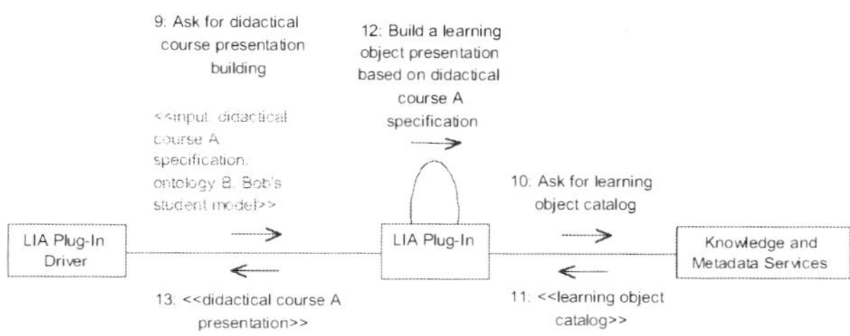

Figure 4 – Step 3.

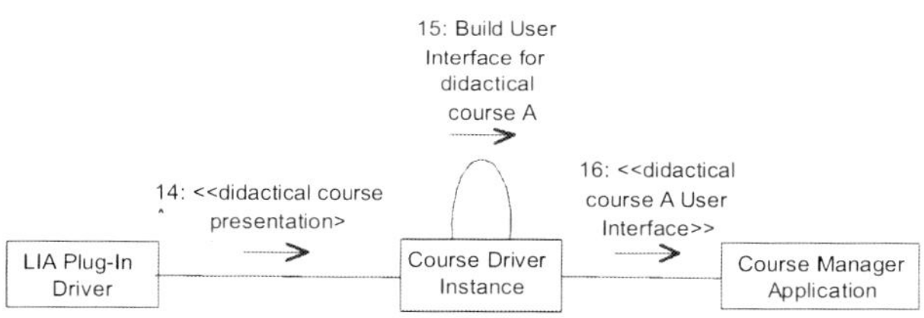

Figure 5 – Step 4.

Moving to the description of the execution flow and software modules involved in the "Delivery of a Didactic Course", we can assume that Student Bob decides to access a didactic course, so he interacts with *Course Manager Application* to obtain a didactic course catalogue and decides to select the course **A**. *Course Manager Application* asks for an instance of a suitable driver to manage the selected course **A** (see figure 2).

The *Course Manager Application* can ask to the obtained course driver instance for the delivery of the course **A**. The course driver instance asks the *Driver Services* to get an instance of a *LIA Plug-In Driver* (i.e. the wrapper used to manage the ITS engine called *LIA*). *LIA* computation needs services provided by *Ontology Plug-In* and *Student Model Plug-In*. (see figure 3 and 4).

When *LIA Plug-In Driver* obtains the result of the needed computation (i.e. the transformation from Didactic Course Specification into Didactic Course Presentation) it sends this result to the *course driver instance*. The delivery of the course **A** presentation is realized by the collaboration between the *course driver instance* and the *Course Application Manager* (see figure 5).

2. Proposed architecture enabling an e-Learning Grid

In deploying the IWT platform into the Grid environment it must be taken into account the new environment in which this platform will be developed and will operate. The new platform will be OGSA compliant, so it will inherit all the features of such architecture. Two aspects, in particular, are important:

- the openness of the architecture, where open means extensibility, vendor neutrality, and commitment to a community standardization process;
- the service orientation and virtualization, where the first is related to the definition of service interfaces and the identification of protocols that can be used to invoke a particular interface, and the second is related to the encapsulation behind a common interface of diverse implementation, so everything (Resources, Learning Objects and so on) in this environment is a service.

This is done by the definition of a Grid Service [2], which is the building block of OGSA. In the figure 6, the architecture of Grid based IWT (GrIWT) is shown.

The platform is built upon a ***Grid-enabling layer***. In our solution, this layer should be based on existing OGSA compliant middleware such as GT3. It is composed of a *core* layer, which implements the interfaces and behaviours described in [3] (e.g. Registration, Factory, Notification) and a *base and collective* layer that implements services for Resource Management, Information Services and Data Transfer in the Grid. It enables single sign-on and security mechanism based on the Grid Security Infrastructure (GSI).

The next layer represents a ***core layer*** that provides the Base Services of the IWT platform, with the addition of a set of services useful for the management of the architecture in a service oriented and highly distributed environment like: *Service Orchestrator* (S.O.) for the coordination of the sub-services; *Service Discovery* (S.D.) for locating and retrieving service description documents; *Failure Handling* (F.H.) to manage the various forms of failure and exceptions that can arise in this environment; *Event Handler* (E.H.) to manage events and notifications between services. These services should be OGSA compliant.

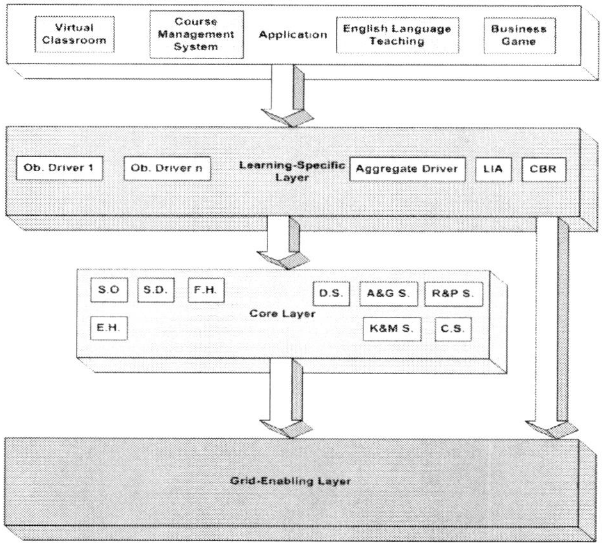

Figure 6 – GrIWT Architecture.

The IWT platform flexibility and extensibility features are a good starting point towards the deployment of the platform in a Grid environment, even if much work must be still done. The IWT services should be wrapped by GSs and extended in order to adapt them to the new environment. For example, the *Account & Group* services of IWT should provide user authentication no more in a stand-alone platform, but in a dynamic and distributed Learning Organization, providing single sign-on mechanisms. Analogously, the IWT *Resource & Permission* services should provide the authorization on the resources distributed across the Grid and belonging to the same Learning Organization, based on the community access policy [4].

In GrIWT the IWT Plug-In mechanism is not required. In the new environment new services can be added and removed dynamically and, furthermore, external services discovered by the use of S.D. can be provided by third parties, distributed across the Grid, taking the role of Content/Service Providers, and can be orchestrated with other services of the platform to build new sophisticated services.

These two layers comprise the minimal set of services that the platform must have. With this set of services a Learning Management System (LMS) is able to access the Grid in a secure way, to discover services and resources and to orchestrate them with its services or resources.

On top of them, there is a ***learning-specific*** layer, including domain specific services. These services comprise Object Drivers and the Aggregate Driver, as well as a set of specific services like LIA. These services should be OGSA compliant, but they could be Web Services invoked by GS too. Like the core layer, there is no need for the plug-in drivers. At the end, there is the ***application*** layer in which the applications can be a composition of GS orchestrated between them.

In the next paragraph, we explain how the scenario, as described in 2.1, changes according to the new Grid based architecture.

3. Delivery of a Didactic Course

The first step of the Didactic Course delivery concerns the selection of a suitable *Course Driver* for the course the student has chosen.

In this case, when the *Driver Services* is invoked by the *Course Manager Application* (step 2 of paragraph 2.1), it queries the S.D. Grid service in order to obtain an appropriate reference (e.g. GSH, see [2] for details) to a Factory of the Driver hosted somewhere on the Grid. After the invocation of the Factory, the *Driver Services* receive a reference to a new instance of the *Course Driver* and returns it to the Application. Now, the Application can invoke the *Course Driver*, which provides the actual delivery of the course.

In this phase (step 2, 3, 4 of paragraph 2.1), the main difference, with respect to the IWT platform, is the introduction of the Orchestration service and the elimination of the *Plug-In Drivers* that become unnecessary with the migration towards a Grid Services based environment.

In order to deliver the course, the *Course Driver* (in this scenario it should be a Grid Service), invokes the *Orchestrator*, transferring to it a description (defined in a specified language) of the workflow between the involved services. The *Orchestrator* runs the workflow definition and manages the interactions between services.

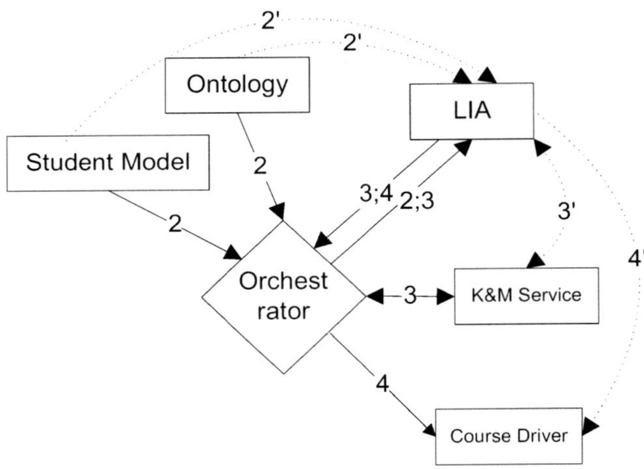

Figure 7 – Workflow for Course Delivery.

The Figure 7 shows how the *Orchestrator* enters in the scenario depicted in 2.1. The numeration of the lines reflects the steps described in 2.1. The dotted lines describe the logical execution flow between the services (it is the same we described in 2.1). While the continuous lines represent the actual execution flow. The *Orchestrator* manages the interactions between the Services. It is a general service, since it simply runs the workflow description, which is generated by the appropriate Driver (in this case the Driver suitable for course A).

We would like to underline the flexibility of this architecture, and the introduction of a modification to the *K&M Service* able to retrieve references to the Learning Objects distributed on the Grid, querying the Service Discovery. This opportunity allows *LIA* to assemble more suitable courses to the student profiles.

4. Conclusions

In this paper we have represented the possibility to use the Grid technologies in order to implement an innovative platform for the distance and collaborative learning. Particular emphasis has been laid on showing the advantages that can derive from deploying the IWT in an OGSA compliant environment. Much work must be done both in the identification and in the implementation of the functionalities peculiar to the new platform. As we have argued, GrIWT can potentially facilitate the birth of new learning models, which are user centred and not content centred, and built upon the Grid technologies.

References

[1] Foster, C. Kesselman and S. Tuecke, "The Anatomy of the Grid"
[2] Foster, C. Kesselman, J. Nick and S. Tuecke, "The physiology of the Grid" 2002
[3] Foster, C.Kesselman, S. Tuecke et al. "Grid Service Specification" draft 05 2002
[4] Foster Kesselmam Tuecke et al. A Community Authorization Service for Group Collaboration, 2002
[5] D. Fensel. Ontologies: a Silver Bullet for Knowledge Management and Electronic Commerce. Springer, 2001.
[6] N. Capuano, M. Marsella, S. Salerno. ABITS: An Agent Based Intelligent Tutoring System for Distance Learning. Proceedings of the International Workshop on Adaptive and Intelligent Web-Based Education Systems. ITS 2000, Montreal, Canada, 2000.
[7] S. Decker, D. Fensel, F. van Harmelen, I. Horrocks, S. Melnik, M. Klein and J. Broekstra: Knowledge Representation on the Web In: Proceedings of the International Workshop on Description Logics (DL2000).
[8] IWT: Intelligent Web Teacher. White Paper. CRMPA. 2002.
[9] N. Capuano, M. Gaeta, A. Micarelli, E. Sangineto. An Integrated Architecture for Automatic Course Generation. Proceedings of the IEEE International Conference on Advanced Learning Technologies. ICALT 2002, Kazan, Russia, 2002.
[10] IMS Learning Resource Meta-data Specification Version 1.2.2. Public Draft Specification. IMS Global Learning Consortium, 2001. http://www.imsproject.org/metadata/index.cfm

Towards the Learning Grid
P. Ritrovato et al. (Eds.)
IOS Press, 2005

A Grid of Remote Laboratories for Teaching Electronics

Andrea Bagnasco and Anna Marina Scapolla
Biophysical and Electronic Engineering Department, University of Genoa, Italy

Abstract. Testing theories through practice is an important approach to teaching, especially for scientific and technical curricula. Lack of resources and logistic problems often make practice impossible. During the last few years, several attempts to find an alternative to in-laboratory experiments have been made by many researchers. In this paper, we present our approach to the challenge of remote laboratories. We outline the model we have created and the prototype we have implemented and validated. Finally, we propose a grid-oriented view of the remote laboratory that could help to support experimental activity in e-learning efforts in a scattered community of users.

Keywords. web-based remote laboratory, e-learning, grid

Teaching Electronics with Remote Labs

Multimedia and network interactivity are leading to new forms of teaching and learning and to new roles for students, who act as participants and not only spectators of their own learning process. Testing theories through practice is an important approach to teaching, especially for scientific and technical curricula. Lack of resources, logistic problems, disabilities, and hazardous or dangerous environment conditions often make practice impossible. During the last few years, riding the e-learning wave, several attempts to find an alternative to in-laboratory experiments have been made, and the literature in this field is vast. Some examples are given in [1, 2, 3, 4, and 5]. Today's lab experiences can be based on simulations or, alternatively, the network can provide an access to remote personal computers that control real instrumentation and physical devices. These solutions are effective for widespread and continuous education (generally limited by time and space constraints) and for special education, based on the use of expensive and rare equipment, geographically scattered. They allow improving the cooperation among researchers from different institutes.

A large amount of work has been done in this field by different groups of researchers, who have presented various solutions. In the next section, we shall illustrate a model called ISILab (pronounced "easy-lab") [6] to share laboratories in the Internet.

1. The ISILab Approach

ISILab is modeled as a distributed environment (see Figure 1) consisting of the main Virtual Laboratory Server (VLS), one or more Real Laboratory Servers (RLSs), and user/client stations. The Internet links all these components.

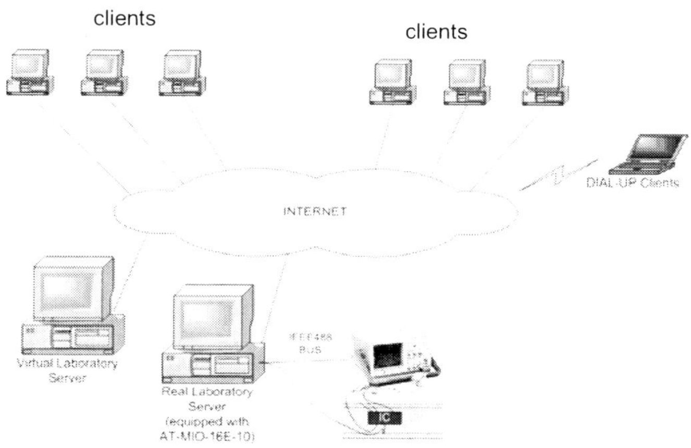

Figure 1. ISILab Architecture

RLSs can be spread over a wide geographic area and control real experiments, managing sets of heterogeneous resources (i.e., measurement instrumentation). No limit exists to the locations of the laboratories, and the only requirement is an Internet connection between clients and servers controlling resources. Users do not need any particular hardware or software, and can carry out experiments through the network. They work transparently to the real location of the device under test in a multi-user concurrent way.

The environment allows users to carry out experiments in two different ways: the guided mode and the independent mode. In the guided mode, a privileged user is the only one able to modify interactively the operating conditions by acting on the instrumentation controls, whereas the other users are only able to see the response of the system on their computer screens. This mode can be very effective in the context of distance education, as teachers can show real laboratory experiments via the Internet. When an experiment is carried out in the independent mode, all users are able to interact with actual instruments in a parallel fashion and see only the results related to their own commands. The coherency of each experimental session is guaranteed by the RLS that takes care of separating different users' data spaces. The RLS also sees to the execution of measurements by applying these settings to the actual instruments in the batch mode.

Another important feature of ISILab is its modular and scaling structure, achieved through the decomposition of the experiment entity into a set of separate, independent, and reusable components, which can be assembled in order to create new and different experiences. Many developers can contribute to increasing the number of experiments.

A prototype for a remote laboratory has been presented and validated. Students, remotely accessing the laboratory, are introduced to a set of experiments/lessons leading to the knowledge of electronic instruments, measurement procedures, and circuits under test. Each experiment is presented as a lecture, characterized by a well-defined objective and a number of exercises that can be carried out via the web. A set of hints, tips and instrument handbooks are available on-line and provide a continuous support to conduct experiments. Figure 2 is a snapshot of the prototype. It is worth noting that it is possible to have both simplified and very realistic virtual panels in order to achieve different didactic targets.

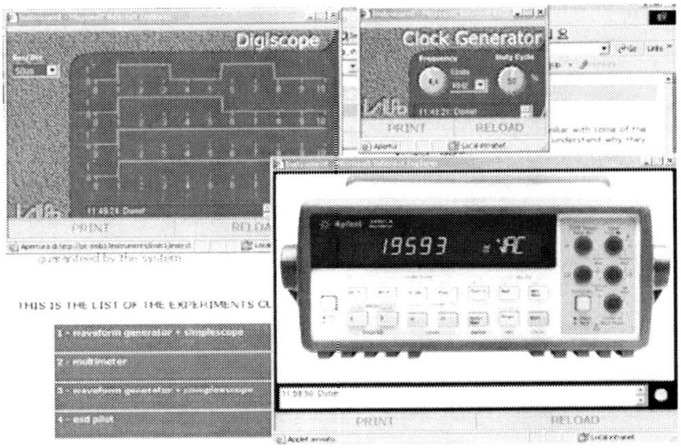

Figure 2. The learning environment

The entire server side of ISILab, both the RLS and the VLS, has been developed by using LabVIEW [7].

The use of HTML and Java on the client side renders the system accessible by use of a common web browser. The XML description of the entire data set associated with the environment ensures the maximum portability.

2. Validation Test

A validation test was carried out according to the work plan of the NetPro project [8], a EU Leonardo da Vinci Programme initiative. ISILab was applied to the teaching of delays in digital circuits, which is part of a course on digital electronics. Both the RLS and the VLS were hosted on an entry level standard PC (Pentium II 350 MHz, 192 MB RAM, Windows 2000) equipped with:

- A multifunction I/O card (National Instruments AT-MIO-16E-10);
- An IEEE488 interface card (National Instrument AT-GPIB) connecting a digital oscilloscope 54645D from HP/Agilent featuring 2 analog channels and 16 digital ones.

The circuits to test were built on an ordinary breadboard. The input to the circuit, for both experiments, was taken from one of the two clock signals available from the I/O card. The output pins of the circuit were connected to the analog channels of the oscilloscope for experiment 1 and to the digital ones for experiment 2.

Three specific user interfaces were built to control the features of:

- the clock generator,
- the analogic oscilloscope,
- the digital oscilloscope.

Students accessed the laboratory from different sites connected via the Internet and over dial-up lines. In order to limit the load of the ISILab server and to better monitor its behavior, the laboratory session was executed in a controlled way, limiting the number of clients able to connect to the RLS. All students worked in the concurrent mode. We settled turns in order to have a maximum of thirteen concurrent accesses at a time. The number of sessions (one hour each) was 16. In this way we were able to guarantee a response time of about one second from the system. The analysis of the log files shows that the average number of actions in each experimental session was about seven per minute, whereas the response time of the system was less than 10 milliseconds, thus proving the feasibility of the system.

3. A Grid View of ISILab

ISILab is characterized by a modular design to guarantee the possibility of extending the environment by including a wide range of equipment, also scattered. We are defining procedures to scale up laboratory experiences, using XML and related technologies to describe resources. Furthermore, the system includes facilities to support the web management of the environment (teacher support, instruments/experiences addition, user administration, activity logs). The target is the cross-institutional integration of experimental resources, an environment where actors of a *virtual organization* [9] cooperate sharing geographically distributed educational resources that become part of a learning grid infrastructure. As a result, referring to the terminology adopted in [10], the VLS acts as a super scheduler. Users discover resources through the VLS. The VLS is responsible for authorizing, filtering and selecting the system where the job must be run. If more than one RLS hosts the same experiment, the VLS has to consider the quality of service available from each candidate RLS. It is expressed in terms of the number of connected users and the provided bandwidth. Once the most appropriate RLS has been chosen, the user starts his/her job. She/he can exploit other features from the VLS to accomplish complementary tasks such as to seeking advice from documentation or recording results. For performance or reliability reasons, the VLS can be duplicated. From the user's point of view, the VLS acts as a provider of learning resources and our target is the alignment of the environment to the standard framework proposed to accessing web services [11]. It is worth noting that we have implemented the entire server side, thus both the RLS and the VLS, using LabVIEW programming language that per se guarantees multi-platform capability. Programs developed with LabVIEW (the so-called VI) are able to run, without modifications, on Microsoft Windows, Linux, Sun Solaris™ and Mac OSs. The use of HTML and Java on the client side renders the system accessible by use of a common web browser. The XML description of the entire data set associated with the environment assures the maximum portability.

To better understand possible matching between ISILab and the Grid model, it can be useful to map the components of the ISILab paradigm on the Grid layer diagram [12], as illustrated in Figure 3. At the lowest level of this model, called "the fabric layer", there are the physical devices or resources that Grid users want to share and access. They can include computers, storage systems, catalogues, networks, and various forms of sensors and devices. Above it, there is the connectivity layer, which contains the core communication and authentication protocols required for Grid-specific network transactions. One step above, the resource layer provides protocols that exploit communications enabling the secure initiation, monitoring, and control of resource-sharing operations. Then, the collective layer contains protocols and services that implement interactions across collections of resources. At the top of the Grid system, there are the user applications that control the components in any layer below. From the perspective of ISILab, in the fabric layer there is the experiment, which is composed of actual instruments and the RLS's software modules that locally control them in order to execute concurrent measurement tasks. The VLS is the module that offers collective management services. It brokers resources for the user, acting as a client for the RLS and as a server for the user application. In the user application layer, there are the interfaces that let the user control the experiment execution.

USER APPLICATIONS	Tools and applications	Instrument GUI
COLLECTIVE SERVICES	Directory brokering, diagnostic and monitoring	VLS
RESOURCE AND CONNECTIVITY PROTOCOLS	Secure access to resources and services	Specific TCP-based protocols
FABRIC	Diverse resources	RLS Actual instrument

Figure 3. Mapping ISILab modules on a Grid model.

At the moment, the schema is developed using proprietary protocols and APIs. We are now investigating the possibility of standardizing our approach by integrating the system with the services offered by the Globus [13] framework. We are also studying the opportunities offered by Microsoft .NET technology.

4. Conclusions

In this paper, we have presented our approach to the challenge of remote laboratories. Furthermore, we have outlined the model we have created and the prototype we have implemented and validated. We have proposed a grid-oriented model for our current work. We think that our approach can be an effective solution to support experimental activity in a scattered community of experiment providers and users.

References

[1] Jose M. Grima Palop and Jose M. Andres Teruel, "Virtual Workbench for Electronic Instrumentation Teaching", IEEE Transactions on Education, Vol. 43, No. 1, Feb. 2000.

[2] Hong Shen et al., "Conducting Laboratory Experiments over the Internet", IEEE Transactions on Education, Vol. 42, No. 3, August 1999.

[3] C. C. Ko et Al., "A Large Scale Web Based Virtual Oscilloscope Laboratory Experiment", Engineering Science and Educational Journal, April 2000.

[4] P. Arpaia, A. Baccigalupi, F. Cennamo, and P. Daponte, "A Measurement Laboratory on Geographic Network for Remote Test Experiments", IEEE Transactions on Instrumentation and Measurement, Vol. 49, No. 5, October 2000.

[5] Chung Ko, Chi et Al., "A Web-Based Virtual Laboratory on a Frequency Modulation Experiment", IEEE Transactions on Systems, Man, and Cybernetics, Vol. 31, No. 3, August 2001.

[6] A. Bagnasco, M. Chirico, A.M. Scapolla "XML Technologies to Design Didactical Distributed Measurement Laboratories, IMTC 2002.

[7] http://www.ni.com/labview.

[8] The NetPro Project, http://netpro.evitech.fi/.

[9] Foster, Kesselman, and Tuecke, "The Anatomy of the Grid: Enabling Scalable Virtual Organizations", International J. Supercomputer Applications, 15(3), 2001.

[10] J.M. Schopf, "Ten Actions When Superscheduling", available on-line at http://www.gridforum.org/Documents/GFD/GFD-I.4.pdf.

[11] http://www.w3.org/2002/ws/.

[12] Ian Foster, "The Grid: A New Infrastructure for 21st Century Science", Physics Today, February 2002.

[13] http://www.globus.org.

Towards the Learning Grid
P. Ritrovato et al. (Eds.)
IOS Press, 2005

The Learning Grid and E-Assessment using Latent Semantic Analysis

Debra Trusso Haley, Pete Thomas, Bashar Nuseibeh, Josie Taylor, Paul Lefrere
Computing Research Centre, The Open University,
Walton Hall, Milton Keynes, UK MK7 6AA
email: [D.T.Haley, P.G.Thomas, B.Nuseibeh, J.Taylor] [at] open.ac.uk

Abstract. E-assessment is an important component of e-learning and e-qualification. Formative and summative assessment serves different purposes and both types of evaluation are critical to the pedagogical process. While students are studying, practicing, working, or revising, formative assessment provides direction, focus, and guidance. Summative assessment provides the means to evaluate a learner's achievement and communicate that achievement to interested parties. Latent Semantic Analysis (LSA) is a statistical method for inferring meaning from a text. Applications based on LSA exist that provide both summative and formative assessment of a learner's work. However, the huge computational needs are a major problem with this promising technique. This paper explains how LSA works, describes the breadth of existing applications using LSA, explains how LSA is particularly suited to e-assessment, and proposes research to exploit the potential computational power of the Grid to overcome one of LSA's drawbacks.

Keywords. Grid, LSA, latent semantic analysis, e-assessment, assessment

Introduction

This paper describes Latent Semantic Analysis (LSA) and presents a research plan for combining the potential computational power of the Grid with LSA's ability to provide immediate, accurate, personalised, and content-based feedback. This electronic feedback, or e-assessment, is an important component of e-learning and e-qualification.

Types of Assessment

Formative assessment provides direction, focus, and guidance concurrent with the learner engaging in some learning process. E-assessment can provide ample help to a learner without requiring added work by a human tutor. A learner can benefit from private, immediate, and convenient feedback. Summative assessment, on the other hand, happens at the end of a learning episode or activity. It evaluates a learner's achievement and communicates that achievement to interested parties. Summative assessment shares the virtues of formative assessment while improving the ability to achieve more objective grading results than those that can occur when many markers are assessing hundreds of students.

LSA and the Grid

The Grid is often described as the next generation of the Web [1]. The success of the Grid depends on useful applications being available [2]. Dahn [3] suggests that a major educational application of the Grid is as a storage medium for learning resources featuring easy location, retrieval, and sharing by students. E-assessment using LSA is another potential Grid application with major pedagogical benefits to learners. It offers immediate feedback to learners exactly when they can most benefit.

1. What is Latent Semantic Analysis?

1.1. About LSA

Researchers at Bellcore developed LSA, a statistical-based method for inferring meaning from a text. Landauer et. al. [4] give a more formal definition: "Latent Semantic Analysis is a theory and method for extracting and representing the contextual-usage meaning of words by statistical computations applied to a large corpus of text". It was first used as an information retrieval technique [5] in the 1980s. By 1997, Landauer and Dumais [6] asserted that LSA could serve as a model for the human acquisition of knowledge. They developed their theory after creating a mathematical information retrieval tool and observing unexpected results from its use. They claimed that LSA solves Plato's problem, that is, *how do people learn so much when presented with so little?* Their answer, oversimplified but essentially accurate, is the inductive process: LSA "induces global knowledge indirectly from local co-occurrence data in a large body of representative text" [6].

From the original application for retrieving information, the use of LSA has evolved to systems that more fully exploit its ability to extract and represent meaning. Recent applications based on LSA compare a sample text with a pre-existing training corpus to judge the quality of the sample. The corpora are very large; for example, Summary Street, an LSA-based instructional software system, uses a corpus of 11 million words [7].

1.2. How LSA Works

Even the developers of LSA understand that its results can seem magical [6]. However, a thorough understanding of the mathematical and statistical underpinnings of the method can provide some clarity.

To use LSA, researchers amass a suitable corpus of text. (Exactly what corpus is most suitable for which purpose is an issue requiring further research.) They create a term-by-document matrix where the columns are documents and the rows are terms [5]. A term is a subdivision of a document; it can be a word or phrase or some other unit. A document can be a sentence, a paragraph, a textbook, or some other unit. In other words, documents contain terms. The elements of the matrix are weighted word counts of how many times each term appears in each document.

After it creates the matrix, LSA decomposes it into three matrices using Singular Value Decomposition (SVD), a well-known technique [8] that is the general case of factor analysis, which decomposes a square matrix with like rows and columns [6]. Deerwester et. al., [5] describe the process as follows.

Let t = the number of terms, or rows
d = the number of documents, or columns
X = a t by d matrix

Then, after applying SVD, X = TSD, where

m = the number of dimensions, $m <= min(t,d)$
T = a t by m matrix
S = an m by m diagonal matrix, i.e., only diagonal entries have non-zero values
D = an m by d matrix

The "magic" performed by LSA is to reduce S, the diagonal matrix created by SVD, to an appropriate number of dimensions resulting in S'. The product of TS'D is the least-squares best fit to X, the original matrix [5].

People often describe LSA as analyzing co-occurring terms when, actually, it does more: Landauer and Dumais [6] explain that the new matrix captures the "latent transitivity relations" among the terms. Terms not appearing in an original document are represented in the new matrix as if they actually were in the original document [6]. LSA's ability to induce transitive meanings is especially important considering that Furnas et. al. [9] report fewer than 20% of paired individuals will use the same term to refer to the same common concept.

LSA exploits what can be named the transitive property of semantic relationships: If $A \rightarrow B$ and $B \rightarrow C$, then $A \rightarrow C$ (where $\rightarrow$ stands for *is semantically related to).* However, the similarity to the transitive property of equality is not perfect. Two words widely separated in the transitivity chain can have a weaker relationship than closer words. For example, LSA might find that copy → duplicate → double → twin → sibling. Copy and duplicate are much closer semantically than copy and sibling.

Finding the correct number of dimensions for the new matrix created by SVD is critical; if it is too small, the structure of the data is not captured. Conversely, if it is too large, sampling error and unimportant details remain, e.g., grammatical variants [5, 7, 8]. Empirical work shows the correct number of dimensions to be about 300 [6, 7].

Creating the matrices using SVD and reducing the number of dimensions, often referred to as training the system, requires a lot a computing power; it can take hours or days to complete the processing [8]. Fortunately, once the training is complete, it takes just seconds for LSA to evaluate a text sample [8].

1.3. Existing Applications using LSA

The earliest application of LSA was Latent Semantic Indexing (LSI) [5, 10]. LSI provided an advantage over keyword-based methods in that it could induce associative meanings of the query [11] rather than relying on exact matches.

Soto [12] suggests another use for LSA: improving the interfaces of software systems. Users more easily learn and remember the function of menu labels when they are related semantically to the users' conceptions. The HCI community uses cognitive walkthroughs, among other things, to assess the learnability and memorability of menu labels. Soto [12] suggests LSA could be a cheaper, faster replacement of cognitive walkthroughs.

Researchers are carrying out some interesting work into medical uses of LSA. Wu et. al. [13], as referenced in Chung & O'Neil [14], are using LSA to classify protein sequences. Skoyle [15] is using the theory of Landauer and Dumais [6] to investigate whether autism results from a failure in an individual's ability to create meaning by an indirect process - the induction modelled by LSA. Campbell and Pennebaker [16] are using LSA to demonstrate linkages between writing about traumatic events and improving health.

Researchers [17] have achieved good results in matching texts to a learner's reading ability using LSA. If a text is too easy, a learner doesn't learn anything; if a text is too hard, it can be incomprehensible. They refer to the Goldilocks principle [17] of using texts at just the right difficulty level – slightly beyond the learner's ability and knowledge.

Much work is being done in the area of using LSA to grade essays automatically and to provide content-based feedback. One of the great advantages of automatic assessment of essays is its ability to provide helpful, immediate feedback to the student without burdening the teacher. This application is particularly suited to distance education, where opportunities for one-on-one tutoring are infrequent or non-existent [18]. Existing systems include Apex [19], Autotutor [20], Intelligent Essay Assessor [17], Select-a-Kibitzer [8], and Summary Street [7, 18]. They differ in details of audience addressed, subject domain, and advanced training required by the system [8]. They are similar in that they are LSA-based, web-based, and provide the scaffolding, feedback, and unlimited practice opportunities without increasing a teacher's workload [18]. See [8] for an excellent analysis of these systems.

2. A Research Agenda

Although research using Latent Semantic Analysis (LSA) to assess essays automatically shows promising results [4, 7, 8, 11, 14, 17-19], not enough research has been done on using LSA for instructional software [19]. Previous studies involved both young students and university-age students, and several different knowledge domains; none of them involved the domain of computer science. An open question is how LSA can be used to improve the learning of university-age, computer science students. The kinds of corpora produced by novice programmers have entirely different characteristics than do the customary expository writing texts usually studied by LSA researchers.

The research aims to combine LSA's ability to provide assessment with the computational power of the Grid, thus avoiding the huge computational demands mentioned by many as a drawback of the method. The goal of the research is to demonstrate that a system based on Latent Semantic Analysis can determine the gaps and/or misconceptions in a computer science student's mental model of the subject thereby allowing immediate and specific content-based feedback customized to a student's personal needs. The initial pilot study, described in section 3, shows promising results.

2.1. LSA and the Grid

The nature of the Grid offers several applications for LSA-related computer science research; exploiting its potentially huge computational power for LSA processing is probably the most obvious. Another use results from the fact that students learning to program, regardless of their native languages, produce programs in the same language – a subset of English-like words. International researchers can share and compare program segments from multi-cultural and multi-lingual students without the need for translation. The Grid could be used to store and retrieve the large training corpora needed for LSA. Its characteristic of easy access could allow researchers to keep their corpora up-to-date with the rapidly changing computer science field.

2.2. Some Research Questions

An examination of the existing LSA-related literature reveals certain unresolved issues. Further research will attempt to answer these questions:

- On what corpus should the LSA system for computer science be trained?
- What is a good size for the corpus? This question is particularly pressing as [21] claim that obtaining a large corpus is "the most relevant problem" when automatically assessing essays.

- How do students feel about using a computer-based grading system? Is there any correlation with learning style or cognitive style?
- How can the Grid be used to solve the heavy computational demands of LSA?

3. A Pilot Study

Thomas et al [22] describe a pilot study carried out to test the feasibility of some of the research proposed in this paper. The study involved answers to three essay questions written by computer science students in a graduate course on computer architectures. The study used the Spearman's rho statistical test [23] to compare the marks given by humans to LSA-generated marks. Only one of the three questions showed a statistical correlation between LSA and human marks.

These results are unacceptable for a real-world application because two out of three questions showed insufficient correlation. However, they are encouraging given the extremely small corpus size of only 17 documents, or about 2,000 words for two of the questions and about 600 words for the third question. This pilot study solidified our understanding of how to use LSA, the importance of a large corpus, and how to approach further research to improve the results and increase the applicability of the results of this pilot study.

4. Summary

This paper introduced and briefly explained LSA and stresses that it can be used to provide e-assessment by both formative and summative assessment. It provided examples of the breadth of existing research that uses LSA for e-assessment. It posed several research questions for which the Grid can be crucial in providing answers. Finally, it discussed a small pilot study conducted to establish the feasibility of the research proposed in this paper.

Acknowledgements

The work reported in this study was partially supported by the European Commission under the Information Society Technologies (IST) programme of the 6th Framework Programme for RTD - project ELeGI, contract IST-002205 and LeGE-WG contract IST-2001-38763.This document does not represent the opinion of the European Community, and the European Community is not responsible for any use that might be made of data appearing therein.

References

[1] S. A. Cerri, "Human and artificial agent's conversations on the Grid," in Proceedings of the 1st International LeGE-WG Workshop, 2002.
[2] V. Reklaitis, "Shaping e-learning applications for a service oriented Grid," in Proceedings of the 2nd International LeGE-WG Workshop, 2003.
[3] I. Dahn, "Software interoperability problems and e-learning," in Proceedings of the 2nd International LeGE-WG Workshop, 2003.
[4] T. K. Landauer, P. W. Foltz, and D. Laham, "An introduction to Latent Semantic Analysis," Discourse Processes, vol. 25, pp. 259-284, 1998.

[5] S. Deerwester, S. T. Dumais, G. W. Furnas, T. K. Landauer, and R. Harshman, "Indexing by Latent Semantic Analysis," Journal of the American Society for Information Science, vol. 41, pp. 391-407, 1990.
[6] T. K. Landauer and S. T. Dumais, "A solution to Plato's problem: the Latent Semantic Analysis theory of acquisition , induction and representation of knowledge," Psychological Review, vol. 104, pp. 211-240, 1997.
[7] D. Wade-Stein and E. Kintsch, "Summary Street: Interactive computer support for writing," University of Colorado, USA 2003.
[8] T. Miller, "Essay assessment with Latent Semantic Analysis," Journal of Educational Computing Research, vol. 28, 2003.
[9] G. W. Furnas, L. M. Gomez, T. K. Landauer, and S. T. Dumais, "Statistical semantics: How can a computer use what people name things to guess what things people mean when they name things?," in Proceedings of the SIGCHI Conference on Human Factors in Computing Systems: ACM, 1982, pp. 251-253.
[10] G. W. Furnas, S. Deerwester, S. T. Dumais, T. K. Landauer, R. A. Harshman, L. A. Streeter, and K. E. Lochbaum, "Information retrieval using a singular value decomposition model of latent semantic structure," ACM, pp. 465-480, 1988.
[11] P. W. Foltz, "Latent semantic analysis for text-based research," Behavior Research Methods, Instruments and Computers, vol. 28, pp. 197-202, 1996.
[12] R. Soto, "Learning and performing by exploration: Label quality measured by Latent Semantic Analysis," in Proceedings of CHI '99. Pittsburgh, PA: ACM, 1999, pp. 418-425.
[13] C. Wu, M. Berry, S. Shivakumar, and J. McLarty, "Neural networks for full-scale protein sequence classification: Sequence encoding with singular value decomposition," Machine Learning, vol. 21, pp. 177-193, 1995.
[14] G. Chung and G. O'Neil, "Methodological approaches to online scoring of essays," Los Angeles 1997.
[15] J. R. Skoyles, "Autistic language abnormality: Is it a second-order context learning defect? - The view from Latent Semantic Analysis," in Proceedings Child Language Seminar, I. Barriere, Chiat, S. G. Morgan, and B. Woll, Eds. London, 1999, pp. 1.
[16] R. S. Campbell and J. W. Pennebaker, "The secret life of pronouns: Flexibility in writing style and physical health," Psychological Science, vol. 14, pp. 60-65, 2003.
[17] P. W. Foltz, D. Laham, and T. K. Landauer, "Automated Essay Scoring: Applications to Educational Technology," in Proceedings of EdMedia '99, 1999.
[18] D. J. Steinhart, "Summary Street: An intelligent tutoring system for improving student writing through the use of Latent Semantic Analysis," Department of Psychology, University of Colorado, Boulder, PhD Dissertation 2001.
[19] B. Lemaire and P. Dessus, "A system to assess the semantic content of student essays." Journal of Educational Computing Research, vol. 24, pp. 305-320, 2001.
[20] P. Wiemer-Hastings, K. Wiemer-Hastings, and A. C. Graesser, "Improving an intelligent tutor's comprehension of students with Latent Semantic Analysis," in Artificial Intelligence in Education, S. P. Lajoie and M. Vivet, Eds. Amsterdam: IOS Press, 1999.
[21] S. Valenti, F. Neri, and A. Cucchiarelli, "An Overview of Current Research on Automated Essay Grading," Journal of Information Technology Education, vol. 2, 2003.
[22] P. Thomas, D. Haley, A. De Roeck, and M. Petre, "E-Assessment using Latent Semantic Analysis in the Computer Science Domain: A Pilot Study," in Proceedings of the eLearning for Computational Linguistics and Computational Linguistics for eLearning Workshop at COLING 2004. Geneva, 2004.
[23] D. C. Howell, Statistical Methods for Psychology, Fourth ed. Belmont, CA: Duxbury Press, 1997.

Towards the Learning Grid
P. Ritrovato et al. (Eds.)
IOS Press, 2005

Learning Agents and Enhanced Presence for Generation of Services on the Grid

Clement Jonquet [a], Marc Eisenstadt [b] Stefano A. Cerri [a]
[a] *LIRMM & Montpellier II University, France*
{jonquet,cerri}@lirmm.fr
[b] *Knowledge Media Institute, The Open University, Milton Keynes, UK*
m.eisenstadt@open.ac.uk

Abstract. Human learning on the Grid will be based on the synergies between advanced artificial and human agents. These synergies will be possible to the extent that conversational protocols among agents, human and/or artificial ones, can be adapted to the ambitious goal of dynamically generating services for human learning. In the paper we highlight how conversations may procure learning both in human and in artificial agents. The STROBE model for communicating agents and its current evolutions shows how an artificial agent may "learn" dynamically (at run time) at the Data, Control and Interpreter level, in particular exemplifying the "learning by being told" modality. The enhanced presence research, exemplified by Buddyspace, in parallel, puts human agents in a rich communicative context where learning effects may occur also as a "serendipitous" side effect of communication.

Keywords. Learning, Grid, e-learning, Social Informatics, Dynamic Service Generation, Agents, Agent Communication Languages, Enhanced Presence, STROBE model.

Introduction[28]

The concept of learning agent is seducing as much as confusing. There is no clear definition of what an artificial agent is, and often, in the best AI tradition, one calls agents both Artificial Agents (AA) and Human Agents (HA) communicating in a network for jointly performing a task. The learning specification for an agent may refer to "learning" (or "elearning") as it occurs for HA within a scenario such as the one of the ELeGI project[29], or else as "machine learning" as it occurs for AA. In this paper we wish to address the issue of learning both for AA and HA on the Grid [2]. The aim is include in a global logic to define a generic architecture, OGHSA, as the successor to OGSA [3]: the Open Grid Human Service Architecture. In this architecture, the concept of agent is fundamental. We assume first that AA are just software programs – and their associated processes – that at least are autonomous, distributed and able to communicate asynchronously with their environment and others agents by means of a communication language that is independent from the content of the communication and from the internals of agents[30]. Objects, for instance, are not AA as they are neither autonomous nor properly communicating, as the communication commands consists just of selectors for methods (interfaces) thus is not independent of the objects

[28] This paper is a revised version of [1].
[29] European Learning Grid Infrastructure project – www.elegi.org.
[30] These languages are called Agent Communication Languages, ACLs, such as KQML or FIPA-ACL. See for example [4].

themselves. Looking at the literature, in spite of the high popularity of the agent literature, one may seldom find agents that really respect all the minimal requirements for agentship. Moreover, the choice of dealing with agents is also explained by considering that Grid and agent need each other [5]. In the ELeGI ambitions [6], perhaps the most challenging one is the personalization of learning services for HAs, that will not be achieved unless a minimal formal, computational model of HA will be exploited during the generation of the corresponding services. We take this challenge by trying to develop a computable model for agents that can also serve the purpose of modelling HA in a deliberately well-circumscribed context.

Therefore, the global topic of this article is how to facilitate the ability of both AA and HA to dynamically generate services to each other. To generate a service s not product delivery. One of the fundamental differences between a product and a service is that when a user asks for a product, he exactly knows what he wants, he knows what the system can give to him and he knows how to formulate his request. A typical procedure call (with good parameters) is then realised as in RPC (Remote Procedure Call) as it is the case in the most widespread Web architecture, i.e. the client-server. In other words, the user asks a fixed algorithm (procedure) to be executed. At the opposite, when a user asks a service to be generated he does not exactly know what he wants and his needs and solutions appear progressively with the dialogue (conversational process) with the service provider until he obtains satisfaction. The service generation approach does not assume the user knows exactly what the service provider can offer him. The user finds out and constructs step by step what he wants as the result of the service provider's reactions. In fact, the service generation is a "nondeterministic" process depending on the conversation between two agents. As an example in everyday life, when somebody looks for clothes, buying ready-to-wear clothes is analogous to asking for a product, whereas having clothes made by a tailor is analogous to requiring a service to be generated. For another example of situation requiring a service generation see the scenario of Clancey [7]. We think that e-learning scenarios have to become stereotypical contexts for such "generated services" putting the learner at the center of the process instead of concentrating on information transfer as is the case in most e-learning environments. We show in [8] that the dynamic generation of service is a process creating new knowledge, particulary fit for e-learning scenarios. That means that making AA learn by interacting with HA today, will make HA learn by having service generated tomorrow.

The dynamic generation of services (See also [9]) can only be done by entities connected together in a network, member of a virtual community and sharing knowledge and resources, as the Grid [10]. Current Web Services or Grid Services [3] do not fulfil the requirements for dynamic service generation. Moreover, both types of agents can not be static, they have to change, learn each time they ask for or generate a service. That is why the paper focuses on learning. Therefore, the issue of learning for HA is put into correspondence with the same for AA. At the risk of oversimplifying, we will initially consider for HA as well as for AA just three types of learning:

6. Learning by being told, the classical instructional effect.
7. Learning by abstracting and generalizing (or by classifying examples, extracting rules or forming theories).
8. Learning as a side effect of communication, what we like to call "serendipitous"[31] learning.

---

[31] The faculty or phenomenon of finding valuable or agreeable things not sought for, by surprise.

Type 2 is often addressed in a number AI papers, including for example [11]. Perhaps what they call induction and abduction in theory construction (or ontology negotiation) may be mapped to our abstraction and generalization. At any rate, most of the machine learning work has been performed in this direction, while type 1 and 3 learning described above - for AA - did not really get much attention in the literature.

The role of conversation is of such great significance to education and learning (conversational processes are the key of arch of services), that we shall take a moment here to provide a theoretical underpinning of our approach.We have been very influenced by the Conversational Framework of Laurillard [12], who argues that learning can be viewed as a series of teacher-learner conversations taking place at multiple levels of abstraction. As summarized in [13]:

At the most general level of description, the learning process is characterized as a 'conversation' between teacher and student (see Figure 1), operating on two levels, discursive and interactive, the two levels being linked by the twin processes of adaptation and reflection.

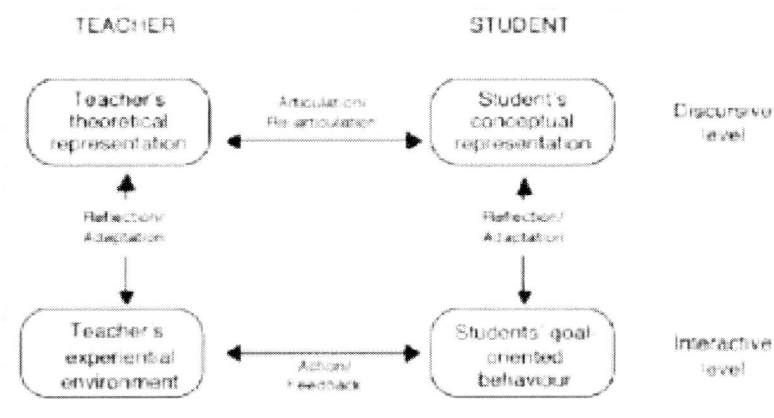

Figure 1. The conversational framework for the learning process (from [12]).

In fact, the framework is more powerful than the simple diagram shows, because multiple styles of interaction are possible, as well as iterations within any type of interaction.

As Laurillard et al describe the framework: Students' work on an interactive resource will take place at the interactive level, where students' adapt their actions in the light of their current conceptual understanding, and discuss and reflect on their practical work in order to develop their conceptual understanding at the discursive level. Similarly, the interactive resource, expressing the 'teacher's experiential environment' is an adaptive response by the teacher who chooses it in the light of discorsive level conversations with students, and a sense of what they need to do in order to learn the topic. Again, the teacher's reflection on what the students do during the interaction will drive their further discussions at the discursive level.

In [14] we extended the model slightly (i) to highlight the iterative nature of every step (e.g. any action or thought process can involve multiple steps at different levels of abstraction); (ii) to add 'Peer-to-peer' (P2P) multiple boxes in the lower right hand corner, to highlight the fact that peer group interactions (not only student-student but also teacher-teacher) are in fact fundamental to many learning scenarios, and (iii) to emphasize that any instance of teacher or student may also be viewed as an agent, and indeed may be either an AA or a HA, in an arbitrary mix.

The rest of the paper is organized as follows: In Section 2 we introduce the STROBE model as a type 1 learning model for AA. In Section 3, we present the concept of Enhanced Presence for type 3 learning, based on practical tools. Section 4 explains why the Grid is a good environment for the integration of the two streams of research; integration unavoidable for developing dynamic service generation systems. Section 5 concludes the article.

1. Learning by being told

1.1. The STROBE model and its evolution

Humans learn facts, rules (or procedures), and languages necessary to understand messages stating facts or procedures, as well as necessary for generating behaviour when applying a particular procedure to parameters. Although we are strong believers in the cognitive constructivist learning paradigm, we nevertheless focus on this highly restricted area of learning, which contains important elements that are so naturally inherited from the computational metaphor. Indeed facts, rules and languages are comparable to Data, Control and Interpreter levels in computing. These three abstractions levels may be found in all programming languages. One may distinguish Data (information) and Control (procedures) levels which correspond to defining new simple data and new procedures abstracting on the existing ones, from the Interpreter level which means to identify the way of evaluating an expression, or defining a special form which cannot be defined at the Control level. Currently, the two first levels could be reached during execution but the challenge is to allow Interpreter level modifications at run time (meta-level modification), in order to generate processes.

In order for conversational processes in ELeGI to be effective, they have to generate services that help HA to learn facts, rules and... languages. That will be possible insofar we model HA by means of AA able to learn dynamically facts, rules and languages. As a resulting side effect, we will have the opportunity to use AA that learn (by being told) during conversations with other AA, thus that show a dynamic behaviour that adapts to the context. The STROBE model (STReams, OBjects, Environments) [15,8] proposes an architecture to support this agent behaviour. The key initial idea is to give to agents an environment as a representation of any type of knowledge and consider them as REPL (Read, Eval, Print, Listen) interpreters[32]. In this model, that inherits most of its features from classical lambda calculus, denotational semantics and the Scheme language [16], we have identified a few basic properties for agents:

[32] Notice that in STROBE, the REPL cycle itself is considered an exemple of control of processes occuring during a HA-AA conversation

1. First class[33] Environments to model memory: linking variable names to values, under the commitment that types are on the values (dynamic typing) and that procedural abstractions are first class.
2. First class OBjects to model the control. As object can be represented by procedures and procedures are first class (in Scheme).
3. First class STReams, modelling the evolving conversational process by using the delayed (lazy) evaluation of values associated to expressions.
4. First class continuations, in order to model non determinism and multiple conversational threads, i.e. a formal expression of the rest of the process consuming the results from the current one once it will be terminated or suspended.
5. First class interpreters, modelling how to generate processes from procedures. They are included in the above described environments.

For the representation of the interlocutor in a conversation, the STROBE agents uses the concept of Cognitive Environments [17] which give to the agent a "partner model" represented by an environment dedicated to this agent. In this environment a dedicated interpreter is stored and used to interpret messages (and their content) sent by this agent. Actually, messages' interpretation is done in a given environment and with a given interpreter. Learning at the Data and Control level consists of modifying the dedicated environment; learning at the Interpreter level (meta-level) consists of modifying the dedicated interpreter. Therefore, if we consider a language as a pair consisting of: i) a language expression evaluation mechanism and ii) a memory to store this mechanism and abstractions constructed with the language. (i.e. Language = Interpreter + Environment) then we can say that the STROBE model allows agents to build a different language for each of their partner. For a formal description of the model see also [8]. Figure 2 illustrates an agent representation.

Within this model, it is not difficult to envison "learning-by-being-told" of variables (Data) or procedural abstractions (Control) insofar as both are acceptable when declared bound to names by an external agent that has the right to "teach me" about facts or rules.

That means that an agent can learn from another one simple information (Data) and procedures (Control) using an interpreter to evaluate assertion typed messages (such as definition or assignment). What is not straightforward is how to learn at run time special forms or any other modification that affect the interpreters. In the HA scenario, it is not difficult to teach a fact or a rule; what is less simple is to teach a piece of language, i.e. teach people how to modify dynamically their interpretation behaviour for new facts or rules. The STROBE model makes it possible by allowing agents dynamically to modify their interpreters.

33 The notion of first-classness in a programming language was introduced by Christopher Strachey . Firstclass objects may be named by variables, may be passed as argument to procedures, may be returned as results and may be included in data structures.

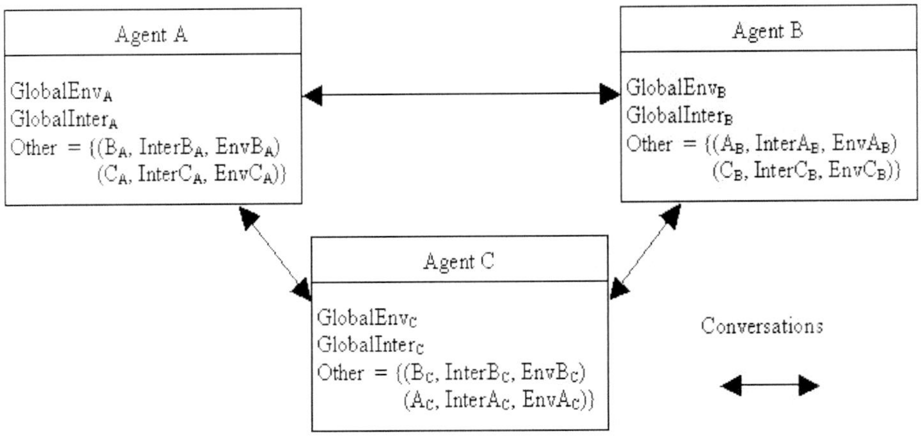

Figure 2. Representation of the others in the STROBE model.

1.2. The meta-level learning architecture

In programming languages, the classic REPL loop interpretation consists of waiting for a user expression, reading (Read) and interpreting (Eval) this expression, sending back the result (Print) and waiting for the next expression (Listen). This represents eventually
a typical Data and Control level modification. The higher level, Interpreter level, is not directly accessible. Our model uses another architecture. Instead of interpreting user expressions with the current interpreter, this one calls a meta-interpreter which itself calls the evaluate procedure (both stored in the dedicated Cognitive Environment) that interprets the user expressions. Thus, user expressions may modify the interpreter which evaluates them by changing the evaluate procedure as any procedure. The idea is to use this architecture with our agents. This feature is quite easily feasible in Scheme, which is an interpreted language such that the evaluate procedure is a feature of the langage itself.

1.3. Example of meta-level learning: "teacher-student" dialogue

We consider that the goal of education is to change the interlocutor's state. This change is done after evaluating new elements brought by the communication. The example in figure 3 shows that a STROBE agent can modify its way of seeing things (i.e. of evaluating messages) by "changing" its dedicated interpreter while communicating. It is a standard "teacher-student" dialogue. An agent teacher asks to another agent student to broadcast a message to all its correspondents. However, student does not initially know the performative[34] used by teacher. So, teacher transmits two messages (assertion and order) clarifying to the student the way of processing this performative by changing the function which interprets the messages (evaluate-kqmlmsg). Finally, teacher formulates

[34] The STROBE model is speech act oriented, such as KQML or FIPA-ACL messages.

again its request to student and obtains, this time, satisfaction. Figure 3 describes the exact dialogue occurring in the experimentation. After the last message process, the student function dedicated to the evaluation of message (evaluate-kqmlmsg) is modified.
Thus a part of its interpreter was dynamically changed. The corresponding code in its environment dedicated to this conversation is changed. Then student agent can process broadcast messages sent by the teacher.

TEACHER	STUDENT
Here is the definition of the square procedure: (kqmlmsg 'assertion teacher student '(define (square x) (* x x)))	Ok, I know now this procedure: (kqmlmsg 'ack student teacher '(*.*))
Broadcast to all your current correspondents: (kqmlmsg 'broadcast teacher student '(order (square 3)))	Sorry, I don't know this performative: (kqmlmsg 'answer student teacher '(no-such-performative broadcast))
Ok, here is the method to add this performative to those you know: Here is the code you have to generate and add to your evaluate-kqmlmsg function: (kqmlmsg 'assertion teacher student learn-broadcast-code-msg) Run this procedure: (kqmlmsg 'order teacher student '(set! evaluate-kqmlmsg learn-broadcast-code)))	 Ok, I have added this code in a binding of my environment: (kqmlmsg 'ack student teacher '(*.*)) Ok, I have just modified my interpreter: (kqmlmsg 'executed student teacher '(*.*))
Broadcast to all your current correspondents: (kqmlmsg 'broadcast teacher student '(order (square 3)))	Ok, I broadcast (kqmlmsg 'order student ... '(square 3))

Figure 3. Learning of the performative broadcast in the *teacher-student* dialogue.

Notice that learn-broadcast-code-msg message indicates how the student agent generates the new function code taking into account the previous student code definition, and to store it in the learn-broadcast-code variable. This is a constructivist method since it is the student, not the teacher who constructs the new knowledge.

This toy-example is very simple but interesting because it shows the potential of such a model. We consider that it is meta-level learning because a part of the agent interpreter is dynamically changed. Another paper [18] describes how to use a nondeterministic interpreter in the STROBE model to do dynamic specification of a problem, in order to fit with dynamic service generation scenarios. The paper gives a typical e-commerce scenario example.

2. Learning as a side effect of communication

The examples provided in the previous section are characteristic of a very narrow spectrum of learning activities, namely those that occur during a particular kind of synchronous (i.e. real time communicative) interaction. Although the overwhelming majority of distance learning and e-learning literature emphasizes either the asynchronous space (particularly via discussion forums) or the one-to-many large-scale synchronous activities afforded by streaming media, there are nevertheless important and indeed profound opportunities that arise during very small-scale synchronous interactions (i.e. one to-one or among very small study groups up to say, three or four participants).We note in particular the opportunistic learning dialogues that can occur in real time in such intensive tutorial situations, and which are precisely suited for the examples presented earlier. Although seemingly small and specialised in nature, it is nevertheless the case that if tutorial dialogues eventually occur between HA and AA, then there are in fact no practical limits to scalability, because every one-to-one interaction that involves an AA can be replicated hundreds, thousands, or even millions of times.

For the time being, our research progresses by studying the nature of synchronous interactions that occur between two, three, or four HA. The ideal paradigm for this is to investigate and facilitate the learning interactions that take place via the world's fastestgrowing software phenomenon: Instant Messaging. In the context of the ELeGI project, we provide a custom environment for learners, called 'BuddySpace' [19] which can be summed up as "Instant Messaging + Smart Maps = Enhanced Presence". It provides continual 'background presence awareness' of peers, by deploying significant extensions to the open-source XML technology from the Jabber Software Foundation. As argued in Smart Mobs [20], tools like BuddySpace leverage the overwhelming power of social cohesiveness that can be brought about by knowledge of the presence and location of others in both real and virtual spaces.We know also from the work of Reffell and Eklund (2001) that this kind of presence awareness is used by students to locate resources, for quick exchange of information and to organize meetings either online or face-to-face.

In reality, enhanced presence is much more than just 'messaging' and 'maps'. In particular, we aim to provide tools that enable us to express the entire situated context of the learner, which is clearly a lot more than just 'location X' and 'online' or 'offline'. The learner's current state of mind, including goals, plans and intentions, must be understood, as well as the way this connects with ongoing activities and devices accessible to the learner. When all these are modelled, plausible inferences can be drawn about what the leaner wants and needs to know, and this gives us an important 'foot in the door' for addressing the problem of delivering the right knowledge to the right people in the right place at the right time. So far, this notion of 'right knowledge' has been nothing more than a Knowledge Management 'slogan', but our belief is that enhanced presence capabilities, linked to the STROBE model, can make this dream a reality.

Putting HA together to generate knowlegde in a serendipitous way in an artificial context (Buddy Space but more generally all computer science feature) is a first step for making them interact with AA. As we know that beyond each AA there is still an human brain, we can imagine that AA will learn by interacting with HA who have themselves learnt by interacting with other HA. The dynamic generation of service is still undone by AA but realised for years by HA, Thus, facilating HA-HA communication and learning through enhanced presence allow us to progressively transmit to AA the faculty of generate services, even if at the beginning theses services will be generated by HA, and just interfaced by AA.

3. Why The Grid?

How does the concept of Grid fit into such a model? To answer this question, we draw a parallel between the essence of our approach and the initial reasons for conceiving and developing Grid technologies in the mid-1990's. The original observation was that facing a major increase of computational needs, for instance in the scientific community (for weather modeling and nuclear physics), there was a parallel increase of computational resources (machines and networks), for which many resources were proprietari and therefore not accessible directly nor on-demand. The original question was how to build a new infrastructure (the Grid) that would satisfy the computational needs in an ondemand fashion by exploiting the computational resources in a seamless way, not requiring 'physical possession' of the resource by the potential clients. That simple observation was based upon an optimization approach: previously idle machines would be used by those who would have needs, satisfying both (in fact, a win-win solution). Our conversational processes and enhanced presence approach proposes, in exactly the same manner, to combine latent and explicit learning needs with potentially available teaching/learning resources able to satisfy those needs in a kind of "human grid" – in this case offer and demand are combined, driven by the demand and enabled by the infrastructure. This is a first approximation to our proposed OGHSA in the ELeGI project, where we study conversational processes among HA (mediated by AA) trying to offer human resources to learners in an on-demand (or 'as needed') manner.

To share services is the intrinsic notion of the Grid. That is why we deal with the Grid for realising the learning paradigm shift of ELeGI. The essence of the Grid concepi is nicely reflected by its original metaphor: the delegation to the electricity network to offer somebody the service of providing him enough electric power as he needs it when he needs it even if he does not know where and how that power is generated. The resource firstly offer by the Grid were computational power and storage but today, recent research on Grid have extended it to the sharing of any kind of ressources and services [3,21]. The Grid has become the platorm for tomorrow's service oriented computing.

The recent evolution of Grid Services research coupled withWeb Services produced the WSRF (Web Services Ressource Framework) specifications [21]. It specifies the association between aWeb Service and one or more named typed state components. In fact, it separates stateless services, that act upon stateful resources from these resources. This view is typically what has been done by the STROBE model since years, which separates the control itself (done by the agent, represented by an object) from the structure keeping the data i.e. the different Cognitive Environments. That is one of the reasons we think that the STROBE model can be an important modelling and implementation element for future Grid Services, its analogy with HA facilitates future OGHSA [2].

4. Conclusion

In this paper we presented the current progress of our work in two domains: the STROBE model both as a model of communication and representation of agents and Enhanced Presence. These are, at a first sight, very different from one another.

Nevertheless we have shown that they may become highly synergic and perhaps also mutually dependent within a rich experimental context such as the one of ELeGI.We perceive their properties as consisting of the identification of models and tools for generating learning services that enable and facilitate co-learning effects, i.e. HA and AA construct their own representations - learn - by exploiting the representation of the partner through conversations.

This social constructivist approach extends to machines the full right membership of societies of learning agents both as "destinations" of knowledge emerging from these societies, and as a continuous source of knowledge digitally represented and stored and potentially consumed by other members through conversations. In these societies, it will be important to partition the responsibilities among members according to their best capacities: exploiting therefore HAs for what they are best in, and, at the same time, AAs for their optimal performance. The consequence is to adopt an approach in Distributed Artificial Intelligence where HA are privileged in their best roles (e.g. motivation, trust, depth of conceptual analysis ...) and AA in other roles (computing fast and reliably, instantaneous transmission of information through the net, storing and retrieving ...).

Acknowledgements

The example cited in section 2 has been developed within the Ph.D research of one of the authors (CJ). Cited papers and current version of the implementation are available on www.lirmm.fr/~ jonquet. The support of the EU project LeGE-WG (Learning Grid Excellence Working Group) is gratefully acknowledged.

This work is partially supported by the European Community under the Innovation Society Technologies (IST) programme of the 6th Framework Programme for RTD - project ELeGI, contract IST-002205. This document does not represent the opinion of the European Community, and the European Community is not responsible for any use that might be made of data appearing therein. For more information about European Learning Grid Infrastructure project: www.elegi.org.

References

[1] Stefano A. Cerri, Marc Eisenstadt, and Clement Jonquet. Dynamic Learning Agents and Enhanced Presence on the Grid. In 3rd International LeGE-WG Workshop: GRID Infrastructure to Support Future Technology Enhanced Learning, Berlin, Germany, December 2003. Electronic Workshops in Computing (eWiC). http://ewic.bcs.org/conferences/2004/3rdlege/.

[2] Stefano A. Cerri. An integrated view of GRID services, Agents and Human Learning. In P. Ritrovato, C. Allison, S. A. Cerri, T. Dimitrakos, M. Gaeta, and S. Salerno, editors, Towards the Learning GRID: advances in Human Learning Services, Frontiers in Artificial Intelligence and Applications. IOS Press, Amsterdam, The Netherlands, September 2005.

[3] Ian Foster, Carl Kesselman, Jeff Nick, and Steve Tuecke. The physiology of the Grid: An Open Grid Services Architecture for distributed systems integration. In Open Grid Service Infrastructure WG, Global Grid Forum. The Globus Alliance, June 2002. Extended version of Grid Services for Distributed System Integration.

[4] Marc-Philippe Huget, editor. Communication in Multiagent Systems, Agent Communication Languages and Conversation Polocies, volume 2650 of Lecture Notes in Computer Science. Springer-Verlag, Berlin Heidelberg New York, 2003.

[5] Ian Foster, Nicholas R. Jennings, and Carl Kesselman. Brain meets brawn: Why Grid and Agents need each other. In 3rd International Joint Conference on Autonomous Agents and Multiagent Systems, AAMAS'04, volume 1, pages 8–15, New York City, New York, USA, July 2004.

[6] Matteo Gaeta, Pierluigi Ritrovato, and Saverio Salerno. ELeGI the European Learning Grid Infrastructure. In P. Ritrovato, C. Allison, S. A. Cerri, T. Dimitrakos, M. Gaeta, and S. Salerno, editors,

Towards the Learning GRID: advances in Human Learning Services, Frontiers in Artificial Intelligence and Applications. IOS Press, Amsterdam, The Netherlands, September 2005.

[7] William J. Clancey. Towards on-line services based on a holistic analysis of human activities. In P. Ritrovato, C. Allison, S. A. Cerri, T. Dimitrakos, M. Gaeta, and S. Salerno, editors, Towards the Learning GRID: advances in Human Learning Services, Frontiers in Artificial Intelligence and Applications. IOS Press, Amsterdam, The Netherlands, September 2005.

[8] Clement Jonquet and Stefano A. Cerri. Agents communicating for dynamic service generation. In 1st International Workshop on GRID Learning Services, GLS'04, pages 39–53, Maceio, Brazil, September 2004.

[9] Abdelkader Gouaich and Stefano A. Cerri. Movement and interaction in semantic grids: dynamic service generation for agents in the MIC* deployment environment. In 4th LeGE-WG InternationalWorkshop: Towards a European Learning Grid Infrastructure: Progressing with a European Learning Grid, Stuttgart, Germany, April 2004. Electronic Workshops in Computing (eWiC). http://ewic.bcs.org/conferences/2003/4thlege/.

[10] Ian Foster and Carl Kesselman, editors. The Grid: Blueprint for a New Computing Infrastructure. Morgan Kaufmann, 1999.

[11] Philippe Lemoisson, Stefano A. Cerri, and Jean Sallantin. Conversational interactions among rational agents. In P. Ritrovato, C. Allison, S. A. Cerri, T. Dimitrakos, M. Gaeta, and S. Salerno, editors, Towards the Learning GRID: advances in Human Learning Services, Frontiers in Artificial Intelligence and Applications. IOS Press, Amsterdam, The Netherlands, September 2005.

[12] Diana Laurillard. Rethinking University Teaching. London: Routledge, 2nd edition, 2002.

[13] Diana Laurillard, Matthew Stratfold, Rose Luckin, Lydia Plowman, and Josie Taylor. Affordances for learning in a non-linear narrative medium. Interactive Media in Education, 2, August 2000. http://www-jime.open.ac.uk/00/2/.

[14] Marc Eisenstadt, Jiri Komzak, and Stefano A. Cerri. Enhanced presence and messaging for large-scale e-learning. In 3rd International Symposium on Tele-Education and Lifelong Learning, TelEduc'04, Havana, Cuba, November 2004.

[15] Stefano A. Cerri. Shifting the focus from control to communication: the STReam OBjects Environments model of communicating agents. In Padget J.A., editor, Collaboration between Human and Artificial Societies, Coordination and Agent-Based Distributed Computing, volume 1624 of Lecture Note in Artificial Intelligence, pages 74–101. Springer-Verlag, Berlin Heidelberg New York, 1999.

[16] Harold Abelson, Geral Jay Sussman, and Julie Sussman. Structure and Interpretation of Computer Programs. MIT Press, Cambridge, Massachusetts, USA, 2nd edition, 1996.

[17] Stefano A. Cerri. Cognitive Environments in the STROBE model. In European Conference in Artificial Intelligence and Education, EuroAIED'96, Lisbon, Portugal, 1996.

[18] Clement Jonquet and Stefano A. Cerri. Agents as scheme interpreters: Enabling dynamic specification by communicating. In 14th Congrès Francophone AFRIF-AFIA de Reconnaissance des Formes et Intelligence Artificielle, RFIA'04, volume 2, pages 779–788, Toulouse, January 2004.

[19] M. Eisenstadt and Martin Dzbor. Buddyspace: Enhanced presence management for collaborative learning, working, gaming and beyond. In JabberConf Europe, Munich, Germany, June 2002.

[20] Howard Rheingold. Smart Mobs: The Next Social Revolution. Perseus, Cambridge, Massachusetts, USA, 2002.

[21] Ian Foster, Jeffrey Frey, Steve Graham, Steve Tuecke, Karl Czajkowski, Don Ferguson, Frank Leymann, Martin Nally, Igor Sedukhin, David Snelling, Tony Storey, William Vambenepe, and Sanjiva Weerawarana. Modeling stateful resources with web services. Whitepaper Ver. 1.1, Web Services Resource Framework, May 2004.

Towards the Learning Grid
P. Ritrovato et al. (Eds.)
IOS Press, 2005

Conversational Interactions among Rational Agents

Philippe LEMOISSON[a], Stefano A. CERRI[a], Jean SALLANTIN[a]

[a] *LIRMM, CNRS & University Montpellier II*
161, Rue Ada 34392 Montpellier Cedex 5, France
lemoisson@lirmm.fr, sallantin@lirmm.fr, cerri@lirmm.fr

Abstract. The new paradigm of "knowledge construction using experiential based and collaborative learning approaches" is an outstanding opportunity for interdisciplinary research. This document is an attempt to introduce and exemplify as much as possible using the lexicon of "social sciences", considerations and tools belonging to "artificial intelligence". In the paper we first draw a conceptual framework for rational agents in conversational interaction; then we use this framework for describing the processes of co-building ontologies, co-building theories, social interactive learning ... as examples of constructive interactions; finally we give a brief description of a conversational protocol aimed at putting a stone in the middle of the gap between human conversation and calculus.

Keywords. SocioConstructivist-Learning, Rational Agents, Ontology Construction, Conversational Protocol

Introduction

The intertwining of cultures in a Society with planetary extension, the progressive fragmentation of every one's daily life, the omnipresence of communication networks and computing machines have induced a radical paradigm shift with an impact on any aspect of today's personal, social, cultural and economic processes:

- people and computers meet through internet, therefore assuming the role of "agents" in conversational interactions;
- the idea of static knowledge which might be enclosed in universal encyclopedias before being delivered to the masses is progressively substituted by the notion of dynamic, interactive, social knowledge construction, based on a consensus reached by means of subsequent cycles of acceptance, refutation and refinement of shared knowledge inside any group;
- learning is therefore no longer considered as "knowledge transfer" – within a behavioristic or cognitive paradigm at choice – rather on "knowledge construction using experiential based and collaborative learning approaches in a contextualized, personalized and ubiquitous way", as it appears in the ELeGI[35] project.

This paradigm shift is an outstanding opportunity for interdisciplinary research. Notions like "interaction", "collaboration" and "learning", that belong historically both

[35] http://www.ELeGI.org/

to "social sciences" and "artificial intelligence" become central. However, it is yet quite unclear if and how there will be a convergence on meanings attributed to which appear as fundamental phenomena for the future of our societies.

This document is an attempt to introduce and exemplify as much as possible using the lexicon of "social sciences", considerations and tools belonging to "artificial intelligence" (e.g.: the machine learning tradition). By doing this, we wish to support the argument, hardly accepted by the general public, that current AI methods and tools, when they respect specific realistic constraints emerging from observing human communities engaged in the construction of shared meanings, indeed are of invaluable help to facilitate, if not enable the convergence of the process and therefore the achievement of important results, among which the learning of complex concepts and skills by humans. This approach may be synthesized by a view of human learning stimulated by doing: the actions being those necessary and sufficient for constructing shared meanings from real observations of experienced phenomena.

The position paper is organized in three parts:

1. an initial scenario introducing a few informal definitions;
2. a conceptual framework exemplified through the processes of co-building ontologies, co-building theories, social interactive learning ...
3. a brief description of a conversational protocol aimed at putting a stone in the middle of the gap between human conversation and calculus.

1. An Initial Scenario Introducing a few Informal Definitions

To start with an elementary scenario let us consider three "agents" looking at a collection of geometrically shaped colored objects. Assume the three agents are motivated and have indeed decided to build a language to describe them.

- "gf1" is an agent able to see shapes (and not colors). "gf1" will naturally classify the objects by shapes and give a name to the resulting classes. A possible classification by "gf1" is: square, triangle
- "gf2" is another agent, equally able to see shapes, and equally unable to see colors. She, or he produces the following class names : carré, triangle
- "rf" is a third agent who cannot see shapes, but can see colors. He identifies and names the following classes: red, green, blue

We wish to settle the basis of a "framework" where protocols can be formally defined, and where the following questions may be discussed in an unambiguous way:

a) will "gf1", "gf2" and "rf" be able to communicate through a language?
b) if YES will they be able to build together a theory concerning the objects (for instance the expression of a particular relation between color and shape)?
c) if YES will they be able to teach this theory to another agent, and how?

In order to start, we assume that:

- there is a "physical world", where real experiences take place. This allows us to say that "gf1", "gf2" and "rf" are looking at the same real objects, although they may see and therefore describe those in different ways.
- there are "intelligent entities", able to put these experiences in order, to link some experiences to others, and to build "meaning" upon all this. AI researchers use to call them "agents" independently from their human or artificial nature. We are going to adopt this habit, not because we have an anthropomorphic view of software (or a mechanistic view of human thought),

but rather for simplicity. Agents and objects are of course part of the real world.

This real or "physical" world is where interaction happens, with or without a communication language: agent "gf1" may select some objects and give them to "rf" without words. Whenever interaction inside a group through real experiences is submitted to a set of rules constraining the behaviors, we shall talk of pragmatic protocols.

But of course, everything becomes easier when the use of a shared communication language is allowed. Such languages have progressively emerged from interactions of intelligent entities; we shall address them from the point of view of syntax which can be described:

- in "social sciences" as the "grammatical relationships among signs, independently of their interpretation or meaning"[36];
- in "artificial intelligence" as the level where "well formed expressions" are built and recognized; when a program is seen as a set of expressions, the syntax is checked by the interpreter or the compiler.

The syntactic level includes almost the totality of "informatics", roughly described as the discipline consisting in defining, using and processing formal languages as abstract models of reality.

One of the powerful paradigms of Artificial Intelligence is "Multi Agents Systems" [1] in which "agents":

- exchange "messages" respecting the (public) rules of "communication languages", so that collaboration may be enjoyed;
- internally use "expressions" respecting the (private) rules of "description languages", so that abstraction may occur;
- for instance, SQUARE, TRIANGLE are concepts in a "description language" for "gf1", and if "gf2" comes to the conclusion that " SQUARE = CARRÉ", then this correspondence may generate a concept belonging to a "communication language" between them.

In order to talk about "interpretation and meaning", we must evocate the SEMANTIC level. SEMANTICS put the focus on the signification of signs or symbols, as opposed to their formal relations. "gf1" interprets the objects as shapes, while «rf» interprets them as colors. One point we wish to outline is that the other agents have NO ACCESS to "gf1's" or "rf's" mind/semantic level, they are just allowed to guess with the help of protocols relying on PRAGMATICS and SYNTAX!

That is to say those agents are not allowed to have direct interaction at the SEMANTIC level; they need the mediation of both the REAL and the SYNTAX levels.

In the simplified framework we need for the purpose of this paper, a RATIONAL AGENT is:

- able to act and react within the REAL world through the mediation of interfaces (eyes, mouth, keyboard, monitor) ... perceptions and actions are the basis for "interaction" between agents;
- able to deal with descriptions of the objects of the real world, as well as to interact inside groups through messages, using structured languages the SYNTAX of which is independent from what is described or exchanged;

[36] Translated from « Le Petit Robert : Dictionnaire de la Langue Française »

- able to keep record of the descriptions of private experiences (perceptions and actions), to classify them, and therefore to develop evolving internal SEMANTICS.

2. A Conceptual Framework for Rational Agents in Interaction

2.1. Analyzing two Simplified Situations

Let us first come back to our initial scenario, and split it in the two simplified situations illustrated in Figure 1 and Figure 2:

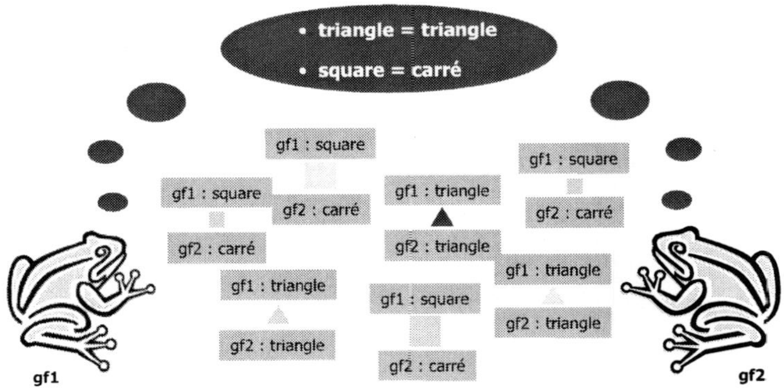

Figure 1. « gf1 » and « gf2 » have identical classifiers

In **Figure 1**, "gf1" is a frog able to see shapes and give them English names, while "gf2" is another frog able to see shapes but who gives them French names.

We imagine a protocol where these two agents are watching the same objects, and sticking labels at them, so that each one can simultaneously see the objects and their associated labels. Because they basically classify the objects in the same way, according to their shapes, we may hope that they are going to understand each other. More precisely, we bet that they will be able to build at the SEMANTIC level a correspondence between English and French labels, which can be described at the SYNTAX level as the first step for sharing ontology[37].

[37] In order to give an informal definition of "ontology", we shall refer to [2] : "In general, an ontology describes formally a domain of discourse. Typically, an ontology consists of a finite list of terms and the relationships between these terms. The terms denote important concepts (classes of objects) of the domain. For example, in a university setting, staff members, students, courses, lecture theaters, and disciplines are some important concepts. The relationships typically include hierarchies of classes. A hierarchy specifies a class C to be a subclass of another class C0 if every object in C is also included in C0. For example, all faculty are staff members. "

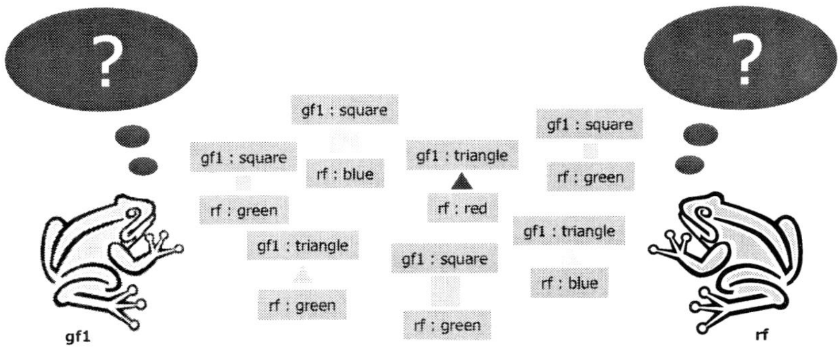

Figure 2. « gf1 » and « rf » have different classifiers

In **Figure 2**, "gf1" is a frog able to see shapes; while "rf" is a frog able to see colors ... then the mutual understanding is much more difficult, simply because classification of the couples (object, label given by other agent) doesn't work here!

We are not intending to give a full discussion of those two cases, but we wish to outline a few points:

- sharing "description languages" and turning them into "communication languages" is the ultimate aim of "ontology building"; the result will belong to the SYNTAX LEVEL, but the "checking" as well as the co-building of ontologies implies PRAGMATIC PROTOCOLS, as illustrated in [3].
- two basic "operations", both implying the semantic level, occur in the building of ontologies; these are classifying and naming:

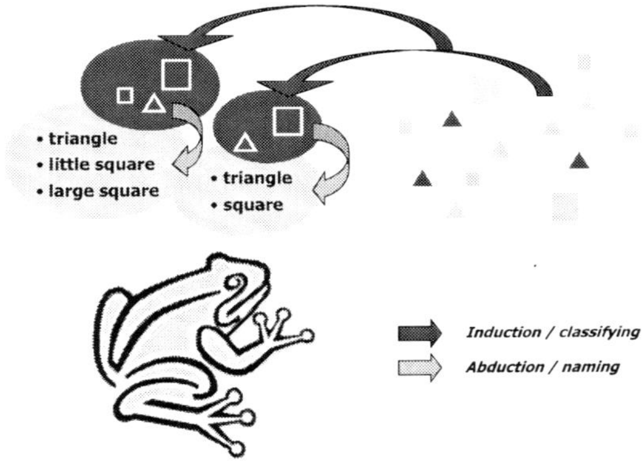

Figure 3. Classifying and naming

- classifying happens in biological brains through the cross-activation of neural networks [4]; it happens in the case of symbolic machine learning through algorithmical analysis of Galois lattice [5]. While human agents classify real experiences, software agents classify only syntactic descriptions, but in both cases, the input is a set of experiences / examples which constitute the local private memory of the agent who classifies; and the output classes keep on transforming as long as this input is fed by new experiences. The logicians call this operation induction[38], because it basically consists in generalizing from peculiar examples. Induction reoccurs as soon as new examples are available; and it may happen than a given object is classified in two different ways at two different moments.

- naming makes a classification visible to other agents; otherwise it would remain confined inside each agent's semantics. Naming is subject to evolution in accordance with the reoccurring induction. In the example given Figure 3 naming the objects "square " or "triangle" is a shortcut for asserting "objects O1, O5, O6, O7, O9 are equivalent and will be referred to as square ; objects O2, O3, O4 are equivalent and will be referred to as triangle". And this can be reconsidered by the agent into "objects O1, O5, O6 are equivalent and will be referred to as little square; objects O7, O9 are equivalent and will be referred to as large square ; objects O2, O3, O4 are equivalent and will be referred to as triangle". So that naming appears as a major step in building a set of logical predicates aimed at describing the real world in the frame of a "theory"[39]. For logicians, the "emission of a set of hypothesis needing validation through further experience" is an abduction. Therefore the basic cycle connecting the private sphere of semantics to the public sphere of syntax is the induction/abduction cycle as illustrated in [6] and [7] through the collaborative construction of a theory by a group of agents.
- the definition of an interaction protocol between a group of rational agents relies on a set of options taken in respect with the following questions :
  - the question of horizon: has each agent a local horizon (can access to only partial information) or a global horizon (can access to complete information)?
  - the question of memory: are all the examples simultaneously given, or are they sequential events which have to be stored by the agent, and for how long?
  - the question of the starting point: do the agents of the group already share a language, is it a formal language derivation rules?

2.2. A More Ambitious Case: Co-Building a Theory

We are now able to put the focus on situations in which a given protocol allows a group to develop a common knowledge, i.e. to build and stabilize a new syntactic corpus through a conversational process involving each agent's semantics. In the following example developed in **Figure 4** and **Figure 5**, two agents are co-building a theory, following a protocol defined by:

- local horizons : "gf1" and "gf2" are not looking at the same objects;
- simultaneous examples : all objects are given at once;
- starting point: "gf1" and "gf2" share an ontology in which the objects are depicted by shapes and colors, and a formal language including epistemic logics.

We consider two steps:

- step1: each agent makes his own abduction, according to his local horizon (Figure 4)

[38] Induction is an inference drawn from all the particulars. [Sir W. Hamilton]

[39] The word "theory" here should be understood as a coherent set of logical assertions

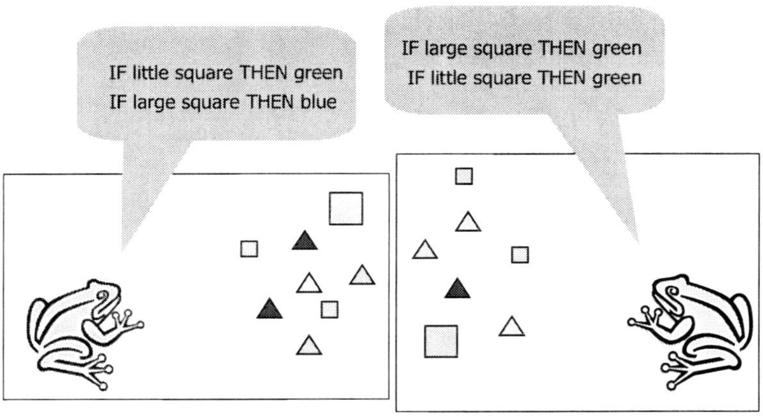

Figure 4. Each agent makes his own abduction, according to his local horizon

- step2: each agent takes into account the other's abduction and proceeds to a revision of one's own theory (Figure 5), since the assertion of the other is not coherent with his own abduction.

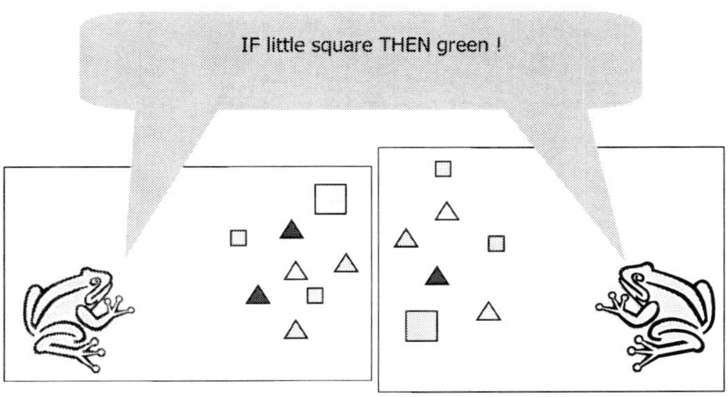

Figure 5. Each agent takes into account the other's abduction and proceeds to a revision of one's theory

Here again, the aim of this paper is not to give a full discussion of the example, which would lead us to the introduction of epistemic logics [8] [9], but rather to give an introduction to the general framework where AI methods and tools can be compared and combined.

In this framework, social supervised learning basically follows the same protocol as co-building of ontologies, the particular point is that the group feeds the learner with examples in order to let him make the correct abductions. A more extensive discussion of this kind of learning can be found in [10] [11].

We could follow the two steps of our "co-building of a theory" through a mock up dialog:

- *[gf1] My own induction about the objects I can see makes me formulate the following hypothesis (abduction): "all little squares are green" & "all large squares are blue"*

- *[gf2] From my own point of view: "all little squares are green" & "all large squares are green"*
- *[gf1] If we consider simultaneously our beliefs, and apply the formal rules of the syntax we share, the only valid hypothesis is "all little squares are green"*
- *[gf2] I agree.*

2.3. A General Framework

The diagram **Figure 6** is a simplified representation of our framework:

- rational agents classify real experiences through INDUCTION
- then they corroborate their interpretations through ABDUCTION

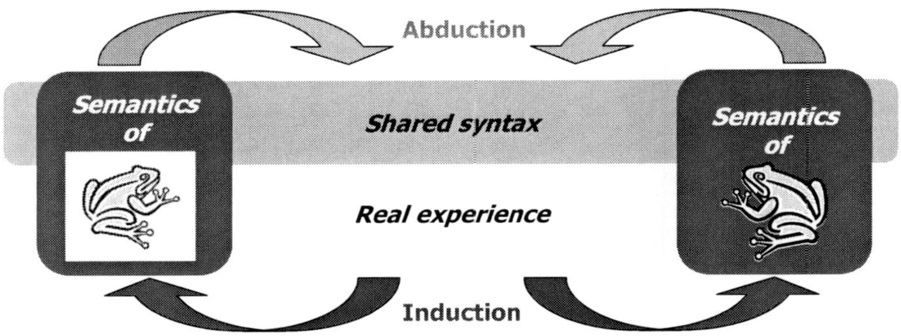

Figure 6. Major flows in conceptual framework

This framework example can apply to more complex scenarios, and then IA tools may become necessary …

For instance, if we try and build a theory about Organic Chemistry instead of geometrically shaped colored objects, we may find it difficult to find out regularities "by hand", that is why we would like to mention here "machine learning", considered as a help for a human learner. [5] directly addresses the induction/abduction cycle through research work on structural machine learning with Galois lattice and graphs.

Moreover, if we want conversational processes to be effective, they have to generate services that help humans to learn facts, rules and ... languages. In [12], artificial agents are able to learn dynamically facts, rules and languages. As a resulting side effect, those artificial agents "learn by being told" during conversations with other artificial agents, and thus show a dynamic behavior that adapts to the context. The strobe model [13] allows artificial agents to modify dynamically their interpreters at the syntax level of our general diagram.

3. E-talk: a Conversational Protocol between Human Conversation and Calculus

3.1. Applying the Framework to Conversations between Humans and Machines

Language based communication happens through conversations in the case of humans, and the metaphor has been kept for communication between a human and a machine, or between two machines; we may therefore talk about "conversations" between rational agents (human or artificial), although "the discourse competences of artificial agents are only a dim shadow of those of humans" [14]. Conversations are always ruled by protocols, but whereas in the case of artificial agents those protocols are "wired", they are merely guidelines in the case of humans.

Referring to our framework:

- a conversation between humans is the creative and unpredictable intertwining of individual induction/abduction cycles relying on a shared syntax but also on private semantics…
- … while a conversation between artificial agents is totally immerged in the world of syntax, and is purely deductive, from the viewpoint of an appropriate logic.

The main purpose of the "e-talk protocol" [15] is to implement the metaphor of a collaborative conversation between rational agents in such a way that:

- each agent is allowed to perform his own induction/abduction cycles
- if each agent is purely deductive, then the global conversation is purely deductive.

An "e-talk interaction" looks like a conversation between human agents inside a room (nobody is allowed to enter after the conversation has started):

- each agent is allowed to formulate questions and assertions in a language using a very expressive syntax, we shall call those: "statements";
- turn-taking in the conversation is automatically controlled in respect with what has been said or asked;
- parallel interactions are allowed;
- each agent is allowed to ask any number of questions before producing his own statements; those are organized in steps so that step N+1 can start as soon as all the questions asked during step N have found an answer;
- each agent has its own privacy: the internal behavior in reacting to a question or to an answer is ignored by the others; in particular, each agent is allowed to choose by abduction one possibility among several when no deterministic algorithm is available.

Yet, it remains a calculus[40]:

- the turn-taking rule, as well as the algorithm giving answers to questions, do not depend on the semantics of the conversation, they only rely on syntactic comparisons between statements;
- the conversation will end in finite time, under some syntactically checkable conditions;
- the issue of the conversation depends only of the initial state (agents including their abduction capability + initial statements);

The purpose of this article is not to enter the technical details of the e-talk protocol; we shall just provide some clues concerning the way we have conciliated the two above viewpoints, and this is by putting two constraints on the agents:

1. "forward specialization" : before interaction starts, agents emit "general statements", and all further statements must be "reductions" or specializations of those, according to a partial order defined on statements ;
2. "no back-tracking on real statements": as soon as a statement is fully "reduced", it becomes "real" and cannot be withdrawn.

[40] A "calculus" here is an algorithm giving a result for any argument value inside the domain in a finite number of steps.

In the following, we shall briefly demonstrate "e-talk" through the example of agenda synchronization between humans assisted by artificial rational agents; we shall see that the artificial agents (that we supposed incorporated in communicating PDAs) interconnect their deductive potentials in order to settle a meeting ... but eventually ask humans to arbitrate when no solution is directly computable.

3.2. A Multi-Agents Conversation Aimed at Organizing a Meeting

The following case has been run on a Java prototype implementing the "e-talk protocol" as well as the language for statements; the behavior of the artificial agents is embedded in Python scripts.

3.2.1. The case

Clement, Jean, Pascal, Philippe and Stefano are possessing PDAs which keep their respective agendas by codifying of each day of the week with a color:

- "green" means "free for meeting"
- "red" means already booked
- "orange" means "not willing, but with no major impossibility"

Besides keeping its owner's agenda, each PDA is programmed in order to negotiate in case of "orange availability"; for instance:

- in case of "orange", Clement's PDA lets Clement arbitrate if he wishes to shift to "green"
- in case of "orange", Jean's PDA waits until Stefano has answered, and will shift to "green" if Stefano is "green"
- in case of "orange", Stefano's PDA waits until all have answered and will shift to "green" if two others come at least

As soon as somebody wishes a meeting for one particular day on a particular subject, the PDAs start a conversation, moderated by another artificial agent called "Palm synchronizer". A meeting will happen only if half the concerned persons at least are present.

In order to illustrate our protocol, we are going to follow the conversation through the "e-talk" interface, which has two mains zones:

- the upper zone, labeled "Pentominos/Invocations", shows the agents. Each of them may be invoked in parallel in several contexts and each invocation will appear as a "child" of the agent. An hourglass appears whenever an invocation is waiting for answers to the questions it has emitted in a previous step of its computation.
- the lower zone, labeled "Syntagmes", displays the statements:
    - o questions, ending by: ";?)"
    - o assertions, ending by: ";)"

3.2.2. Initial state of the conversation: **Figure 7**

6 agents appear in the upper zone, having not yet started to talk:

- the first 5 are the PDAs : Clements's PDA; Jean's PDA; Pascal's PDA; Philippe's PDA; Stefano's PDA
- the 6th is the Palm Synchronizer which moderates the conversation
    - * by computing the different meeting propositions in parallel (if several demands meet on the same day, then their order of emission gives priority)

- * by asking the concerned persons (PDAs) for availability
- * by summarizing the answers

The initial statements appear in the lower zone:

- everybody is orange on the 16/09/2008 (lines 1 to 5)
- Stefano, Philippe, Pascal and Clement are concerned by "Social Informatics" (lines 6 to 9); Stefano, Philippe, and Jean are concerned by "Machine Learning" (lines 10 to 12)
- a proposition of meeting on the 16/09/2008 about "Social Informatics" has been emitted at time "1.0", (line 15); another one on the 16/09/2008 about "Machine Learning" has been emitted at time "2.0", (line 16)

3.2.3. Intermediate state of the conversation: **Figure 8**

The upper zone shows the parallel invocations of each agent, who have all started to talk:

- Clement is only concerned by Social Informatics; so his PDA has been invoked once only. This PDA has finished "talking" after Clement has arbitrated: "red"
- Jean is only concerned by Machine Learning; so his PDA has been invoked once only. His PDA is waiting for Stefano's answer
- Pascal is only concerned by Social Informatics; so his PDA has been invoked once only. His PDA is waiting for Pascal to arbitrate through a dedicated window where the information concerning the other attendants is displayed
- Philippe is concerned by both subjects; so his PDA has been invoked twice. His PDA has already shifted to "green" for "Social Informatics" and has not yet been asked for "Machine Learning", because if the first meeting did not happen, he could free himself for the second
- Stefano's PDA has also been invoked twice, waiting for the others' answers about "Social Informatics" (step 2/3) and having not yet enquired for the others' answers about "Machine Learning" (step 1/3)
- "Palm synchronizer" is moderating in parallel the two conversations, and is more advanced about "Social Informatics" (step 3/4) then about "Machine Learning" (step 2/4, for priority reasons

3.2.4. Final state of the conversation: **Figure 9**

The upper part of the window shows that all invocations have finished talking. The lower part shows the final statements:

- Stefano, Philippe and Pascal have arbitrated "green" for Social Informatics (lines 6, 7, 8) and then turned to "red"(line 1 to 3) to indicate that are not free for other meetings on the same day
- The meeting about " Social Informatics" has been successfully organized (line4) because 3 persons were available out of 5 invited
- The meeting about "Machine Learning" could not be organized because of no participants at all (even Jean would not have come since Stefano had turned to red)

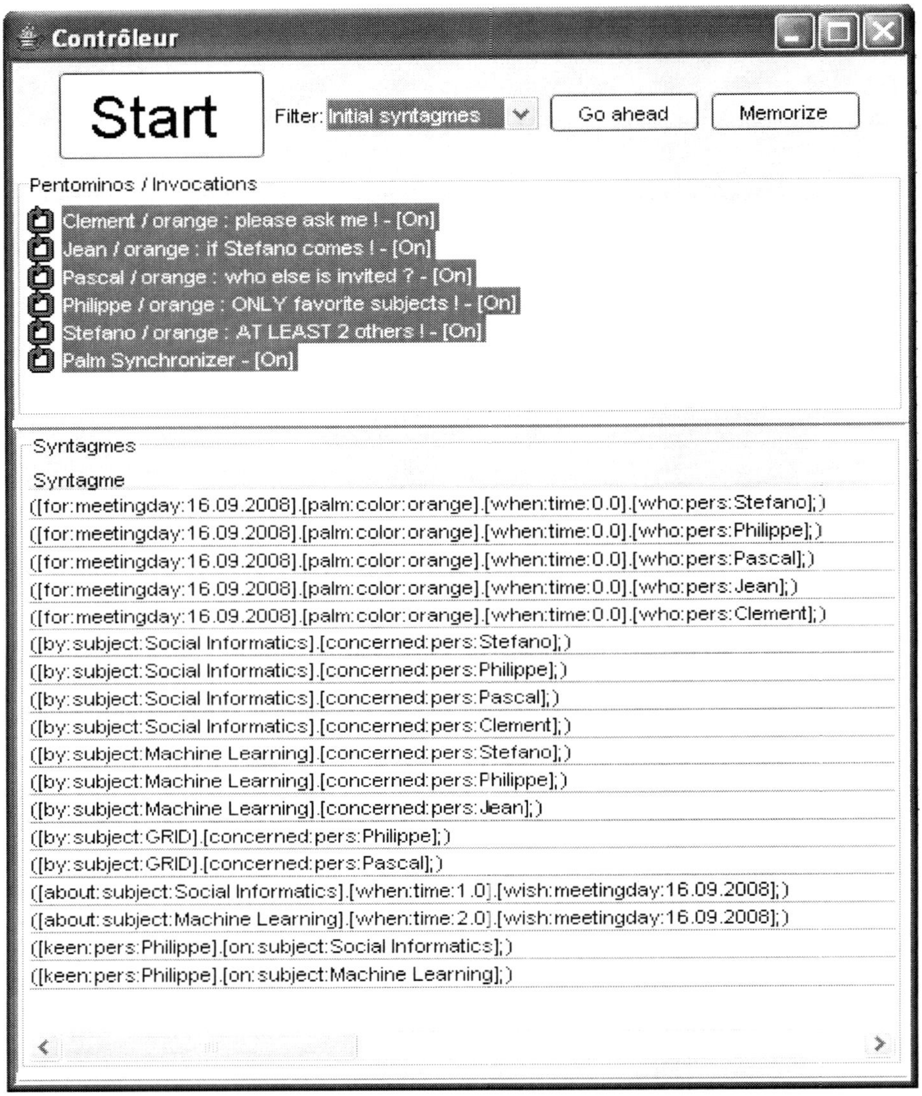

Figure 7. Initial state before conversation

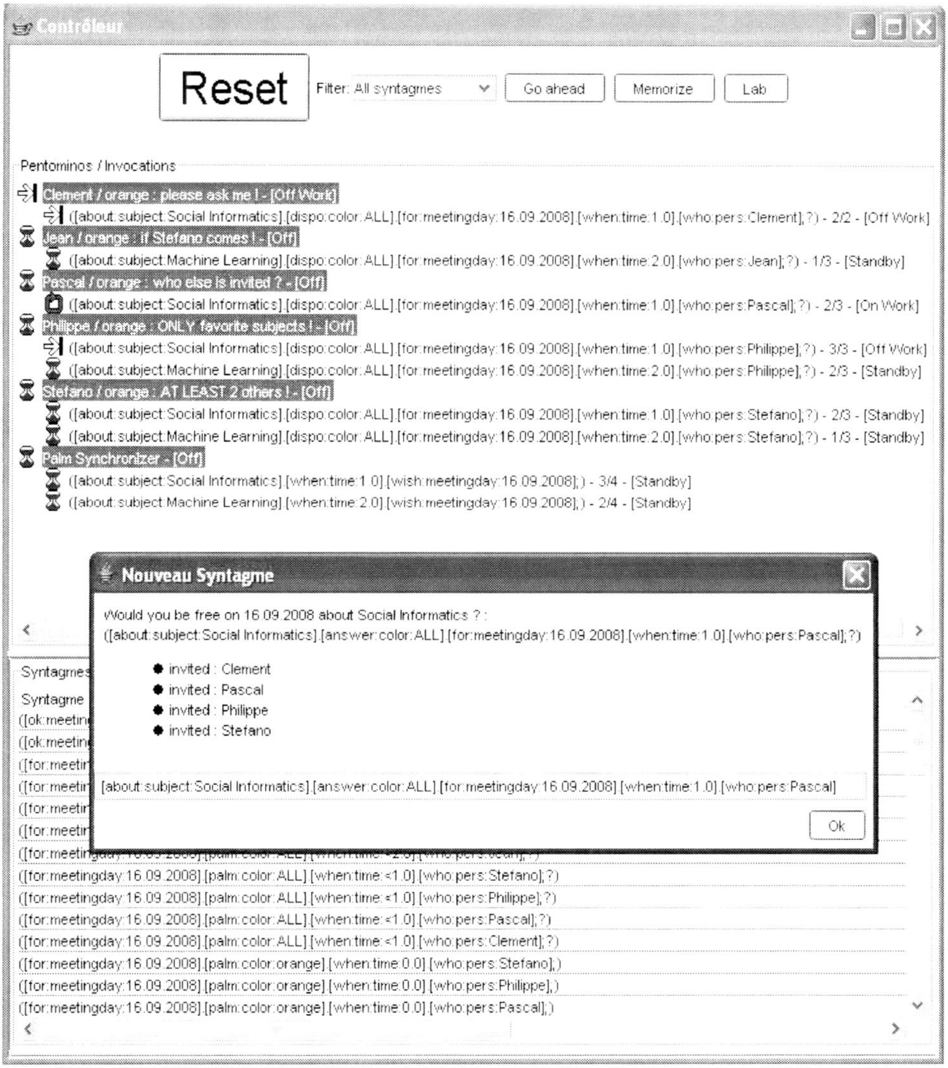

Figure 8. Intermediate state

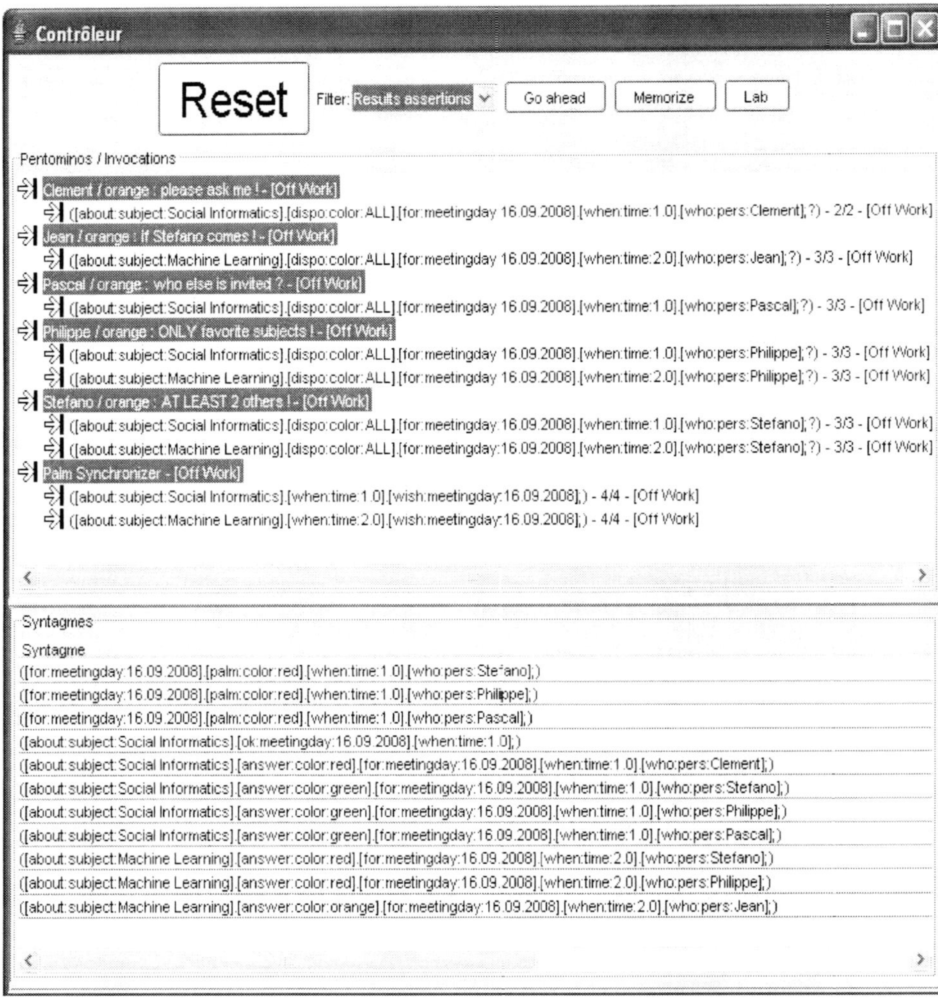

Figure 9. Final state after conversation

3.3. Discussion

Being a distributed algorithm, the global conversation is SYNTACTICALLY controlled through comparisons between the statements:

- Control of question answering: "does statement x answer to statement y?" relies on the syntactical comparison: "is x a specialization of y?"
- Control of turn taking: "does statement z invoke agent A?" relies on the syntactical comparison: "is z a specialization of A's trigger?"

But it is the meaning of statements which governs those SYNTACTICAL expression above which are computed turn-taking and questions answering, therefore the conversation is in fact SEMANTICALLY synchronized!

This also means that the global conversation is subject to eventual SEMANTIC "dead-locks", a well known phenomenon in multi-agents interactions, when several wait for each other in a loop.

For instance, if in the previous case "Machine Learning" had been proposed before "Social Informatics", Jean and Stefano would have endlessly waited for each other... not because of a computational problem, but because of a conceptual problem embedded in the semantics of the case!

Of course the constraint of "waiting endlessly for pertinent answers" could be released ... but then the issue of the global conversation would depend on the resulting turn-taking, and could not be qualified of PURELY DEDUCTIVE any longer!

Whenever a dead-lock occurs, the constructive attitude is to make the system evolve; meaning that at least one of the agents has to update his behavior; this is highly facilitated by "e-talk":

- the SYNTACTICAL loop is automatically put out by the protocol;
- its highly expressive syntax allows easy SEMANTIC interpretation.

The other point to outline is that such a protocol allows Clement as well as Pascal to freely arbitrate whether they will come or not, yet the way they arbitrate does not interfere with the computational properties of the conversation! As it has been said before, although each agent is allowed to perform his own INDUCTION/ABDUCTION CYCLES, their conversation remains a calculus.

4. Conclusion

The conceptual framework we have drawn for rational agents in interaction has allowed us to represent some of the major ingredients of social interactive learning:

- co-building ontologies
- co-building theories
- collaboration in problem solving

As we have pointed out, these constructive interactions inside groups rely on protocols allowing dynamic consensus by means of subsequent cycles of acceptance, refutation and refinement of shared knowledge.

An experimental protocol has been presented; it allows conversational interactions between human and artificial agents, and the synchronization of their conversations is guided by semantic coherence, not just by the syntactic respect of a classical protocol.

Acknowledgements

This work was partially supported by the European Community under the Information Society Technologies (IST) programme of the 6th Framework Programme for RTD - project ELeGI, contract IST-002205. This document does not represent the opinion of the European Community, and the European Community is not responsible for any use that might be made of data appearing therein.

References

[1] J. Ferber "Multi Agents Systems: an introduction to distributed artificial intelligence". Addison-Wesley

[2] G. Antoniou & F. van Harmelen. « A Semantic Web Primer ». Technical Report 03009, The MIT Press, 2005.
[3] J. Sallantin, J. Divol and P. Duroux. "Conceptual Framework for interactive ontology building". In Second IEEE International Conference on Cognitive Informatic ICCI 2003 London 18-20 August 2003 pp 179-186
[4] G. M. Edelman "Neural Darwinism: The Theory of Neuronal Group Selection». Basic Books, 1988
[5] M. Liquière and J. Sallantin. "Structural machine learning with gallois lattice and graphs". In 5th International Conference on Machine Learning, pages 305–313, Madison, Wisconsin (USA),1998. Morgan Kaufmann.
[6] G. M. da Nóbrega, S. A. Cerri, and J. Sallantin. "A contradiction-driven approach to theory formation: Conceptual isssues pragmatics in human learning". In Journal of the Brazilian Computer Society November 2003 Volume 9 Number 2 pp 37-55
[7] S. Charron « Un protocole pour l'étude d'un processus social de découverte : le jeu Nobel-Eleusis » Mémoire de DEA, université de Montpellier II, 2004
[8] R. Fagin, J. Y. Halpern, Y. Moses, and M. Y. Vardi. "Reasoning About Knowledge". MIT-Press, 1995.
[9] J. Gerbrandy. "Bisimulations on Planet Kripke». PhD thesis, Institute of Logic, Language and Computation, University of Amsterdam, Amsterdam, The Netherlands, 1999
[10] G. M. da Nóbrega, S. A. Cerri, and J. Sallantin. "On the Social Rational Mirror: learning e-commerce in a Web-served Learning Environment". In S.A. Cerri, G. Gouardères, and F. Paraguaçu, editors, Intelligent Tutoring Systems 6th International Conference - ITS 2002, Biarritz (France), June 5-8 2002. LNCS 2363, pp. 41-50. Springer-Verlag Berlin Heidelberg 2002
[11] L. F. Martins, E. Ferneda, G. M. da Nóbrega, and J. Sallantin. "A discovery support system based on Interactive Asynchronous Reasoning Advances in intelligent system and robotic" LAPTEC 2003 Edited by Germano Lambert Torres, Jair Minoro Abe Marcos Luiz Mucheroni Paulo Estevao Cruvinel IOS Press 2003 pp87 –95
[12] S. A. Cerri, M. Eisenstadt, C. Jonquet. "Learning Agents and Enhanced Presence for Generation of Services on the Grid". THIS BOOK
[13] S. A. Cerri. "Shifting the focus from control to communication: the STReams Objects environments model of communicating agents". In Padget, J.A. (ed.) Collaboration between Human and Artificial Societies, pages 74–101, Berlin, Heidelberg, 1999. New York: Springer-Verlag, Lecture Notes in Artificial Intelligence.
[14] J. Breuker. « Towards a conceptual framework for conversation and services». ELeGI Technical Report D12 : Preliminary version of Grid Service Architecture for conversational and collaboration processes / 2.3., Internal Deliverable on http://portal.sema.es/ October 2004
[15] P. Lemoisson. « E-talk : un protocole de résolution distribuée ». Technical Report 03009, université de Montpellier II, www.lirmm.fr/bibli/DocumentPrint. htm?numrec=031974857915660 , Juin 2003.

Towards the Learning Grid
P. Ritrovato et al. (Eds.)
IOS Press, 2005

EnCOrE (Encyclopédie de Chimie Organique Electronique) : an Original Way to Represent and Transfer Knowledge from Freshmen to Researchers in Organic Chemistry

Catherine COLAUX-CASTILLO [a,41], Alain KRIEF [a]
[a] *Département de chimie, Facultés Universitaires Notre-Dame de la Paix, Namur, Belgium*

Abstract. EnCOrE is an original proposal which is expected to allow the sharing and the transfer of knowledge in organic chemistry. The system will use MIDES software, whith a peer-to-peer architecture, which will allow setting up a technological and methodological frame to allow collaborative building of knowledge in between chemists. Learning Grid's services will help for Experimental Electronic Laboratory "LabCOrE" as well as for predictive computational tools.

Keywords. E-Learning, Grid, Social Informatics, Chemical Information Technology, Grids for chemistry

1. Organic Chemistry experiments and representation of data

Chemistry is the sciences of change: "La Chimie crée son objet" (Berthelot) [1]. Matter is part of our day life and belongs to chemistry. Compounds as mixture or as pure products are found in nature or prepared de nuovo by chemical synthesis have often specific properties (dyes, pesticides, health care, material sciences ...) [2]. Useful products which are present in nature but in poor quantities or are unknown, have to be prepared (synthesized) by chemists from less elaborated compounds. The choices of the starting material, the number of subsequent reactions which have to be used are determined by a strategic plan elaborated by the chemist according to his knowledge [3].

Use of less expensive ingredients and the shortest route, has a dramatic impact on the final cost of the product. In order to determine such plan, the chemist works by analogy and use rules which have been dictated by observations and physical principles. In fact the chemist works conceptually on molecules which are ideally the smallest part of a compound having the properties of the whole compound [4]. Those possess a structure, a design involving atoms and bonds, usually in three dimensions, which can be determined by several physical methods such as X-ray crystallography [4]. The structure consists of substructures which belong either to the skeleton (chains or cycles, hindrance constraints ...) or to the arrangement of atoms (functional group). Those

[41] Laboratoire de Chimie Organique de synthèse, Facultés Universitaires Notre-Dame de la Paix, 61 rue de Bruxelles, 5000 Namur, Belgium ; E-mail: catherine.colaux@fundp.ac.be

confer specific physical and chemical behaviours to all the compounds which possess them.

Reactions imply one or several products which when mixed, in a close environment, spontaneously or under the action of applied energy (heat, light...) are transformed to one or several new compounds. The chemist represent these events as "chemical equations" in which the structure of the starting materials and products formed are respectively presented at the left or the right side of an arrow, which symbolizes the time elapsed, the human "actions" (heating, cooling, addition of a product, ...) and the observations made during the chemical process [4]. Keywords related to the products, to the structures or to the reaction characteristics are linked to the "chemical equation".

Chemists think, work, represent, organise and transfer their knowledge in three main distinct ways: Experiments [5, 6], Chemical equations and texts linked to references [7-10]. Predictions using computational tools are now available and more and more used by experimentalists in organic chemistry [11].

Databases involving structures (more than 17 millions) and "chemical equations" (several millions) are available from early 1900 [12]. Electronic versions are available since 1985 and widely distributed since 2000 [13].

Basic knowledge is disclosed in manuals (textbooks) [4, 7, 8] and more elaborated or specific one are found in dedicated books, 9 series of books [6,10a] and encyclopaedias [10b]. In general those describe, in textual environment, mainly generic "chemical equations" and a few specific "chemical equations" with comments about their generalisation, limitation, and rationalization. No media to display those data in an integrated format is up to now available.

2. Organic Chemists and knowledge in Organic Chemistry

Organic chemists perceive their subject as intellectually highly structured, with many interconnected ideas. There are many quite different ways of teaching it, because there are many starting points, but the end result is often the same: a broad understanding and a shared but opaque language to outsiders. The sense of logic to the interconnected ideas disguises the fact that there is a serious problem in making the subject truly systematic. Classifying all the known organic reactions, for example, into conceptually recognizable groups sounds as though it would be easy, but in fact, apart from some straightforward seeming groups, like oxidation, reduction, addition and elimination, the categories are not well defined. Even some of those reactions pose problems.

Many concepts, very well accepted and used, cannot, as yet, be rendered into a format that computers can manipulate, although most organic chemists will be blind to the difficulties, and probably surprised how little can be done beyond the calculations, the handling of chemical structure databases and the word processing that they are familiar with. One of our aims is to try to reveal the underlying structure, and to achieve some systematic understanding of what organic chemists actually mean.

For this reason and others, this is an immensely ambitious project, for we are not simply entering the data to be found already in the secondary chemical literature, and providing an index to it. There are already more or less effective ways of searching large chemical databases like *Chemical Abstracts* [12a] and *Beilstein* [12b]. Instead, we shall collect afresh the fundamental chemical information needed, as one would if one were writing a book or series of books, and enter it into the encyclopaedia, in order to format it and structure it to suit more flexible computer-based retrieval. We expect that our finished product will allow students at all levels from first degree upwards to make connections that books and indexed databases are not designed for. We expect that it will contribute to the design of new ways of teaching, especially of organic chemistry, which has complex problems of having to handle words, chemical structures, mathematical formulae and experimental techniques, all equally important. We also expect that, by revealing connections that are not currently recognised, it will even expose areas of ignorance we are not aware of.

3. Goals to Achieve and architecture of our Program

We want to achieve two goals related to Organic Chemistry and based to online transfer of knowledge:

3.1. Experimental electronic laboratory "LabCOrE":

The objective is to teach experimental Organic Chemistry using exactly the same environment as the one of the most sophisticated research laboratories in universities or industries. This will be possible using a reaction flask which is connected to a robot [14], like those used in combinatorial chemistry, and linked to the net. It is also necessary, for an optimal process, to link these robots to equipments which permit to follow the reactions, to isolate pure products (Chromatography: TLC, GC, HPLC) and to allow their structure determination.

Moreover this project will allow the "student" to adjust the conditions to get the best results. Background information, conceptual approach to the most adequate solution (ratio of starting materials, solvents, experimental conditions, temperature, and reaction time) will be helped by the concomitant use of EnCOrE.

3.2. Electronic Encyclopaedia EnCOrE

3.2.1. Architecture of EnCOrE

EnCOrE (Encyclopédie de Chimie Organique Electronique) tends to integrate and organize all the existing knowledge in organic chemistry. It should provide the average user all the information he needs. For that purpose we planned to manage interconnected huge databases of texts, chemical equations and references. The system will be built (Figure 1) according the conceptual view of the chemist (what do we want to include) and the need of the user (what and how the user wants to get the information).

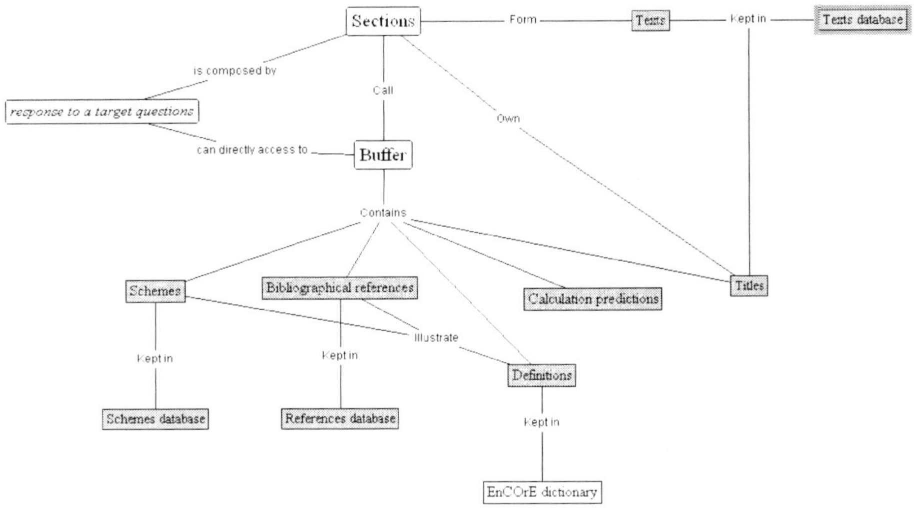

Figure 1: Architecture of EnCOrE

The huge interconnected databases of texts, plans, chemical equations (Scheme database in Figure), references, and dictionaries, described above, will be linked to a "buffer zone" where all the information could be retrieved using integrated software's. These include predictive computational tools which require the Grid to work optimally (Figure 2). This kind of architecture will assure rapidity and efficiency of our system.

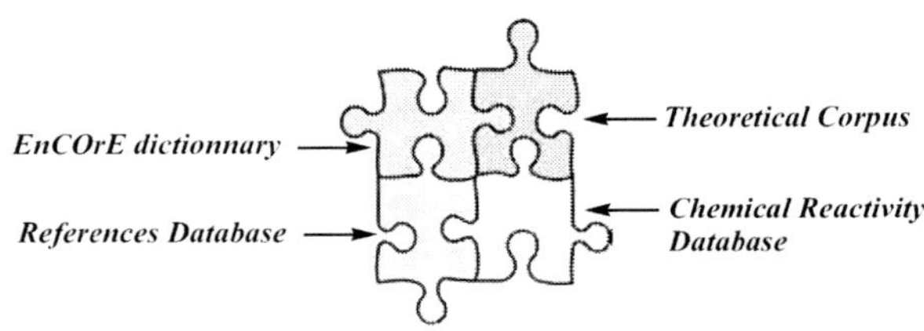

Figure 2: Imbrications of the different parts of EnCOrE

3.2.2. Unitex Software

We have selected Unitex software to manipulate, treat and search the texts [15, 16]. It will help us to find most of the chemical words in our corpus using electronic standard dictionaries. These dictionaries are lists of words associated with coded grammatical indications which can be used by the syntax analyser. They will be employed to extract unrecognized chemical words which will be included in our electronic chemical dictionaries associated to grammatical and specific indications. Local grammars (graphs) should be therefore drawn particularly useful descriptor of "syntax motives". In a first approach, graphs will be used to cut each text into pertinent sections, later the same program should be employed as an efficient search engine.

3.2.3. IUPAC and MIDES Chemical Dictionaries

At the beginning we propose to use IUPAC (International Union of Pure and Applied Chemistry) dictionary which contains basic chemical definitions [17] to structure and analyze the texts, but we plan to use as soon as possible our own dictionary "EnCOrE electronic dictionary" which will describe the meaning of each word according to his each context in which it is used with adequate references and Schemes [18, 19].

3.2.4. Construction of EnCOrE and the Grid infrastructures

We aim to create the Encyclopedia of Organic Chemistry by collaborative building of knowledge in between chemists using a peer-to-peer architecture communicating on the Web. Its relevance for Grid scenarios will depend on motivates and influences the improving availability of conversational services on future Grid infrastructures. Current major result is the computational architecture, but perhaps more interesting is the chain of arguments for each architectural choices made, and the emerging conceptual model supporting human learning within a socio-constructivist approach, consisting of cycles of deductions, inductions and abductions upon facts (the shared reality) and concepts (their subjective interpretation) submitted to negotiations, and finally converging to a consensus.

3.2.5. The three main components of EnCOrE

We consider three principal components to construct an encyclopedia of Organic Chemistry [20]:

An ontological nucleus [21] containing domain-specific scientific terms defined and organized with explicit relations between them. On a consensual basis, terms will describe shared concepts (e.g.: Chemicals, substances, structure, functional group, chemical equation, named reaction, reaction steps, transformations, retro-synthesis, etc.), using typical Semantic Viewpoints aimed at classifying theoretical situations, and therefore at contextualizing the meaning. In the same time, a collection of Pragmatic Viewpoints will be stored and managed in order to take into account the questions raised during the knowledge acquisition process. The roles of the ontological nucleus are:

- to gather the shared vocabulary of the community, to explicit formal representation modes;
- to achieve a coherent integration of contents for their reusability and their recovery by artificial agents;
- to serve as a reference for those willing to construct new ontologies around it, by providing a reusable shared conceptual framework to describe meaning.

A preliminary proposition to organize the ontological nucleus content relies upon the following sub-ontologies: Ontology of Concepts (e.g. Chemical structure, Element, Functional group, Connectors ...) Ontology of Techniques (e.g. Equipment, Methods, Document types, Document organization ...) Ontology of pragmatic viewpoints (e.g. Strategic, Stereo chemical, Reactivity ...) , Ontology of semantic viewpoints (as a starting point, six semantic viewpoints are proposed, three to consider primary objects, and three to consider secondary objects: Equation/Redistribution, Taxonomy/Examples, and Strategy/Practice).

An EXPERIMENTAL CORPUS containing chemical reactions stored with their original description represented using terms and viewpoints from the ontological nucleus. The experimental corpus is a collection of facts in their experimental description based on the notion of Vessel Reaction. The value of the experimental corpus will reside in the selection of reaction examples following a chart defined by EnCOrE editors, and in its data structure refereeing to the ontological nucleus. Experimental facts (Vessel Reactions) represent the "hard" reality less prone to controversy, and are a good basis to construct a stable ontological nucleus that will be reused in the theoretical corpus.

A THEORETICAL CORPUS made of scientific articles conceptualizing the experimental corpus. Article content will be "indexed" by the terms and viewpoints of the ontological nucleus. Based on the hard reality of the experimental corpus, the theoretical corpus will be the ground to construct a soft reality, in line with the Popperian [29] approach of conjecture/refutation. The semantic viewpoints and pragmatic viewpoints from the ontological nucleus will help formalizing the Synthetic Organic Chemistry theories.

The following illustration (Figure 3) shows the components of the encyclopedia, and the relations between them.

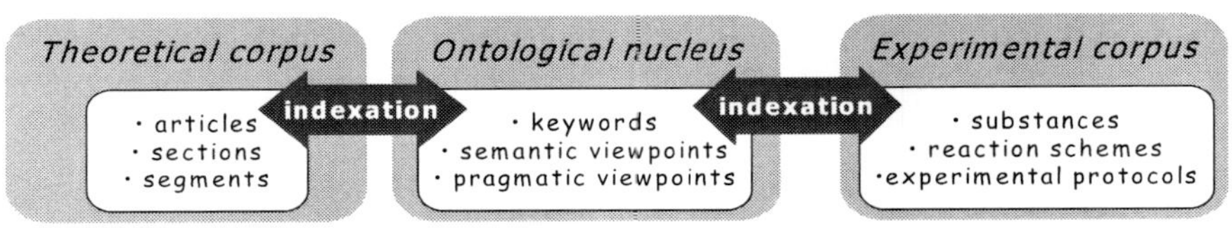
Theoretical corpus
· articles
· sections
· segments
indexation
Ontological nucleus
· keywords
· semantic viewpoints
· pragmatic viewpoints
indexation
Experimental corpus
· substances
· reaction schemes
·experimental protocols

Figure 3: Indexation relationship between the ontological nucleus and both the theoretical and experimental corpuses.

The building block of the theoretical corpus is the encyclopedia "article"; while the "segment" is defined as an editorial "atom", to which pragmatic and semantic viewpoints are attached. Each article is composed of "sections", themselves composed of segments. Each segment is indexed by both pragmatic and semantic viewpoints; therefore, the organization of the domain into formal structures will occur on a bi-dimensional way, corresponding respectively to the encyclopedia and dictionary modality of utilization of EnCOrE. Articles, as well as experimental protocols, include some terms of the ontological nucleus and the indexation link is established with the definition of the term in accordance with the relevant semantic viewpoint.

Acknowledgements

This work has been supported by the FNRS (Fonds National de la recherche Scientifique, Bruxelles, Belgique), by the CNRS (Centre de la Recherche Scientifique, Paris, France). The authors thank Prof. I. Fleming (Cambridge University, United Kingdom), Dr E. Untersteller (Institut de Chimie des Substances Naturelles ICSN-CNRS, Gif sur Yvette France and FUNDP, Belgium), Ms M.A.Marchal (Facultés Universitaires Notre Dame de la Paix, Namur, Belgium, and Université Catholique de Louvain, Louvain la neuve, Belgique) for their helpful contribution.

Encore is a collaborative project involving five active sites: (a) Facultés Universitaires Notre Dame de la Paix (FUNDP), Namur, Belgium, (b) Institut de Chimie des Substances Naturelles ICSN-CNRS, Gif sur Yvette, France) (c) Laboratoire d'Informatique, de Robotique et de Microélectronique de Montpellier (LIMM), Montpellier, France (d) Ecole nationale Supérieure de Chimie de Montpellier (ENSCM), Montpellier, France (e) Université Catholique de Louvain, Louvain la neuve, Belgique).

References

[1] Berthelot, M. "La synthèse chimique", Librairie Germer Baillière et Cie, 1876
[2] (a) Selinger, B. "Chemistry in the Marketplace" HarcourtBrace and Company, London, 1998 (b) Pybus, D. H.; Sell, C. S. "The Chemistry of Fragrances" Royal Society of Chemistry 1999 (c) Coultate, T. P. "Food" The Chemistry of its Components Royal Society of Chemistry, Fourth edition, 2002.
[3] Corey, E.J.; Xue-Min Cheng "The logic of Chemical Synthesis" John Wiley and Sons, New York, 1989.
[4] (a) Atkins, P. W. "Physical Chemistry", Oxford University Press, Oxford, Fift edition 1994 (b) Sykes P. "A guidebook to mechanism in organic chemistry" Longman, Fourth edition, 1975.
[5] (a) Lowenthal, H. J. E. "A Guide for the Perplexed Organic Experimentalist" 2nd edition, John Wiley and Sons, New York, 1990 (b) Harwood, L. M.; Moody, C. M. "Experimental Chemistry, Principles and Practice Backwell Scientific Publications, Oxford, 1989.
[6] Organic Syntheses Series John Wiley and Sons, New York.
[7] (a) March, J. "Advanced Organic Chemistry: Reactions, Mechanisms, and Structures" John Wiley and Sons, New York, Fourth edition, 1992 (b) Smith, M.A. " Organic Synthesis" McGraw-Hill, Inc., 1994.
[8] Carey, F. A.; Sunberg, R. J. "Advanced Organic Chemistry" Part A: Structure and Mechanism; Part B: Reactions and Synthesis, Kluwer Academic/Plenum Publishers, New York, 2001.
[9] (a) Davis, A. G. "Organotin Chemistry" VCH, Weinheim, 1997 (b) Tsuji, J. "Organic Synthesis with Palladium Compounds" Reactivity and Structure Concepts in Organic Chemistry 10, Springer-Verlag, Berlin, 1980 (c) Krief, A; Hevesi, L. "Organoselenium Chemistry I" Springer-Verlag, Berlin, 1988.
[10] (a) Organic reactions Series Wiley and Sons, New York (b) Comprehensive Organic Chemistry, Pergamon Press, Ed. Trost, B.M.; Fleming, I. 1991.
[11] "Cache Software" from Fujitsu Company for example: http://www.cachesoftware.com/
[12] (a) Chemical abstracts, American Chemical Society, http://www.cas.org/ (b) Beilstein, Beilstein Institute, http://www.beilstein-institut.de
[13] (a) Scifinder and SciFinder Scholar http://www.cas.org/SCIFINDER/SCHOLAR/index.html (b) STN: http://www.cas.org/casdb.html (c) Crossfire for Beilstein MDL Information Systems GmbH, http://www.beilstein.com/beilst_2.shtml.
[14] Robots for parallel synthesis. (a) Chempseed: http://www.chemspeed.com/VLT100.html (b) ProSense Laboratory & Process equipment: http://www.prosense.net/
[15] Gross, M. Ann. Télécommun., 5, 44, n°1-2, 1989.
[16] http://www-igm.univ-mlv.fr/~unitex/
[17] IUPAC Compendium of Chemical Terminology: http://www.chemsoc.org/chembytes/goldbook/
[18] Paraguaçu, F.; Cerri, S. A.; Costa, C; Untersteller, E.; IEEE/ITRE2003, August 10-13, 2003, Newark, New Jersey, USA.
[19] Paraguaçu F. ; Untersteller E. (2003) Interactive Model for Scientific Discovery Application to the Conception and Realisation of a Dictionary in Organic Chemistry. Technical Report LIRMM Univ. Montpellier II, ICSN CNRS, FUNDP, and FNRS. May 15th, 2003.
[20] Lemoisson P. ; Untersteller E. ; Nunes M.A. ; Cerri S.A. ; Krief A. ; Paraguaçu F. ITS'04: International Conference on Intelligent Tutoring Systems (ACT-I 04), Workshop on Grid Learning Services (GLS'04 at ITS'04, Maceio, Alagoas, Brazil, August 30 - September 3, 2004)) Acte :11459, 2004, 78-93 : http://pckaty.lirmm.fr/Document.htm&numrec=031982057916480
[21] http://protege.stanford.edu

Author Index